Morie A. Gertz · Philip R. Greipp

Hematologic Malignancies: Multiple Myeloma and Related Plasma Cell Disorders

Springer
Berlin
Heidelberg
New York
Hong Kong
London
Milan
Paris
Tokyo

Morie A. Gertz · Philip R. Greipp

Hematologic Malignancies: Multiple Myeloma and Related Plasma Cell Disorders

With 65 Figures and 59 Tables

Contributors

Angela Dispenzieri · Rafael Fonseca · Morie A. Gertz · Philip R. Greipp
Suzanne R. Hayman · Robert A. Kyle · Martha Q. Lacy · Donna J. Lager
Nelson Leung · John A. Lust · S. Vincent Rajkumar · Guillermo A. Suarez
Dietlind L. Wahner-Roedler · Jerry M. Winkler · Thomas E. Witzig
Steven R. Zeldenrust

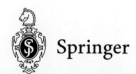

Springer

Edited by
Morie A. Gertz, M.D.
Chair, Division of Hematology and Internal
Medicine, Mayo Clinic; Professor of Medicine,
Mayo Medical School; Rochester, Minnesota, USA

and

Philip R. Greipp, M.D.
Consultant, Division of Hematology and Internal
Medicine, Mayo Clinic; Professor of Medicine
and of Laboratory Medicine, Mayo Medical School;
Rochester, Minnesota, USA

ISBN 3-540-00811-X Springer-Verlag Berlin Heidelberg New York

Library of Congress Cataloging-in-Publication Data
Hematologic malignancies: multiple myeloma and related plasma cell disorders / Morie A.
    Gertz, Philip R. Greipp (eds.)
        p.; cm.
    Includes bibliographical references and index.
    ISBN 3-540-00811-X (alk. paper)
    1. Multiple myeloma. 2. Plasma cell diseases. I. Title: Multiple myeloma and related
plasma cell disorders. II. Gertz, Morie A. III. Greipp, Philip R., 1943–
    [DNLM: 1. Multiple Myeloma. 2. Paraproteinemias. WH 540 H487 2003]
    RC280.B6H46 2003
    616.99′418–dc22

The triple-shield Mayo logo and the words MAYO and MAYO CLINIC are marks of Mayo Foundation for Medical Education and Research.

Care has been taken to confirm the accuracy of the information presented and to describe generally accepted practices. However, the authors, editors, and publisher are not responsible for errors or omissions or for any consequences from application of the information in this book and make no warranty, expressed or implied, with respect to the contents of the publication. This book should not be used apart from the advice of a qualified health care provider.

The authors, editors, and publisher have exerted efforts to ensure that drug selection and dosage set forth in this text are in accordance with current recommendations and practice at the time of publication. However, in view of ongoing research, changes in government regulations, and the constant flow of information relating to drug therapy and drug reactions, the reader is urged to check the package insert for each drug for any change in indications and dosage and for added warnings and precautions. This is particularly important when the recommended agent is a new or infrequently used drug.

Some drugs and medical devices presented in this publication have U.S. Food and Drug Administration (FDA) clearance for limited use in restricted research settings. It is the responsibility of health care providers to ascertain the FDA status of each drug or device planned for use in their clinical practice.

Production: PRO EDIT GmbH, 69121 Heidelberg, Germany
Typesetting: K+V Fotosatz GmbH, Beerfelden
Cover design: Erich Kirchner, 69121 Heidelberg, Germany

21/3150/beu-göh – 5 4 3 2 1 0 – Printed on acid-free paper

Preface

The monoclonal gammopathies and related disorders represent fewer than 10% of all hematologic malignancies and approximately 1% to 2% of all disorders seen by practicing clinicians in the fields of hematology and oncology. In view of the small number of patients seen with these relatively unique disorders, many practicing clinicians are uncomfortable in the diagnosis, management, and assessment of prognosis for patients with these disorders. The genesis of this handbook was to call on the clinical expertise of the Dysproteinemia Clinic at Mayo Clinic to develop a practical approach to the recognition and management of these disorders. The Dysproteinemia Clinic at Mayo Clinic, which was started by Dr. Robert A. Kyle, now has more than 5,000 patient visits per year, spanning the gamut of plasma cell dyscrasias. The physician authors of this handbook have a cumulative experience of 115 years in the clinical management of plasma cell dyscrasias. All of the authors have significant clinical commitment (know of what they speak) when it comes to the assessment of these patients.

The fundamental underpinning of all plasma cell dyscrasias is the assessment of the patient with monoclonal gammopathy of undetermined significance. Dr. Kyle reviews the laboratory evaluation of patients with monoclonal gammopathies and outlines differential diagnosis, long-term outcome, and association with nonhematologic disorders, in particular, rare skin disorders that are well recognized to be associated with monoclonal gammopathies.

Dr. Rajkumar reviews the particularly frustrating and complex topic of progressive sensorimotor peripheral neuropathy associated with monoclonal gammopathy of undetermined significance. This difficult to treat disorder is discussed with a practical working diagnostic algorithm and practical treatment recommendations.

Multiple myeloma is clearly the most frequent and most serious of all of the monoclonal gammopathies, and Dr. Dispenzieri extensively reviews the history, pathogenesis, clinical diagnosis, and up-to-date therapies for this disorder. The variants of multiple myeloma, including solitary plasmacytoma and extramedullary plasmacytoma, are comprehensively reviewed by Dr. Lust, including monitoring these patients with the newest laboratory techniques, appropriate use of radiation therapy, and predicting outcomes. Plasma cell leukemia, primary and secondary, is an important subset of multiple myeloma that requires specific recognition, aggressive management, and awareness of some of the unique complications. These are reviewed by Dr. Hayman.

Several more obscure plasma cell dyscrasias are reviewed because it is our experience that without awareness of these disorders the diagnosis is frequently overlooked and the patient is not correctly managed. Dr. Wahner-Roedler reviews gamma, mu, and alpha heavy chain disease, their clinical manifestations and laboratory diagnosis. Amyloidosis, which is a life-threatening subset of the monoclonal gammopathies, is extensively reviewed, including the latest data on the use of stem cell transplantation. Other forms of immunoglobulin deposition disorders, including light chain deposition disease, its recognition and management, are covered by Dr. Zeldenrust, with emphasis on the differential diagnosis of an otherwise difficult to recognize problem.

Dr. Winkler provides comprehensive background on Waldenström macroglobulinemia, the rarest of the malignant monoclonal gammopathies, that strikes almost 1,500 patients per year, with new insights into its molecular biology, genetics, classification, staging, and therapy. A subset of patients with IgM monoclonal gammopathies have cryoprecipitable proteins. Dr. Dispenzieri reviews the clinical presentation of this multisystemic disorder in patients who frequently present to rheumatologists, neurologists, and dermatologists because of the diverse clinical presentation involving skin ulcers, joint pain, and peripheral neuropathy. Finally, Dr. Lacy reviews the clinical criteria to diagnose the rarest of the kappa light chain disorders, Fanconi syndrome, with its impact on skeletal structures.

We hope that by comprehensively covering both frequently and rarely seen monoclonal gammopathies this book can serve as a long-lasting reference volume for practicing clinicians and scientists directly involved in the care of patients with multiple myeloma and associated disorders, ultimately benefiting the patient by shortening the diagnostic evaluation and allowing appropriate timing of systemic therapy.

MORIE A. GERTZ, M.D.
PHILIP R. GREIPP, M.D.
Division of Hematology
and Internal Medicine
Mayo Clinic
Rochester, Minnesota

Contents

1 Monoclonal Gammopathies
of Undetermined Significance
and Smoldering Multiple Myeloma .   1
Robert A. Kyle, M.D.,
and S. Vincent Rajkumar, M.D.

2 Neuropathy Associated
With Plasma Cell Proliferative
Disorders   35
S. Vincent Rajkumar, M.D.,
Robert A. Kyle, M.D.,
Guillermo A. Suarez, M.D.,
and Angela Dispenzieri, M.D.

3 Multiple Myeloma   53
Angela Dispenzieri, M.D., Martha Q.
Lacy, M.D., and Philip R. Greipp, M.D.

4 Solitary Plasmacytoma of Bone
and Extramedullary Plasmacytoma . 111
John A. Lust, M.D., Ph.D.

5 Plasma Cell Leukemia 119
Suzanne R. Hayman, M.D.

6 Heavy Chain Diseases 133
Dietlind L. Wahner-Roedler, M.D.,
Robert A. Kyle, M.D.,
and Thomas E. Witzig, M.D.

7 Immunoglobulin Light Chain
Amyloidosis
(Primary Amyloidosis, AL) 157
Morie A. Gertz, M.D.,
Martha Q. Lacy, M.D.,
and Angela Dispenzieri, M.D.

8 Light Chain Deposition Disease   . . . 197
Steven R. Zeldenrust, M.D., Ph.D.,
Donna J. Lager, M.D.,
and Nelson Leung, M.D.

9 Waldenström Macroglobulinemia . . 205
Jerry M. Winkler, M.D.,
and Rafael Fonseca, M.D.

10 Cryoglobulinemia 227
Angela Dispenzieri, M.D.,
and Morie A. Gertz, M.D.

11 Acquired Fanconi Syndrome
Associated With Monoclonal
Plasma Cell Disorders 257
Martha Q. Lacy, M.D.,
and Morie A. Gertz, M.D.

Subject Index 265

Contributors

Angela Dispenzieri, M.D.
Consultant, Division of Hematology and Internal
Medicine, Mayo Clinic, Assistant Professor
of Medicine, Mayo Medical School, Rochester,
Minnesota, USA

Rafael Fonseca, M.D.
Consultant, Division of Hematology and Internal
Medicine, Mayo Clinic, Associate Professor
of Medicine, Mayo Medical School, Rochester,
Minnesota, USA

Morie A. Gertz, M.D.
Chair, Division of Hematology and Internal
Medicine, Mayo Clinic, Professor of Medicine,
Mayo Medical School, Rochester, Minnesota, USA

Philip R. Greipp, M.D.
Consultant, Division of Hematology and Internal
Medicine, Mayo Clinic, Professor of Medicine
and of Laboratory Medicine, Mayo Medical
School, Rochester, Minnesota, USA

Suzanne R. Hayman, M.D.
Consultant, Division of Hematology and Internal
Medicine, Mayo Clinic, Instructor in Medicine,
Mayo Medical School, Rochester, Minnesota, USA

Robert A. Kyle, M.D.
Consultant, Division of Hematology and Internal
Medicine, Mayo Clinic, Professor of Medicine
and of Laboratory Medicine, Mayo Medical
School, Rochester, Minnesota, USA

Martha Q. Lacy, M.D.
Consultant, Division of Hematology and Internal
Medicine, Mayo Clinic, Assistant Professor
of Medicine, Mayo Medical School, Rochester,
Minnesota, USA

Donna J. Lager, M.D.
Consultant, Division of Anatomic Pathology,
Mayo Clinic, Associate Professor of Pathology,
Mayo Medical School, Rochester, Minnesota, USA

Nelson Leung, M.D.
Senior Associate Consultant, Division
of Nephrology and Internal Medicine,
Mayo Clinic, Instructor in Medicine, Mayo
Medical School, Rochester, Minnesota, USA

John A. Lust, M.D., Ph.D.
Consultant, Division of Hematology and Internal
Medicine, Mayo Clinic, Associate Professor
of Medicine, Mayo Medical School, Rochester,
Minnesota, USA

S. Vincent Rajkumar, M.D.
Consultant, Division of Hematology and Internal
Medicine, Mayo Clinic, Associate Professor
of Medicine, Mayo Medical School, Rochester,
Minnesota, USA

Guillermo A. Suarez, M.D.
Consultant, Department of Neurology,
Mayo Clinic, Assistant Professor of Neurology,
Mayo Medical School, Rochester, Minnesota, USA

DIETLIND L. WAHNER-ROEDLER, M.D.
Consultant, Division of Area General Internal
Medicine, Mayo Clinic, Assistant Professor
of Medicine, Mayo Medical School, Rochester,
Minnesota, USA

JERRY M. WINKLER, M.D.
Fellow in Hematology, Mayo Graduate School
of Medicine, Instructor in Medicine
and in Oncology, Mayo Medical School,
Rochester, Minnesota, USA

THOMAS E. WITZIG, M.D.
Consultant, Division of Hematology and Internal
Medicine, Mayo Clinic, Professor of Medicine,
Mayo Medical School, Rochester, Minnesota, USA

STEVEN R. ZELDENRUST, M.D., Ph.D.
Senior Associate Consultant,
Division of Hematology and Internal Medicine,
Mayo Clinic, Assistant Professor of Medicine,
Mayo Medical School, Rochester, Minnesota, USA

Monoclonal Gammopathies of Undetermined Significance and Smoldering Multiple Myeloma

Robert A. Kyle, M.D., S. Vincent Rajkumar, M.D.*

Contents

1.1	Introduction	2
1.2	Monoclonal Gammopathy of Undetermined Significance	5
	1.2.1 Mayo Clinic Study	6
	1.2.1.1 Laboratory Studies	6
	1.2.1.2 Serum and Urine Studies	6
	1.2.1.3 Follow-up	6
	1.2.1.4 Analysis by Immunoglobulin Type	8
	1.2.1.5 Long-Term Follow-up in 1,384 MGUS Patients From Southeastern Minnesota	9
	1.2.1.6 Outcomes	11
	1.2.1.7 Risk Factors for Progression	15
	1.2.1.8 Follow-up in Other Series	16
	1.2.2 Predictors of Malignant Transformation in MGUS	16
	1.2.2.1 Amount of M Protein	16
	1.2.2.2 Type of Immunoglobulin	17
	1.2.2.3 Bone Marrow Plasma Cells	17
	1.2.2.4 Other Predictors	17
	1.2.3 Life Expectancy and Cause of Death in Patients With MGUS	17
	1.2.4 Differentiation of MGUS From Multiple Myeloma and Macroglobulinemia	18
	1.2.5 Management of MGUS	20
	1.2.6 Variants of MGUS	21
	1.2.6.1 Smoldering (Asymptomatic) MM	21
	1.2.6.2 Risk of Progression in Smoldering MM	21
	1.2.6.3 Predictors of Progression in Smoldering MM	22
	1.2.6.4 Management of Smoldering MM	22
	1.2.6.5 Biclonal Gammopathy	22
	1.2.6.6 Triclonal Gammopathy	23
	1.2.7 Benign Monoclonal Light Chain Idiopathic (Bence Jones) Proteinuria	23
	1.2.7.1 IgD MGUS	24
	1.2.8 Association of Monoclonal Gammopathy With Other Diseases	24
	1.2.8.1 Lymphoproliferative Disorders	24
	1.2.8.2 Leukemia	26
	1.2.8.3 Other Hematologic Diseases	26
	1.2.8.4 Connective Tissue Disorders	27
	1.2.8.5 Osteosclerotic Myeloma (POEMS)	27
	1.2.8.6 Dermatologic Diseases	28
	1.2.8.7 Immunosuppression	28
	1.2.8.8 Miscellaneous Conditions	29
	1.2.8.9 M Proteins With Antibody Activity	30
References		30

* This work was supported in part by grant CA62242 from the National Cancer Institute.

1.1 Introduction

The monoclonal gammopathies are a group of disorders characterized by the proliferation of a single clone of plasma cells that produces a homogeneous monoclonal (M) protein (Table 1.1). Each M protein consists of 2 heavy polypeptide chains of the same class and subclass and 2 light polypeptide chains of the same type. Polyclonal immunoglobulins are produced by many clones of plasma cells. The population of polyclonal immunoglobulins is heterogeneous with respect to heavy-chain classes and includes both light-chain types. The various types of immunoglobulins are designated by capital letters that correspond to the isotype of their heavy chains, which are designated by Greek letters: gamma (γ) constitutes immunoglobulin G (IgG), alpha (α) is found in IgA, mu (μ) is present in IgM, delta (δ) occurs in IgD, and epsilon (ε) characterizes IgE. IgG1, IgG2, IgG3, and IgG4 are the subclasses of IgG, and the subclasses of IgA are IgA1 and IgA2. Kappa (κ) and lambda (λ) are the 2 types of light chain.

One must distinguish between a monoclonal and a polyclonal increase in immunoglobulins because a monoclonal increase results from a clonal process that is malignant or potentially malignant, whereas a polyclonal increase in immunoglobulins is caused by a reactive or inflammatory process. In a group of 148 patients with a polyclonal gamma globulin concentration of 3.0 g/dL or more, liver disease was the most common association (61%), followed by connective tissue diseases (22%), chronic infections (6%), hematologic disorders (5%), and nonhematologic malignancies (3%) (Dispenzieri et al. 2001a).

Analysis of the serum or urine requires a sensitive, rapid, dependable screening method to detect the presence of an M protein and a specific assay to identify it according to its heavy-chain class and light-chain type. Agarose gel electrophoresis is more sensitive than cellulose acetate and is the preferred method of detection. After recognizing a localized band on electrophoresis, immunofixation or immunoelectrophoresis must be done to confirm the presence of an M protein and to determine its immunoglobulin heavy-chain class and its light-chain type. Immunofixation or immunoelectrophoresis should also be done when multiple myeloma (MM), Waldenström macroglobulinemia (WM), primary systemic amyloidosis (AL), or a related disorder is suspected, because small M proteins may be missed with serum protein electrophoresis (Keren et al. 1999).

Table 1.1. Classification of monoclonal gammopathies

I. Monoclonal gammopathy of undetermined significance

  A. Benign (IgG, IgA, IgD, IgM, and, rarely, free light chains)

  B. Associated with neoplasms of cell types not known to produce M proteins

  C. Biclonal gammopathies

  D. Idiopathic Bence Jones proteinuria

II. Malignant monoclonal gammopathies

  A. Multiple myeloma (IgG, IgA, IgD, IgE, and free κ or λ light chains)

    1. Overt multiple myeloma

    2. Smoldering multiple myeloma

    3. Plasma cell leukemia

    4. Nonsecretory myeloma

    5. IgD myeloma

    6. POEMS: polyneuropathy, organomegaly, endocrinopathy, M protein, and skin changes (osteosclerotic myeloma)

  B. Plasmacytoma

    1. Solitary plasmacytoma of bone

    2. Extramedullary plasmacytoma

  C. Malignant lymphoproliferative disorders

    1. Waldenström macroglobulinemia (primary macroglobulinemia)

    2. Malignant lymphoma

    3. Chronic lymphocytic leukemia or lymphoproliferative disorders

  D. Heavy-chain diseases

    1. Gamma heavy-chain disease

    2. Alpha heavy-chain disease

    3. Mu heavy-chain disease

  E. Amyloidosis

    1. Primary amyloidosis

    2. With multiple myeloma (secondary, localized, and familial amyloidosis have no M protein)

From Kyle RA, Rajkumar SV (2002) Monoclonal gammopathies of undetermined significance. Rev Clin Exp Hematol 6:225–252. By permission of Blackwell Publishing.

Serum protein electrophoresis should be done when MM, WM, or AL is suspected. In addition, electrophoresis is indicated in any patient with unexplained weakness or fatigue, elevation of the erythrocyte sedimentation rate, anemia, unexplained back pain, osteoporosis, osteolytic lesions or fractures, hypercalcemia, Bence Jones proteinuria, renal insufficiency, or recurrent infections (Kyle 1999). Serum protein electrophoresis should also be performed in adults with unexplained sensorimotor peripheral neuropathy, carpal tunnel syndrome, refractory congestive heart failure, nephrotic syndrome, orthostatic hypotension, or malabsorption, because a localized band or spike strongly suggests AL. Weight loss, change in the tongue or voice, paresthesias, numbness, increased bruising, bleeding, and steatorrhea are additional indications for the performance of serum protein electrophoresis. Even when the serum protein electrophoretic pattern is nondiagnostic, immunofixation should be performed whenever MM, AL, or related disorders are suspected clinically.

An M protein is usually visible as a localized band on the agarose gel electrophoretic strip or as a tall, narrow spike or peak in the β or γ regions or, rarely, in the α_2-globulin area of the densitometer tracing (Fig. 1.1). The agarose gel should always be examined directly by the interpreter. A polyclonal increase in immuno-globulins produces a broad band or broad-based peak and migrates in the γ region.

Immunofixation to determine the type of monoclonal protein may be performed by using commercial kits or systems such as Sebia Pentafix and 9-IF (Fig. 1.2) (Kyle et al. 2002a). An alternative is for laboratory personnel to pour their own plates and perform immunofixation. An M protein is characterized on immunofixation by the presence of a sharp, well-defined band associated with a single heavy-chain class and a sharp, defined band of the same mobility, which reacts with either κ or λ antisera. A biclonal gammopathy consists of 2 heavy chains and 2 monoclonal light chains that match the mobility of the heavy chains. This occurs in more than 5% of patients with monoclonal gammopathies. In all patients with a monoclonal light chain in the serum and no corresponding γ, α, or μ heavy chain, the possibility of IgD or IgE monoclonal gammopathy must be considered. One can screen by Ouchterlony immunodiffusion for an increased amount of IgD or IgE. Immunofixation with IgD or IgE antisera must be done if the concentration of either immunoglobulin is elevated on nephelometry or immunodiffusion to determine whether the increase is monoclonal. Immunoelectrophoresis may also be used for the detection of an M protein, but it is not as sensitive as immunofixation and it is more labor intensive, so most laboratories no longer perform it.

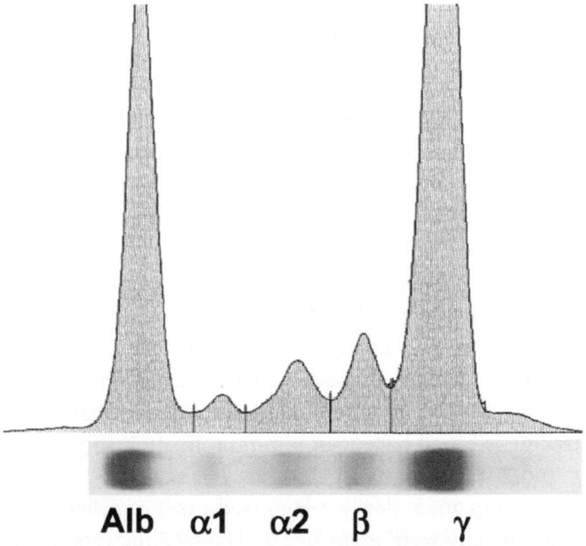

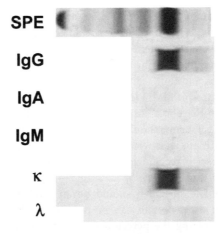

Fig. 1.1. *Top,* Monoclonal pattern of serum M protein by densitometry after electrophoresis on agarose gel. Note tall, narrow-based peak of fast gamma mobility. *Bottom,* Monoclonal pattern from electrophoresis of serum on agarose gel (anode on left; dense localized band in fast gamma area)

Alb α1 α2 β γ

IgG κ

Fig. 1.2. Immunofixation of serum with antisera to IgG, IgA, IgM, kappa, and lambda shows a localized band with IgG and kappa in the gamma region. *SPE,* serum protein electrophoresis

SPE
IgG
IgA
IgM
κ
λ

Quantitation of immunoglobulins is best performed with a rate nephelometer, because it is not affected by molecular size and accurately measures 7S IgM, polymers of IgA, and aggregates of IgG. However, values for IgM obtained by nephelometry may be 1,000 to 2,000 mg/dL higher than those expected on the basis of the serum protein electrophoretic tracing. The quantitative IgG and IgA levels may be increased similarly (Riches et al. 1991). If an M protein value is small, the use of quantitative immunoglobulins also reflects the amount of polyclonal immunoglobulin in the serum. To monitor the amount of the M protein, we recommend use of serum protein electrophoresis with densitometry. If the M protein value is large and there is little polyclonal immunoglobulin, nephelometry can be used to monitor the amount of the M protein. Because the results of the 2 methods are not identical, sequential monitoring must be done with either the densitometry tracing or nephelometry or both techniques.

Analysis of urine is essential for patients with monoclonal gammopathies. Sulfosalicylic acid or Exton reagent is best for detection of protein. Dipsticks, which are used in many laboratories to screen for protein, are often insensitive to Bence Jones protein and should not be used. Screening tests have been used for the detection of Bence Jones protein since the discovery of their unique thermal properties. The heat test produces false-positive and false-negative results and should not be used for the detection of Bence Jones proteinuria. Recognition of Bence Jones proteinuria depends on the demonstration of monoclonal light chain by electrophoresis and immunofixation of an adequately concentrated aliquot from a 24-hour urine specimen. All patients with a serum M-protein concentration of more than 1.5 g/dL should have urine electrophoresis and immunofixation. In addition, electrophoresis should be done in all instances of MM, WM, AL, and heavy-chain diseases or when there is a suspicion of these entities. Immunofixation of urine should also be done in the evaluation of older patients with a nephrotic syndrome of unknown cause to recognize the presence of AL or light-chain deposition disease.

A 24-hour urine specimen should be collected so that the amount of M protein can be measured. This is done by multiplying the percentage of the M spike in the densitometer tracing by the total protein in the 24-hour specimen. The amount of M protein in the urine provides an index of the tumor's mass and consequently is useful in monitoring the course of the pa-

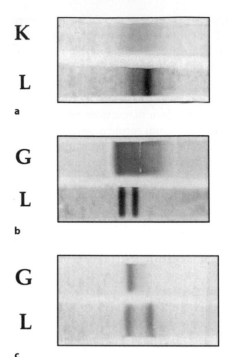

Fig. 1.3. *a,* Immunofixation of concentrated urine specimen with antisera to κ (K) and λ (L) shows discrete λ band. This indicates a monoclonal λ light chain. *b,* Immunofixation of urine with antisera to IgG (G) and λ (L) shows 2 discrete λ bands. The reaction with IgG is polyclonal. The 2 discrete bands represent monomers and dimers of the monoclonal λ light chain. *c,* Immunofixation of urine with antisera to IgG (G) and λ (L). The findings indicate a monoclonal λ protein plus IgG λ fragment. (*a–c* From Kyle et al. [2002a]. By permission of the American Society for Microbiology.)

tient's disease. A urinary M protein is seen as a dense localized band on the agarose gel or a tall narrow homogeneous peak on the densitometer tracing. Occasionally, 2 discrete globulin bands are seen on the agarose gel. These bands may represent monomers and dimers of a monoclonal light chain or a monoclonal light chain plus a monoclonal immunoglobulin fragment from the serum M protein (Fig. 1.3). A polyclonal increase of light chains is seen as a broad band on electrophoresis, extending through much of the γ region. The densitometer tracing is broad based, and immunofixation shows both κ and λ bands.

During 2002, newly recognized cases of monoclonal gammopathy were identified at Mayo Clinic (Fig. 1.4*a*). The type of monoclonal gammopathy is shown in Figure 1.4*b*. The term "monoclonal gammopathy of undetermined significance" (MGUS) denotes the presence of an M protein in persons without evidence of MM,

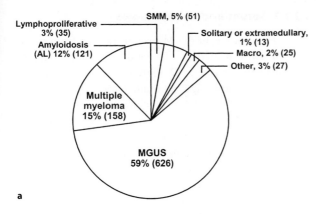

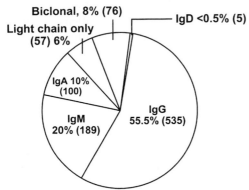

Fig. 1.4. *a*, Monoclonal gammopathies, Mayo Clinic, 2002. *b*, Monoclonal serum proteins. *MGUS*, monoclonal gammopathy of undetermined significance. *SMM*, smoldering multiple myeloma. (From Kyle RA, Rajkumar SV [2003] Monoclonal gammopathies of undetermined significance: a review. Immunol Rev 194:112–139. By permission of Blackwell Munksgaard.)

WM, AL, lymphoproliferative disorders, plasmacytoma, or related conditions.

1.2 Monoclonal Gammopathy of Undetermined Significance

MGUS indicates the presence of a monoclonal protein (M protein) in persons without evidence of MM, macroglobulinemia, amyloidosis, lymphoma, or other related diseases. MGUS is characterized by a serum M-protein concentration of less than 3 g/dL, less than 10% plasma cells in the bone marrow, no or only small amounts of M protein in the urine, the absence of lytic bone lesions, anemia, hypercalcemia, renal insufficiency related to the M protein, and, most importantly, stability of the M protein and failure of development of additional ab-

normalities. The proliferative (growth) rate of the plasma cells (plasma cell labeling index) is low. The finding of MGUS is an unexpected event in the laboratory testing of an apparently normal person or may occur during the evaluation of an unrelated disorder.

The term "benign monoclonal gammopathy" is misleading because it is not known at diagnosis whether an M protein will remain stable and benign or will develop into symptomatic MM, macroglobulinemia, amyloidosis, or a related disorder. Since Waldenström's introduction of the term "essential hyperglobulinemia" in 1952, many terms have been used, including "idiopathic, asymptomatic, benign, nonmyelomatous, discrete, cryptogenic, and rudimentary monoclonal gammopathy, dysimmunoglobulinemia, lanthanic monoclonal gammopathy, idiopathic paraproteinemia, and asymptomatic paraimmunoglobulinemia." Waldenström emphasized the constancy of the amount of the M protein, contrasting it to the increasing quantity of the M protein in myeloma.

MGUS has been found in approximately 3% of persons older than 70 years in Sweden (Axelsson et al. 1966), the United States (Kyle et al. 1972), and France (Saleun et al. 1982). In 6,995 persons from Sweden older than 25 years, an M protein was found in 1% (Axelsson et al. 1966). In a community cluster of cases of MM in a small Minnesota community (Kyle et al. 1972), M protein was detected in 15 of 1,200 persons 50 years or older (1.25%), and in France, in 303 of 17,968 persons 50 years or older (1.7%) (Saleun et al. 1982). The incidence of MGUS is higher in older patients. In 111 patients older than 80 years, 10% had an M protein. Of 4,039 persons aged 75 to 84 years, 23% had an M protein. In a study of persons in North Carolina (Cohen et al. 1998), the incidence of MGUS was 3.6% in 816 persons 70 years or older.

The incidence of M proteins is higher in African Americans than in whites. In the study by Cohen et al. (1998), the prevalence of an M protein was 8.4% in 916 African Americans compared with 3.6% in whites. On the other hand, only 2.7% of elderly Japanese patients had a monoclonal gammopathy. Recently, Kurihara et al. (2000) found an M protein in 71 of 2,007 inpatients and outpatients (3.5%) in a Japanese university hospital. Excluding the 13 patients with myeloma and macroglobulinemia, the incidence was 2.9%, which is greater than previously reported.

An M protein was found in 1.2% of 73,630 hospitalized patients. In a study of 118,130 nonhospitalized patients in Italy, 0.63% had an M protein (Sala et al.

1989), whereas 0.7% of 102,000 persons in an Italian general hospital had an M protein.

MGUS is a common finding in medical practice. It is important for the patient and the physician to determine whether the M protein will remain benign or will progress to MM or related disorders.

1.2.1 Mayo Clinic Study

We reviewed the medical records of all patients with monoclonal gammopathy who were evaluated at Mayo Clinic from 1956 through 1970. Patients with MM, macroglobulinemia, amyloidosis, lymphoma, or related disorders were excluded. Two hundred forty-one patients remained for long-term study. Only 4% of patients were younger than age 40 years at the time of recognition of the M protein, and one-third were age 70 years or older. The median age was 64 years. Fifty-eight percent were male. The liver was palpable in 15% and the spleen was palpable in 4%, but hepatosplenomegaly was not directly related to the M protein.

1.2.1.1 Laboratory Studies

The hemoglobin concentration at initial evaluation ranged from 7.2 to 16.6 g/dL. Melena, myeloid metaplasia, myeloproliferative disease, Wegener granulomatosis, hypoplasia of bone marrow, chronic cold agglutinin disease, and hypernephroma accounted for the anemia in the 9 patients whose hemoglobin was <10 g/dL. Leukopenia ($<2\times10^9$/L) occurred in a patient with a myeloproliferative process and in another with myeloid metaplasia. Thrombocytopenia ($<100\times10^9$/L) occurred in only 5 patients, and they had myeloid metaplasia, acute leukemia, idiopathic thrombocytopenic purpura, lupus erythematosus, or bone marrow hypoplasia. Thrombocytosis ($>500\times10^9$/L) occurred in 2 patients – 1 had pneumonia and the other had rectal bleeding. Serum creatinine was >2.0 mg/dL in 5 patients. Three had nephrosclerosis, 1 had diabetes mellitus, and another had uric acid nephropathy. Two patients (1 with Wegener granulomatosis and the other with hypernephroma) had a serum albumin value <2 g/dL. The 2 patients with hypercalcemia (>11 mg/dL) had hyperparathyroidism.

1.2.1.2 Serum and Urine Studies

The concentration of the M protein ranged from 0.3 to 3.2 g/dL, with a median of 1.7 g/dL. Of those samples with a visible spike, 77% migrated in the γ area and 20% in the β area. IgG accounted for 73%; IgA, 11%; and IgM, 14%; a biclonal gammopathy was found in 2%. The monoclonal light-chain type was κ in 62% and λ in the remainder. Twenty-nine percent of the 181 patients who had measurement of their immunoglobulins had a decrease in uninvolved immunoglobulins. Eighty-seven percent of the patients had IgG1 subclass, 4% had IgG2, 4% had IgG3, and 5% had IgG4.

Electrophoresis of a 24-hour urine specimen was performed in less than one-half of patients because proteinuria is found infrequently on routine urinalysis and consequently the physician does not collect a 24-hour specimen. Thirty-four percent of the 74 patients who were tested with immunoelectrophoresis had a monoclonal light chain. In all but 3 patients the M protein was less than 1 g/24 h. The number of bone marrow plasma cells ranged from 1% to 10% (median, 3%) in the 109 patients in whom a bone marrow study was performed at the time of recognition of the M protein.

1.2.1.3 Follow-up

At 24 to 38 years of follow-up after recognition of the M protein, the number of patients who were still living and whose M protein had remained stable and whose disease could be classified as "benign monoclonal gammopathy" was 25 (10%). The M protein disappeared without apparent cause from the serum of 2 patients. The concentration of hemoglobin, amount of serum M protein, type of serum heavy and light chains, decrease in uninvolved immunoglobulins, subclass of IgG heavy chain, and number of plasma cells in the bone marrow did not differ substantially in the benign group compared with the remainder. One patient had IgGκ and an M protein of approximately 2.6 g/dL for 26 years and a monoclonal κ light chain in the urine >1 g/24 h for the 25 years of follow-up. He had grade 3–4 proteinuria for 7 years before the recognition of the light chain in the urine. This patient remained well. Six patients with a small M protein value in the urine, which was discovered after recognition of the serum M protein, remained stable during 13+ years of follow-up.

Twenty-six patients (11%) had an increase of the M protein to >3 g/dL but did not develop symptomatic

MM, macroglobulinemia, or amyloidosis. The median interval from the recognition of the M protein to an increase of 3 g/dL was 9 years. Five patients are still living and continue to be followed. One patient with smoldering macroglobulinemia had an IgM protein >3 g/dL for more than 13 years. He had not required chemotherapy. The M protein increased gradually over 8 to 18 years before reaching 3 g/dL; 6 had a fluctuating M protein for 6 to 18 years before reaching 3 g/dL. One patient had a sudden increase in the M protein. The remaining 5 patients' data were insufficient to ascertain the pattern of increase. Eight of the 26 patients had a monoclonal light chain in the urine, and in 1 patient the urine M protein disappeared after removal of a parathyroid adenoma, but the serum M protein remained stable. The λ light chain reappeared after 19 years, but multiple biopsies showed no evidence of amyloidosis.

One hundred twenty-seven patients (53%) died without development of myeloma or related disorders. The median interval from the recognition of the serum M protein to death was 7 years. Thirty-one patients were followed for more than 10 years. Fourteen patients had a monoclonal protein in the urine. The most frequent cause of death was cardiac (37%), followed by cerebrovascular disease (15%). Fifteen patients died of a nonplasma cell malignancy.

MM, macroglobulinemia, amyloidosis, or lymphoproliferative disease developed in 63 patients; actuarial rate at 10 years was 17%, at 20 years it was 33% (Fig. 1.5), and at 25 years it was 40%. Forty-three of the 63 patients (68%) with progression had MM. All but 4 with a diagnosis of MM had a bone marrow aspirate or biopsy specimen that contained more than 15% abnormal plasma cells. In 2 of the 4 patients, the diagnosis of MM was made at their local hospital and we were unable to obtain the bone marrow slides. Both patients had extensive lytic lesions and severe anemia. The 3rd patient had a large destructive plasmacytoma of the sacrum, stenosis of the spinal canal, and an M protein of 2.4 g/dL. Results of the bone marrow examination were not available. The 4th patient had severe anemia, hypercalcemia, and an M protein of 3.7 g/dL, but this patient refused a bone marrow examination. Three of the 8 patients with an M protein <3 g/dL had a large urinary M-protein value and all 8 had skeletal involvement. Of the 25 patients who were studied, 20 had a urinary M protein. Lytic bone lesions were found in 73%. Three other patients had osteoporosis. Thus, the diagnosis of MM is secure.

Intervals from the recognition of the M protein to the diagnosis of MM ranged from 2 to 29 years (median, 10 years) (Table 1.2). In 9 patients, the diagnosis was made 20 years after recognition of the serum M protein. Median survival after diagnosis of MM was 33 months, which is similar to the expected survival.

The M-protein value increased gradually or abruptly (Table 1.3). In 11 patients, it remained stable for a median of 8 years and then gradually increased over 3 years until the diagnosis of symptomatic myeloma. In 7 patients, the serum M-protein concentration was stable

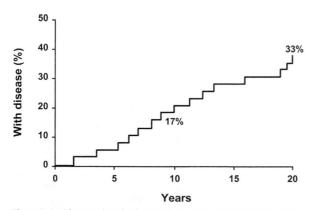

Fig. 1.5. Incidence of multiple myeloma, macroglobulinemia, amyloidosis, or lymphoproliferative disease after recognition of monoclonal protein. Actuarial analysis. (From Kyle RA, Lust JA [1990] The monoclonal gammopathies [paraproteins]. Adv Clin Chem 28:145–218. By permission of Elsevier Science.)

Table 1.2. Development of myeloma or related diseases in 63 patients with monoclonal gammopathy of undetermined significance

Disease	Patients		Interval to diagnosis, y*	
	No.	%	Median	Range
Multiple myeloma	43	68	10	2–29
Macroglobulinemia	7	11	8.5	4–20
Amyloidosis	8	13	9	6–19
Lymphoproliferative	5	8	10.5	6–22
Total	63	100		

* Actuarial rate was 17% at 10 years and 33% at 20 years.

From Kyle RA, Rajkumar SV (2002) Monoclonal gammopathies of undetermined significance. Rev Clin Exp Hematol 6:225-252. By permission of Blackwell Publishing.

Table 1.3. Pattern of increase in M protein in 39 patients with monoclonal gammopathy of undetermined significance in whom multiple myeloma developed

Patients, no.	Pattern of increase, y	Duration, y
11	Stable 4–18 (median, 8)	Then gradual ↑, 1–4 (median, 3)
7	Stable 2–25 (median, 8)	Then rapid ↑
7	Stable 1–16 (median, 2)	Then 2–10 without data (median, 4)
7	Gradual (fluctuating)	5–29 (median, 12)
7	Insufficient data	Insufficient data

for a median of 8 years and then increased rapidly as myeloma developed. Seven patients had a fluctuating but gradually increasing serum M-protein spike until MM was diagnosed at a median of 12 years. In 7 patients, serum M protein was stable for a median of 4 years, but data were not available to determine the mode of development of myeloma. For the remaining 7 patients, no M-protein values were available between the recognition of the M protein and the diagnosis of myeloma 3 to 10 years later.

WM developed in 7 patients. All had a serum IgMκ protein ranging from 3.1 to 8.5 g/dL and other typical features during the course of the disease.

Systemic amyloidosis was found in 8 patients 6 to 19 years after the recognition of an M protein in the serum (median, 9 years). Amyloidosis was recognized at autopsy in 3 patients, renal biopsy in 2, lymph node biopsy in 1, and rectal biopsy in 1 at the same time as operation for carcinoma of the colon. Two patients had nephrotic syndrome and 1 had cardiomegaly. Amyloidosis was not clinically suspected in the 3 patients in whom the diagnosis was made at autopsy, and it would have been overlooked if a postmortem examination had not been done. One of these patients developed acute pulmonary edema and died in the emergency department; another had weakness, weight loss, and gastrointestinal tract symptoms, without apparent cause; and the 3rd had symptomatic cryoglobulinemia, congestive heart failure, and sensorimotor peripheral neuropathy.

A malignant lymphoproliferative process developed in 5 patients 9 to 22 years (median, 10.5 years) after detection of the M protein. One patient had a biclonal gammopathy and lupus erythematosus, and an aggressive, diffuse undifferentiated malignant lymphoma developed 9 years later. Anorexia, weight loss, and generalized bone pain developed in another patient 22 years after the recognition of an IgMλ M protein. Extensive retroperitoneal lymphadenopathy, bone marrow evidence of immunoblastic lymphoma, and lymphocytes in the cerebrospinal fluid were consistent with lymphoma. Chronic lymphocytic leukemia developed in 1 patient. The M protein did not change and was probably unrelated to the chronic lymphocytic leukemia. Another patient had a diffuse mixed lymphoma of the jejunum at surgical exploration for abdominal pain 10 years after the detection of the serum M protein.

1.2.1.4 Analysis by Immunoglobulin Type

The actuarial rate of development of myeloma and related disorders in patients with an IgG or an IgA protein was 13% at 10 years and 29% at 20 years (Fig. 1.6); those with an IgM protein had an actuarial rate of 21% at 10 years and 49% at 20 years (Fig. 1.7). There was no statistical difference in progression on the basis of the type of M protein. Survival of patients with IgG, IgA, or IgM M proteins was also similar. Either MM or a related disorder or an increase of the serum M protein >3 g/dL occurred in 82 of the 241 patients (34%). Survival of the

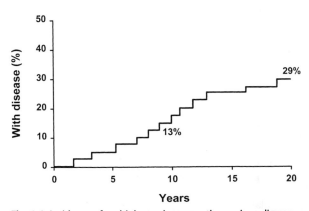

Fig. 1.6. Incidence of multiple myeloma or other serious disease after recognition of IgG or IgA monoclonal gammopathy. Actuarial analysis. (From Kyle RA, Lust JA [1990] The monoclonal gammopathies [paraproteins]. Adv Clin Chem 28:145–218. By permission of Elsevier Science.)

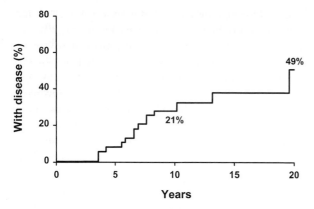

Fig. 1.7. Incidence of macroglobulinemia, amyloidosis, or lympho-proliferative disease after recognition of IgM monoclonal gammo-pathy. Actuarial analysis. (From Kyle RA, Lust JA [1990] The mono-clonal gammopathies [paraproteins]. Adv Clin Chem 28:145–218. By permission of Elsevier Science.)

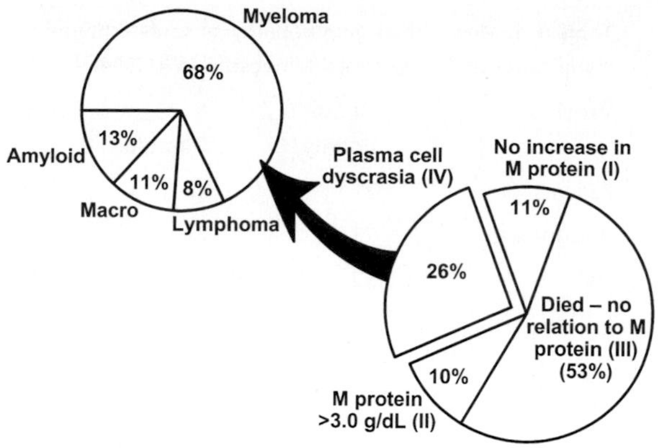

Fig. 1.9. Evolution of monoclonal gammopathies in 241 patients from Mayo Clinic, 1956–1970. *Macro*, macroglobulinemia. (Modified from Kyle RA, Rajkumar SV [2002] Monoclonal gammopathies of undetermined significance. Rev Clin Exp Hematol 6:225–252. By permission of Blackwell Publishing.)

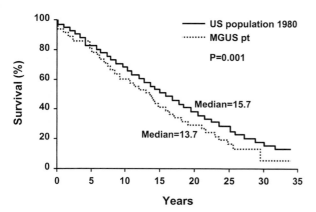

Fig. 1.8. Survival among 241 patients with a monoclonal gammo-pathy of undetermined significance (*MGUS*) and the age- and sex-adjusted 1980 US population. (From Kyle [1993]. By permission of Mayo Foundation for Medical Education and Research.)

Table 1.4. Monoclonal gammopathy of undetermined significance in southeastern Minnesota

Age at diagnosis of MGUS*, y	Patients, %
<40	2
40–49	4
50–59	11
60–69	24
70–79	35
80–89	21
≥90	3
Total	100

MGUS, monoclonal gammopathy of undetermined significance.
* Median, 72 years; range, 24-96 years.

241 MGUS patients was 13.7 years compared with 15.7 years for the age- and sex-adjusted US population of 1980 (Fig. 1.8). Results of long-term follow-up of the 241 MGUS patients are shown in Figure 1.9.

1.2.1.5 Long-Term Follow-up in 1,384 MGUS Patients From Southeastern Minnesota

A population-based study was done to confirm the find-ings of the original Mayo Clinic study, which consisted mainly of patients referred to a tertiary care center. One thousand three hundred eighty-four persons who re-sided in the 11 counties of southeastern Minnesota were

identified as having MGUS with a serum M protein val-ue of 3.0 g/dL or less; ≤10% plasma cells in the bone marrow, if the test was done; no or only modest amounts of M protein in the urine; and the absence of lytic bone lesions, anemia, hypercalcemia, or renal in-sufficiency related to the M protein. The patients were evaluated at Mayo Clinic from January 1, 1960, through December 31, 1994 (Kyle et al. 2002b). The median age at diagnosis of MGUS was 72 years. There were 753 males (54%) and 631 females (46%). Only 24 patients (2%) were younger than 40 years of age at diagnosis

Table 1.5. Monoclonal gammopathy of undetermined significance in southeastern Minnesota (N=1,384)

Variable	Olmsted County	Non-Olmsted	Total
Patients, %	37	63	100
Age, median, y	73	72	72
Male, %	52	60	54
IgG, %	69	70	70
M spike, median g/dL	1.3	1.2	1.2

compared with 810 (59%) who were age 70 years or older (Table 1.4). Other than a slightly older age of Olmsted County residents (median, 73 vs. 72 years; $P=0.04$) and a higher M-protein value (median, 1.3 vs. 1.2 g/dL; $P=0.01$), there was no statistically or clinically significant difference between the 2 groups, so they were combined for the analysis (Table 1.5).

The M protein at diagnosis ranged from unmeasurable to 3.0 g/dL (Fig. 1.10). On the basis of heavy-chain type, 70% of the M proteins were IgG; 12%, IgA; and 15%, IgM. A biclonal gammopathy was found in 45 patients (3%). The light chain was κ in 61% and λ in 39%. The electrophoretic mobility of the M protein and its heavy-chain type and light-chain class were unchanged throughout the period of observation. A reduction of uninvolved (normal or background) immunoglobulins was found in 38% of 840 patients in whom immunoglobulins were quantified. The median levels of the reduced immunoglobulins were 40 mg/dL for IgA, 50 mg/dL for IgM, and 580 mg/dL for IgG. Electrophoresis, immunoelectrophoresis, and immunofixation of urine were performed in 418 patients. Twenty-one percent had a monoclonal κ light chain and 10% had λ at the time of recognition of the abnormal monoclonal gammopathy; 69% were negative. Only 17% of the patients had an M protein >150 mg/24 h (Fig. 1.11).

One hundred sixty patients (12%) had a bone marrow examination performed at the time of detection of the M protein. The median percentage of bone marrow plasma cells was 3% (range, 0% to 10%). The initial hemoglobin values ranged from 5.7 to 18.9 g/dL. The hemoglobin value was <10 g/dL in 7% and ≤12 g/dL in 23%. The anemia was from causes other than the plasma cell proliferative process (such as iron deficiency, renal insufficiency, or myelodysplasia) in each instance. The median platelet value was 264×10⁹/L, and only 3% of patients had values <100×10⁹/L. The serum creatinine concentration was >2 mg/dL in 6% of the patients and was attributable to unrelated causes such as diabetes, hypertension, and glomerulonephritis. Unrelated hypercalcemia (serum calcium >11 mg/dL) was present in 0.5% of the MGUS patients at diagnosis.

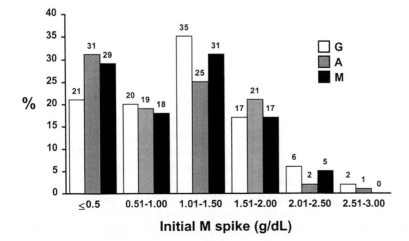

Fig. 1.10. Amount of serum M protein at time of diagnosis of 1,384 patients with monoclonal gammopathy of undetermined significance from southeastern Minnesota. *A*, IgA; *G*, IgG; *M*, IgM

Fig. 1.11. Amount of urine M protein at time of diagnosis of 1,384 patients with monoclonal gammopathy of undetermined significance from southeastern Minnesota.

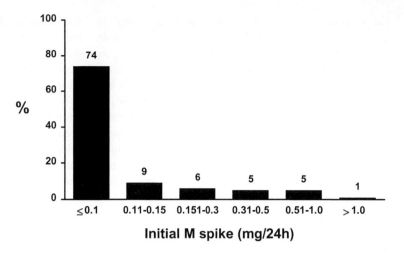

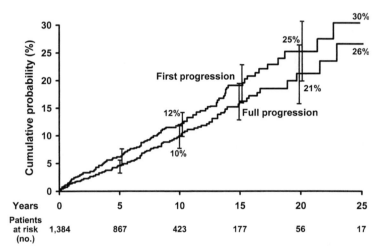

Fig. 1.12. Probability of progression among 1,384 residents of southeastern Minnesota in whom monoclonal gammopathy of undetermined significance (*MGUS*) was diagnosed from 1960 through 1994. The top curve represents the probability of progression to a plasma cell cancer (115 patients) or of an increase in the monoclonal protein concentration to more than 3 g/dL or the proportion of plasma cells in the bone marrow to more than 10% (32 patients). The bottom curve shows only the probability of progression of MGUS to multiple myeloma, IgM lymphoma, primary amyloidosis, macroglobulinemia, chronic lymphocytic leukemia, or plasmacytoma (115 patients). The bars show 95% confidence intervals. (From Kyle et al. [2002b]. By permission of the Massachusetts Medical Society.)

Table 1.6. Duration of follow-up of patients with monoclonal gammopathy of undetermined significance in southeastern Minnesota

Variable	Finding
Person-years	11,009
Range, y	0–35
Median, y	15.4
Deaths, no. (%)	963 (70)

1.2.1.6 Outcomes

These 1,384 patients were followed for a total of 11,009 person-years (median, 15.4 years; range, 0 to 35 years) (Table 1.6). Nine hundred sixty-three patients (70%) have died. During follow-up, 115 patients (8%) developed MM, AL, lymphoma with an IgM serum M protein, macroglobulinemia, plasmacytoma, or chronic lymphocytic leukemia (Table 1.7). The cumulative probability of progression to 1 of these disorders was 10% at 10 years, 21% at 20 years, and 26% at 25 years (Fig. 1.12). The risk of progression was about 1% per year; patients were at risk for progression even after 25 years or more of stable MGUS. In addition, 32 patients were identified in whom the M-protein value increased to >3 g/dL or the percentage of bone marrow plasma cells increased to >10% but in whom symptomatic MM did not develop. Because patients who die are removed, this curve reflects the probability that a patient who has not died of other causes will experience plasma cell progression at each point in the follow-up; it therefore represents the natural history of the disease. The cumulative probability of progression to MM or a related disorder plus an increase in M protein to >3 g/dL or >10% in bone marrow plasma cells was 12% at 10 years, 25% at 20 years, and 30% at 25 years.

MGUS patients survived less well than expected for Minnesota residents of similar age and sex (8.1 vs. 11.8 years, $P \leq 0.001$) (Fig. 1.13). The rate of death at 10 years was 6% from plasma cell disorders and 53% from non-plasma cell disorders such as cardiovascular and cerebrovascular diseases and nonplasma cell cancers (Fig. 1.14). At 20 years, the rates were 10% for plasma cell disorders and 72% for nonplasma cell disorders. At 25 years, the rate for plasma cell disorders was 11% compared with 76% for nonplasma cell diseases. These findings confirmed the results of the initial Mayo Clinic study (Fig. 1.15).

The number of patients with progression to a plasma cell disorder (115 patients) was 7.3 times the number expected on the basis of the incidence rates for those conditions in the general population (Table 1.7). The risk of developing MM was increased 25-fold, macroglobulinemia 46-fold, and AL 8.4-fold. The risk of development of lymphoma was increased only modestly at 2.4-fold, but this risk is underestimated because only lymphomas associated with an IgM protein counted in the observed number, whereas the incidence rates for lymphomas associated with IgG, IgA, and IgM proteins were used to calculate the expected number. The risk of development of chronic lymphocytic leukemia was only slightly increased (Table 1.7) when all 6 cases were included.

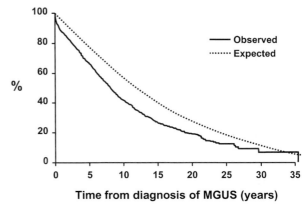

Fig. 1.13. Survival of 1,384 patients with monoclonal gammopathy of undetermined significance (*MGUS*) in southeastern Minnesota compared to a normal population (8.1 vs. 11.8 years, respectively; *P* <0.001). (From Kyle RA, Rajkumar SV [2003] Monoclonal gammopathies of undetermined significance: a review 194:112–139. Immunol Rev 194:112–139. By permission of Blackwell Munksgaard.)

Table 1.7. Relative risk of progression among 1,384 southeastern Minnesota residents diagnosed with monoclonal gammopathy of undetermined significance

Disease	Progression			
	Obs	Exp	RR	95% CI
Multiple myeloma	75	3[*]	25	20, 32
Lymphoma	19[†]	7.8[*]	2.4	2, 4
Amyloidosis	10	1.2[‡]	8.4	4, 16
Macroglobulinemia	7	0.2[*]	46	19, 95
Chronic lymphocytic leukemia	3	3.5[*]	0.9	0.2, 3
Plasmacytoma	1	0.1[*]	8.5	0.2, 47
Total	115	15.8	7.3	6, 9

CI, confidence interval; exp, expected; obs, observed; RR, relative risk. [*] Iowa SEER registry. [†] All had IgM serum monoclonal protein. [‡] Kyle et al. 1992. From Kyle et al. (2002b). By permission of the Massachusetts Medical Society.

Fig. 1.14. Rate of death from nonplasma cell disorders compared to progression to plasma cell disorders in 1,384 patients with monoclonal gammopathy of undetermined significance from southeastern Minnesota. (From Kyle RA, Rajkumar SV [2003] Monoclonal gammopathies of undetermined significance: a review. Immunol Rev 194:112–139. By permission of Blackwell Munksgaard.)

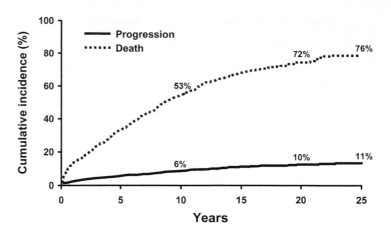

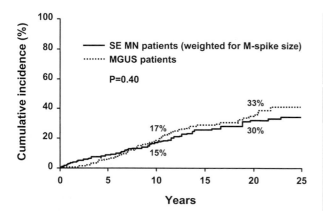

Fig. 1.15. Comparison of survival of 241 patients with monoclonal gammopathy of undetermined significance (*MGUS*) and 1,384 MGUS patients from southeastern Minnesota (*SE MN*).

Table 1.8. Clinical features of patients with monoclonal gammopathy of undetermined significance in southeastern Minnesota who developed multiple myeloma during follow-up

Characteristic	SE MN (N=75)	Mayo referral (N=1,027)
Age, median, y	76	66
Males, %	47	59
Hgb <12 g/dL, %	72	69
Calcium >11 mg/dL, %	7	13
Creatinine ≥2 mg/dL, %	14	19
Lytic, %	46	66
BMPC <10%, %	6	4
Median BMPC, %	40	50
Serum M spike, median g/dL	3.2	3.2
Urine M protein present, % of patients	81	78

BMPC, bone marrow plasma cells; SE MN, southeastern Minnesota.

The 75 patients who developed MM accounted for 65% of the 115 patients who had progression to a plasma cell disorder. Four of the patients with MM had an initial plasmacytoma, and 3 other myeloma patients also had AL. In 24 patients (32%), the diagnosis of MM was made more than 10 years after detection of the M protein, and 5 (7%) were recognized only after 20 years of follow-up.

The characteristics of these 75 myeloma patients are comparable to those 1,027 newly diagnosed patients with myeloma referred to Mayo Clinic from 1985 to 1998, except that the southeastern Minnesota patients were older (median, 76 vs. 66 years) and less likely to be male (47% vs. 59%) (Table 1.8). The degree of anemia, presence of renal insufficiency, number of bone marrow plasma cells, serum M-protein concentration, occurrence of urine light chains, and reduction of unin-volved immunoglobulins were not different in the 2 groups, but lytic bone lesions (66% vs. 46%) and hypercalcemia (13% vs. 7%) were more frequent in the referral patients. Light chain myeloma was also more common in the referral group (16% vs. 0.3%), as expected, because all patients in the southeastern Minnesota group had a preceding serum M protein measurement, and patients with idiopathic Bence Jones proteinuria were excluded. The median survival for MM patients was short-

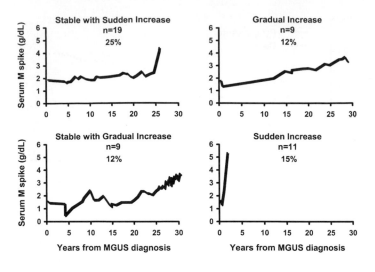

Fig. 1.16. Mode of development of multiple myeloma among southeastern Minnesota patients with monoclonal gammopathy of undetermined significance (*MGUS*). (From Kyle RA, Rajkumar SV [2003] Monoclonal gammopathies of undetermined significance: a review. Immunol Rev 194:112–139. By permission of Blackwell Munksgaard.)

er in the southeastern Minnesota group (16 vs. 33 months). This may, at least partially, be explained by their older age at diagnosis (median, 76 vs. 66 years).

The mode of development of MM among the MGUS patients varied (Fig. 1.16). The M protein increased within 2 years of the recognition of MGUS in 11 patients (Fig. 1.16), whereas the serum M protein was stable for more than 2 years and then increased within 2 years in 19 patients; in 9 others, the M protein increased grad-

ually after having been stable for at least 2 years. In 9 patients, the M protein gradually increased during follow-up until the diagnosis of symptomatic MM was made. In 10 patients, the serum M protein remained essentially stable; the diagnosis of MM was unequivocal in these 10 patients because of an increase in bone marrow plasma cells, development of lytic lesions, or occurrence of anemia, renal insufficiency, or an increased amount of urine M protein. Seventeen patients had an insufficient number of serum M-protein measurements to determine the pattern of increase. In macroglobulinemia, the M-protein value showed a gradual increase in 3 patients, stable levels followed by a sudden increase in 2, and insufficient data in 2 patients (Table 1.9).

The M protein disappeared during follow-up in 66 patients (5%). All of these patients had low initial values of M protein; only 17 had a value > 0.5 g/dL at diagnosis. However, treatment of patients who had progressed to MM or lymphoma or who had other disorders such as idiopathic thrombocytopenic purpura and vasculitis unrelated to the monoclonal gammopathy caused the disappearance of the M protein in 39 cases. The M protein disappeared without an apparent cause in 27 patients (2%). Only 6 of these 27 patients (0.4% of all patients) had a discrete spike on the densitometer tracing of the initial electrophoresis (median 1.2 g/dL), whereas the remaining 21 patients had a small M-protein value that could not be measured by the densitometer. In addition to the 66 patients, in 19 other patients the results of immunofixation or immunoelectrophoresis were initially thought to represent an M protein, but subsequent studies showed no evidence of M protein, suggesting

Table 1.9. Patterns of protein increase in monoclonal gammopathy of undetermined significance in southeastern Minnesota

Pattern	Multiple myeloma, pt, no.	Macro-globulinemia, pt, no.
Stable with sudden increase	19	2
Stable with gradual increase	9	0
Gradual increase	9	3
Sudden increase	11	0
Stable	10	0
Indeterminate	17	2
Total	75	7

Pt, patients. From Kyle et al. (2002b). By permission of the Massachusetts Medical Society.

that it was not present initially. Nevertheless, patients with a small M protein concentration (0.5 g/dL or less) had a 14% actuarial risk of progression at 20 years. Thus, spontaneous disappearance of M protein after the diagnosis of MGUS is rare.

1.2.1.7 Risk Factors for Progression

Among the baseline variables evaluated with respect to predicting progression of the monoclonal gammopathy (age; sex; hepatosplenomegaly; hemoglobin; serum creatinine; serum albumin; concentration of serum M protein; type of serum M protein [IgG, IgA, IgM]; presence, type, and amount of monoclonal urinary light chain; number of bone marrow plasma cells; and reduction in uninvolved immunoglobulins), only the concentration and type of M protein were independent predictors of progression. The presence of an M protein (κ or λ) in the urine and reduction of 1 or more uninvolved immunoglobulins were not risk factors for progression

(Tables 1.10 and 1.11). Patients with IgM or IgA M protein had an increased risk of progression to disease compared with patients who had IgG M protein (P <0.001) (Fig. 1.17).

However, the initial concentration of the serum M protein was the most important risk factor for progression to a plasma cell disorder. The relative risk of progression was related directly to the concentration of M protein in the serum at the time of diagnosis of MGUS (Fig. 1.18). The risk of progression to MM or a related disorder 10 years after diagnosis of MGUS was 6% for an initial M-protein value of 0.5 g/dL or less, 7% for 1 g/dL, 11% for 1.5 g/dL, 20% for 2 g/dL, 24% for

Table 1.10. Rates of full progression by urinary light chain in monoclonal gammopathy of undetermined significance in southeastern Minnesota

Light chain	Rate of full progression, %			
	10 y	20 y	25 y	P
κ or λ	12	28	NA	0.12
Negative	11	34	34	

NA, not available. Modified from Kyle et al. (2002 b). By permission of the Massachusetts Medical Society.

Table 1.11. Rates of full progression by reduction of uninvolved immunoglobulins in monoclonal gammopathy of undetermined significance in southeastern Minnesota

Uninvolved immunoglobulin reduction, no.	Rate of full progression, %			
	10 y	20 y	25 y	P
1	12	33	33	0.15
2	22	22	22	0.09
0	8	17	30	

Modified from Kyle et al. (2002 b). By permission of the Massachusetts Medical Society.

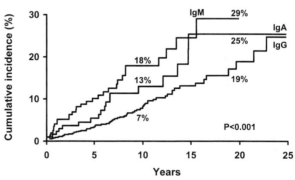

Fig. 1.17. Risk of progression by type of M protein in 1,384 patients with monoclonal gammopathy of undetermined significance. (From Kyle RA, Rajkumar SV [2002] Monoclonal gammopathies of undetermined significance. Rev Clin Exp Hematol 6:225–252. By permission of Blackwell Publishing.)

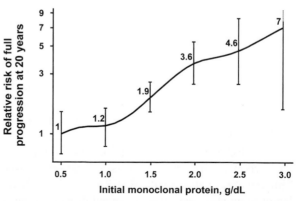

Fig. 1.18. Relative risk of full progression by amount of serum M protein at diagnosis. (Modified from Kyle RA, Rajkumar SV [2002] Monoclonal gammopathies of undetermined significance. Rev Clin Exp Hematol 6:225–252. By permission of Blackwell Publishing.)

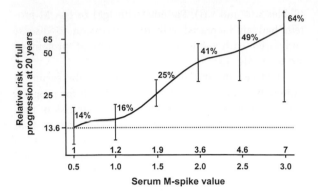

Fig. 1.19. Actuarial risk of full progression by serum M-protein value at diagnosis. (From Kyle RA, Rajkumar SV [2003] Monoclonal gammopathies of undetermined significance: a review. Immunol Rev 194:112–139. By permission of Blackwell Munksgaard.)

2.5 g/dL, and 34% for 3.0 g/dL. Corresponding rates for progression at 20 years were 14, 16, 25, 41, 49, and 64%, respectively (Fig. 1.19). The risk of progression with an M-protein value of 1.5 g/dL was almost 2-fold greater than the risk of progression for a patient with an M protein of 0.5 g/dL, whereas the risk of progression with an M protein of 2.5 g/dL was 4.6 times that of a 0.5 g/dL spike.

1.2.1.8 Follow-up in Other Series

In the 20 years of follow-up, 2 of 64 MGUS patients had died of MM and 1 of lymphoma. Three of the 19 surviving patients had had an increase in the M protein and a 4th patient had a large monoclonal IgAκ protein and then developed a high degree of Bence Jones proteinuria (5 g/L). Thus, 11% of the 64 patients with long-term follow-up had some evidence of progression of their benign monoclonal gammopathy. In another study, 6.2% of 64 patients developed MM after a long period of stability. Others reported malignant transformations in 14% of 213 persons followed for 5 to 8 years and in 18% of 100 patients with MGUS who were followed for 13 years. The actuarial risk of development of MM, macroglobulinemia, or AL in 213 patients with MGUS was 4.5% at 5 years, 15% at 10 years, and 26% at 15 years. Thirteen of 128 patients with MGUS followed for a median of 56 months developed malignant disease (Bladé et al. 1992). The actuarial probability of the development of malignant disease was 8.5% at 5 years and 19.2% at 10 years. The median interval from the recognition of the

M protein to diagnosis of malignant transformation was 41.6 months (range, 12–155 months).

In another study with a short follow-up, 3.3% of 243 patients with MGUS progressed to MM. Others found that 6.6% of 334 patients with MGUS developed a malignant transformation after a median follow-up of 8.4 years. Baldini et al. (1996) noted that 6.8% of 335 patients with MGUS had progression during a median follow-up of 70 months. In a series of 263 cases of MGUS, the actuarial probability of development of malignancy was 31% at 20 years (Pasqualetti et al. 1997). Eleven of 2,192 persons (0.5%) older than age 21 years in a New Zealand town had an M protein. Seven of the 11 patients developed a hematologic malignancy (MM, 4; macroglobulinemia, 2; and lymphoma, 1) after a 31-year follow-up of the 2,192 persons, 1,065 of whom were ≥age 50 years. In a group of 1,104 MGUS patients, >5% bone marrow plasmacytosis, presence of Bence Jones proteinuria, polyclonal immunoglobulin reduction, and high erythrocyte sedimentation rate were independent factors influencing MGUS transformation (Cesana et al. 2002). In summary, all studies essentially confirm that the risk of progression from MGUS to MM or related disorders is about 1% per year. They also demonstrate that the risk does not disappear, even after long-term follow-up.

1.2.2 Predictors of Malignant Transformation in MGUS

No findings at diagnosis of MGUS distinguish the patients who will remain stable from those who go on to develop a malignant condition (Kyle 1993). When MM develops, the type of M protein is always the same as it was in MGUS.

1.2.2.1 Amount of M Protein

In a series of 1,384 patients with MGUS, the concentration of the M protein at recognition of MGUS was the most important predictor of progression. Among the baseline variables evaluated with respect to predicting progression of the monoclonal gammopathy (age; sex; hepatosplenomegaly; hemoglobin; serum creatinine; serum albumin; amount of serum M protein; type of serum M protein [IgG, IgA, IgM]; presence, type, and amount of monoclonal urinary light chain; number of bone marrow plasma cells; and reduction in uninvolved

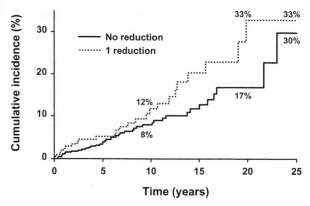

Fig. 1.20. Risk of full progression in 1,384 patients with monoclonal gammopathy of undetermined significance on the basis of reduction of uninvolved immunoglobulin.

immunoglobulins), only the concentration and type of M protein were independent predictors of progression. The presence of a monoclonal urine protein (κ or λ) and reduction of 1 or more uninvolved immunoglobulins were not risk factors for progression (Fig. 1.20).

The initial concentration of the serum M protein was the most important risk factor for progression to a plasma cell disorder. The relative risk of progression was related directly to the concentration of M protein in the serum at the time of diagnosis of MGUS (Fig. 1.19).

On the other hand, others noted that one-third of their patients with MGUS had an M protein >3 g/dL but showed no greater risk for malignant evolution. Bladé et al. (1992) also reported no increase in transformation in patients with an M protein greater than 3 g/dL. They suggested that limits to define MGUS should be more flexible.

1.2.2.2 Type of Immunoglobulin

In the southeastern Minnesota series, patients with IgM or IgA M protein had an increased risk of progression compared with those who had IgG M protein ($P=0.001$) (Fig. 1.17). Bladé et al. (1992) noted that patients with an IgA M protein had a greater probability of developing MM than the others.

1.2.2.3 Bone Marrow Plasma Cells

The number of plasma cells in the bone marrow may be of some help in the prediction of progression. Cesana et al. (2002) reported that more than 5% bone marrow plasma cells was an independent risk factor for progression. Others reported that a value of 20% bone marrow plasma cells was a reasonable level for differentiation of MGUS from MM. Baldini et al. (1996) reported that the malignant transformation rate was 6.8% when the bone marrow plasma cell level was less than 10% and 37% in the group with MGUS who had a bone marrow plasma cell value of 10 to 30%.

1.2.2.4 Other Predictors

In the 263 patients with MGUS reported by Pasqualetti et al. (1997), a multivariate regression analysis showed that only age was significantly associated with the risk of a malignant immunoproliferative disease developing. Increased bone resorption is an early sign of malignancy in patients with an apparent MGUS (Bataille et al. 1996). Bence Jones proteinuria and high erythrocyte sedimentation rate have been reported as independent factors in progression of MGUS (Cesana et al. 2002).

The majority of patients with MM have most likely had a previous monoclonal gammmopathy. In our experience, 32 of 55 patients (58%) with MM in Olmsted County, Minnesota, had MGUS, smoldering myeloma, or a plasmacytoma before the diagnosis of myeloma (Kyle et al. 1994).

1.2.3 Life Expectancy and Cause of Death in Patients With MGUS

It is important to know whether the presence of MGUS shortens the patient's life expectancy. Bladé et al. (1992) found no significant differences between survival of patients with MGUS and that of a control population, but there was a trend toward a shorter survival of the MGUS population. In another study, the long-term survival of 334 patients with MGUS was slightly shorter than the expected survival of an age- and sex-adjusted population. The survival of 241 patients with MGUS diagnosed before 1971 was significantly less than that of an age- and sex-adjusted 1980 US population (13.7 vs. 15.7 years) (Kyle 1993). The median survival of the 1,384 patients with MGUS was 8.1 years compared with 11.8 years ($P<0.001$) expected for Minnesota residents of matched age and sex (Fig. 1.13). The rates of death at 10 years were 6% from plasma cell disorders and 53% from non-plasma cell disorders, such as cardiovascular and cerebrovascular diseases and nonplasma cell cancers. At 20 years, the rates for plasma cell disorders were 10% and for nonplasma cell disorders, 72%. At 25 years, the rate for plasma cell disorders was 11% compared with 76% for nonplasma cell diseases.

1.2.4 Differentiation of MGUS From Multiple Myeloma and Macroglobulinemia

The differentiation of MGUS from MM may be difficult. The amount of the M protein, hemoglobin value, percentage of bone marrow plasma cells, amount of M protein in the urine, presence of hypercalcemia or renal insufficiency, and lytic bone lesions are often helpful. The concentration of the serum M protein is of help because higher values are associated with a greater likelihood of malignancy. The presence of a serum M protein >3 g/dL usually indicates overt MM or macroglobulinemia, but some exceptions such as smoldering MM or WM do exist.

Values of the IgG class not associated with the M protein (normal polyclonal or background immunoglobulins) are not helpful in differentiating benign from malignant monoclonal gammopathies. In patients with MM, the values of uninvolved immunoglobulins are reduced in more than 90% of patients (Kyle et al. 2003). However, reduction of uninvolved immunoglobulins occurs in patients with MGUS. In our series of 241 patients with MGUS, uninvolved immunoglobulins were reduced in 29%, and in our 1,384 patients with MGUS, uninvolved immunoglobulins were reduced in 38%. The reduction of uninvolved immunoglobulins, however, did not identify patients in whom progression subsequently developed (Kyle et al. 2002b).

An M protein in the urine (Bence Jones proteinuria) may be suggestive of a neoplastic process, but in a study of 42 patients with benign monoclonal gammopathy, the presence of Bence Jones proteinuria was reported in 11 patients. Others reported that 40% of their patients with benign monoclonal gammopathy had a monoclonal light chain in the urine. In our MGUS cohort from southeastern Minnesota, 31% of the 418 tested patients had a monoclonal light chain in the urine. The value was >150 mg/24 h in only 17%. However, the presence of a monoclonal light chain in the urine was not a risk factor for the subsequent development of MM.

The presence of more than 10% plasma cells in the bone marrow is suggestive of MM, but patients with a higher level of plasmacytosis may remain stable for long periods. The plasma cells in MM are often atypical; however, these morphologic features may also be seen in MGUS and smoldering MM. The assessment of nuclear cytoplasmic asynchrony has been proposed to help differentiate benign from malignant disease. In our experience, plasma cell nucleolar size, grade, and asynchrony are of limited use in differentiating MGUS from MM.

Milla et al. (2001) reported that the presence of nucleoli was the most important feature in differentiating MM from MGUS. The percentage of plasma cells, cytoplasmic contour irregularities, and isocytosis also predicted a diagnosis of MM in multivariate analysis. Using these criteria, they correctly identified 36 of 41 MGUS cases and all 21 cases of MM. The light-chain ratio may be helpful in the differentiation of MM from MGUS, but it is not useful when the number of plasma cells is small. Others reported that the presence of more than 20% plasma cells in the bone marrow differentiated stage I myeloma patients from those with MGUS. Laroche et al. (1996) performed histomorphometric studies of bone biopsy specimens in 34 patients with a monoclonal gammopathy. Patients with MGUS had normal bone remodeling, whereas bone resorption increased and bone formation decreased in patients with stage III myeloma.

The presence of osteolytic lesions is strongly suggestive of MM, but metastatic carcinoma may also produce lytic lesions as well as plasmacytosis and be associated with an unrelated serum M protein. If fewer than 10% plasma cells are present, the M protein is modest in amount, and constitutional symptoms are present, it is more likely that metastatic carcinoma is present with an unrelated MGUS.

The plasma cell labeling index for detection of synthesis of DNA is useful in differentiating the patient with MGUS or smoldering MM from the patient with MM (Greipp et al. 1987). We use a monoclonal antibody (BU-1) reactive with 5-bromo-2-deoxyuridine (BrdUrd). A bone marrow specimen is exposed to BrdUrd for 1 h. Cells synthesizing DNA incorporate the BrdUrd, which is recognized by a monoclonal antibody (BU-1) conjugated to goat antimouse immunoglobulin-rhodamine complex. Because this antibody does not require denaturation for its activity, fluorescein-conjugated immunoglobulin (κ and λ) antisera identify the population of monoclonal plasma cells. An increased plasma cell labeling index is strong evidence that MM is present or that it will soon develop. However, approximately one-third of patients with symptomatic MM have a normal plasma cell labeling index.

A good correlation exists between the plasma cell labeling index of peripheral blood and the bone marrow labeling index (Witzig et al. 1988). Mononuclear cells are separated on Ficoll-Hypaque and the T cells are removed with magnetic beads. The cells are then incubated with BrdUrd, and cytospin slides are made. They are stained with κ and λ antisera after staining with BU-1 and goat antimouse IgG labeled with rhodamine isothiocyanate. A 500-cell count is done of peripheral blood cells bearing the same cytoplasmic light-chain isotype as the M protein. The median peripheral blood labeling index was 0.2% for MGUS or smoldering MM and 0.8% for patients with newly diagnosed MM. Four patients had an increased peripheral blood labeling index but clinically inactive disease at the time of the study; within 6 months all developed active MM that required chemotherapy (Witzig et al. 1988).

The presence of circulating plasma cells in the peripheral blood is a good marker of active disease. Monoclonal plasma cells are frequently present in the peripheral blood of patients with active MM, even though they are not detectable in routine peripheral blood smears. Plasma cells are infrequently present in patients with MGUS or smoldering MM. The presence of 3×10^6/L or more peripheral blood plasma cells in persons with MGUS or smoldering MM indicates that the patient is likely to develop symptomatic myeloma within a few months. Peripheral blood plasma cells are detected in approximately 60% of patients with newly diagnosed myeloma and in more than 90% of patients with relapsed or refractory disease.

An increase in the number of circulating monoclonal plasma cells or their proliferative rate is a good predictor of development of symptomatic myeloma. In a series of 57 patients with newly diagnosed smoldering MM, 16 had progression within 12 months. Sixty-three percent of them had abnormal peripheral blood plasma cells. By contrast, only 10% of the patients who remained stable had an increased number of peripheral blood plasma cells. The median time to progression was 9 months in patients with abnormal peripheral blood plasma cells and 30 months for those without abnormal peripheral blood plasma cells. Thus, the presence of increased numbers of circulating peripheral blood plasma cells or an increase in the labeling index indicates symptomatic disease (Witzig et al. 1994).

Conventional cytogenetic studies are not useful in the differentiation of MGUS from MM because abnormal karyotypes are rarely seen in MGUS as a result of the small number of plasma cells and the low proliferative rate. Fluorescence in situ hybridization studies showed that abnormalities can be detected in bone marrow plasma cells from most patients with MGUS (Avet-Loiseau et al. 1999 a, b; Fonseca et al. 1998). In a study using interphase fluorescence in situ hybridization, chromosome abnormalities were found in 53% of 36 patients with MGUS. Trisomy was found in at least 1 of chromosomes 3, 7, 9, and 11 in 12% to 72% of bone marrow plasma cells in 12 of 14 hyperdiploid patients with MGUS. Deletion of chromosome 13q was detected in 45% of 29 patients with MGUS. Nine of 17 patients (53%) with MM progressing from a preexisting MGUS had deletion of 13q14 on fluorescence in situ hybridization. Deletion of 13q14 is an early event in the development of monoclonal gammopathies. However, in contrast to myeloma, deletions of 13q are less common in MGUS (Avet-Loiseau et al. 1999 a, b). Deletions of chromosome 13q may be involved in the progression from MGUS to myeloma.

The most common chromosome abnormalities in MGUS are translocations involving chromosome 14q32, which is the immunoglobulin heavy-chain locus (Avet-Loiseau et al. 1999 a, b). Fonseca et al. (1999) found that the translocations involving chromosome 14q32 were present in more than 75% of patients with MGUS. It appears that chromosome abnormalities frequently found in myeloma are present even at the MGUS stage.

Magnetic resonance imaging (MRI) may be helpful in differentiating MGUS from MM. Bellaiche et al. (1997) reported that the MRI was normal in all 24 patients with MGUS, whereas abnormalities were found in 86% of 44 patients with MM.

Ocqueteau et al. (1998) found a population of polyclonal plasma cells with CD38 expression and low forward light scatter. The plasma cells expressed CD19 but were negative for CD56. The monoclonal plasma cell population showed a lower CD38 expression and a higher forward light scatter population and expressed CD56 but not CD19. Ninety-eight percent of patients with MGUS had >3% normal polyclonal plasma cells, but only 1.5% of patients with MM had the same findings.

The amount of C-terminal telopeptide of type I collagen was increased in 34% of 35 patients with MGUS. Serum osteocalcin values were increased in 31%, and serum bone-specific alkaline phosphatase was increased in 17%. This suggests that abnormal bone metabolism occurs in MGUS (Vejlgaard et al. 1997).

Increased telomerase activity was found in 21 of 27 patients with MM, but in 1 of 5 with MGUS. Thus, MGUS cells may not be immortalized, and activation of telomerase may have a role in the transformation from MGUS to MM (Xu et al. 2001). The percentage of granular lymphocytes in the bone marrow was increased in 27% of patients with MGUS and in only 15% of patients with MM. Natural killer cells (CD57$^+$, CD16$^+$) were more abundant in MGUS than in MM.

Methylation of p15 (INK4b) and p16 (INK4a) was found in similar frequencies in MGUS and MM. This suggests that methylation of these genes is an early event and not associated with progression of MGUS to MM. Methylation of p15 (INK4b) and p16 (INK4a) may contribute to immortalization of plasma cells rather than to malignant transformation (Guillerm et al. 2001).

Interleukin (IL)-1β is produced by plasma cells in virtually all cases of MM but is undetectable in most patients with MGUS. IL-1β has strong osteoclast-activating factor activity that increases the expression of adhesion molecules and induces paracrine IL-6 production. This parallels the development of osteolytic bone lesions, homing of myeloma cells to bone marrow, and IL-6 induced cell growth. IL-1β may play an important role in the homing of plasma cells to the bone marrow. Lytic lesions may result from stimulation of osteoclasts through the production of IL-1β, as well as paracrine IL-6 secretion. IL-6 also stimulates osteoclasts through the production of IL-1β (Lacy et al. 1999).

Using immunohistochemical techniques to identify microvessels, Vacca et al. (1994) reported that bone marrow angiogenesis was increased in MM but not in MGUS. Studies done at our institution confirm these findings, although this test has limited value in differentiating MGUS from MM because angiogenesis is not increased in approximately one-third of patients with MM (Rajkumar et al. 2000). In studies done with the chick embryo chorioallantoic model, sorted bone marrow samples were angiogenic in 76% of patients with myeloma and 20% of patients with MGUS.

The serum level of IL-6 may aid in the differentiation of monoclonal gammopathies. In 1 study, the serum IL-6 value was increased in 35% of patients with overt MM but in only 3% of patients with MGUS. In another report, the serum IL-6 value was increased in 42% of 210 patients with MM. The expression of a multidrug-resis-

tant phenotype (MDR-1), the absence of CD56 expression, and a low proliferative rate may be useful in differentiating MGUS from smoldering MM.

β_2-Microglobulin concentration is not helpful in differentiating MGUS from low-grade MM because there is too much overlap between the 2 entities. Neither the presence of J chains in malignant plasma cells nor the acid phosphatase values in plasma cells are reliable for differentiation. The leukocyte alkaline phosphatase score is increased in myeloma in contrast to MGUS and may be helpful in differentiation. Decreased numbers of OKT4$^+$ T cells, increased numbers of monoclonal idiotype-bearing peripheral blood lymphocytes, and increased numbers of immunoglobulin-secreting cells in peripheral blood are characteristic of MM, but overlap exists with MGUS.

Ellis et al. (2001) found that relative numbers of CD30$^+$ T cells were increased and activated lymphocytes from normal-aged individuals and in MGUS patients. It was postulated that these cells may contribute to chronic activation of B cells through the production of IL-6.

1.2.5 Management of MGUS

Regardless of the results of sophisticated laboratory tests, the differentiation between MGUS and MM is made on the basis of clinical factors such as symptoms, anemia, hypercalcemia, renal insufficiency, and lytic bone lesions. However, the presence of a high plasma cell labeling index in a patient with MGUS or smoldering MM needs to be followed more frequently for other evidence of progression. No single factor can differentiate a patient with a benign monoclonal gammopathy from one in whom a malignant plasma cell disorder will subsequently develop. The serum M protein must be measured periodically and clinical evaluation conducted to determine whether serious disease has developed.

If a patient has no features of myeloma or amyloidosis and the serum M-protein value is less than 1.5 g/dL, serum protein electrophoresis should be repeated at annual intervals. Skeletal radiography, bone marrow examination, and 24-hour urine immunofixation are rarely necessary in this situation.

If the asymptomatic patient has an M-protein value of 1.5 to 2.0 g/dL, one should quantify IgG, IgA, and IgM and collect a 24-hour urine specimen for electrophoresis and immunofixation. The serum protein electrophoretic pattern should be determined again in 3 to 6 months and, if stable, should be repeated in 6 months and then annually, or sooner if any symptoms occur. If the IgG or IgA serum M protein value is >2.0 g/dL, a radiographic bone survey should be done, including views of the humeri and femora. Bone marrow aspirate and biopsy should also be performed. Cytogenetic studies, performance of the plasma cell labeling index, and a search for circulating plasma cells in the peripheral blood should be done if possible. Values of β_2-microglobulin and C-reactive protein should be determined. If the patient has an IgM M protein, aspiration and biopsy of the bone marrow and a computed tomographic scan of the abdomen may be useful for recognizing macroglobulinemia or a related lymphoproliferative disorder. If results of these tests are satisfactory, serum protein electrophoresis should be repeated in 3 months, and if the results are stable, the tests should be repeated at 6- to 12-month intervals.

1.2.6 Variants of MGUS

1.2.6.1 Smoldering (Asymptomatic) MM

Patients with smoldering MM have a serum M-protein value ≥3 g/dL or ≥10% plasma cells in the bone marrow (Table 1.12). Frequently, a reduction of uninvolved immunoglobulins in the serum and a small amount of M protein in the urine are found. These findings are consistent with MM, but anemia, renal insufficiency, and skeletal lesions are not present. In addition, the plasma cell labeling index is low. Biologically, these patients have a benign monoclonal gammopathy or MGUS but

it is not possible to make this diagnosis when the patient is initially evaluated because most patients with this amount of M protein in the serum or with this level of bone marrow plasma cell infiltration have symptomatic MM (Kyle and Greipp 1980).

Smoldering MM accounts for approximately 15% of all cases of newly diagnosed MM (Dimopoulos et al. 2000). Ninety-five of 635 patients (15%) with MM were considered to have asymptomatic MM. Other investigators have found a higher proportion of patients with smoldering or asymptomatic myeloma, but the sample size in those studies was small. The prevalence estimates of smoldering MM are variable because many reports include asymptomatic patients with lytic lesions on skeletal survey. Some exclude skeletal lesions on radiographic studies but include patients who have lytic lesions on MRI. A true prevalence derived from strict criteria for smoldering MM is not available.

1.2.6.2 Risk of Progression in Smoldering MM

Most patients with smoldering MM progress eventually to symptomatic disease, and the risk of progression is higher than with MGUS (Dimopoulos et al. 2000). Some patients can remain free of progression for many years (Kyle and Greipp 1980). The median time to progression to symptomatic disease is approximately 1 to 3 years. A recent study found only a 20% risk of progression at 6 years (Cesana et al. 2002). However, patients were considered to have smoldering MM only if they demonstrated no disease progression after 1 year of follow-up.

Table 1.12. Mayo Clinic criteria for the diagnosis of MGUS, SMM, and MM

Disorder	Criteria
MGUS	Serum monoclonal protein <3 g/dL *and* bone marrow plasma cells <10% *and* absence of anemia, renal failure, hypercalcemia, and lytic bone lesions
SMM	Serum monoclonal protein ≥3 g/dL *or* bone marrow plasma cells ≥10% *and* absence of anemia, renal failure, hypercalcemia, and lytic bone lesions
MM	Presence of a serum or urine monoclonal protein, bone marrow plasmacytosis, *and* anemia, renal failure, hypercalcemia, or lytic bone lesions; patients with primary systemic amyloidosis and ≥30% bone marrow plasma cells are considered to have both multiple myeloma and amyloidosis

MGUS, monoclonal gammopathy of undetermined significance; MM, multiple myeloma; SMM, smoldering multiple myeloma. Modified from Rajkumar SV, Dispenzieri A, Fonseca R, Lacy MQ, Geyer S, Lust JA, Kyle RA, Greipp PR, Gertz MA, Witzig TE (2001) Thalidomide for previously untreated indolent or smoldering multiple myeloma. Leukemia 15:1274-1276. By permission of Nature Publishing Group.

1.2.6.3 Predictors of Progression in Smoldering MM

The assessment of prognostic factors for smoldering MM is hampered by varying diagnostic criteria used to define the cohort. Several studies include patients with lytic lesions as well. Future studies of smoldering MM will need to use more uniformly accepted criteria so that results can be compared.

Patients with abnormal peripheral blood monoclonal plasma cell studies, defined as an increase in the number or proliferative rate of circulating plasma cells by immunofluorescent assays, are at higher risk for earlier progression to myeloma. An increased plasma cell labeling index has been shown to be an adverse prognostic factor.

In a study conducted at the M.D. Anderson Cancer Center (Weber et al. 1997), the 3 most important prognostic factors for progression in smoldering MM included serum monoclonal protein concentration more than 3.0 g/dL, immunoglobulin IgA subtype, and urinary monoclonal protein excretion more than 50 mg/day. Patients with more than 2 of these features had a median time to progression of 17 months, those with 1 risk factor had a median time to progression of 40 months, and patients who had none of these factors had a time to progression of 95 months. This study excluded patients with abnormalities on bone survey but did include patients with abnormal MRI results, which were present in 40% of patients. Abnormal MRI findings were associated with a shortened time to progression of 21 months.

Other studies have also found value in MRI abnormalities as a predictor of rapid disease progression in patients with smoldering MM (Dimopoulos et al. 2000). Patients who undergo MRI studies in the absence of lytic lesions for skeletal survey often have abnormalities detected as a result (Dimopoulos et al. 2000). In such patients, an abnormality depicted on MRI is an adverse prognostic factor for progression (Mariette et al. 1999). Whether patients who have MRI abnormalities should be considered as having smoldering MM is debatable. Nevertheless, these patients can be considered to have low-grade MM and observed without therapy, similar to smoldering MM.

1.2.6.4 Management of Smoldering MM

The current standard of care in smoldering MM is close follow-up once every few months without any chemotherapy. This recommendation results from trials that demonstrated no significant improvement in overall survival in patients who received immediate treatment with melphalan plus prednisone compared with those who received treatment at progression for stage I or asymptomatic myeloma. Hjorth and colleagues (1993) randomly assigned 50 patients with asymptomatic stage I myeloma to observation versus melphalan plus prednisone chemotherapy. No differences were observed in overall survival between the 2 groups. Grignani and colleagues (1996) reported similar survival time with immediate or deferred therapy in a series of 44 patients with asymptomatic myeloma. The recommendation to observe closely without treatment until progression is also derived from the toxicity of therapy and the fact that for many patients the disease may not progress for months to years (Kyle and Greipp 1980).

Investigational approaches may be considered for selected patients in appropriate clinical trials. Thalidomide is being studied as a single agent, with a preliminary partial response rate of approximately 35%. Other studies are evaluating the role of bisphosphonates, interleukin-1β inhibitors, clarithromycin, and dehydroepiandrosterone in an attempt to delay progression to symptomatic myeloma. In a Mayo Clinic study, 30 patients have been enrolled and 16 patients are evaluable. However, because the main goal of therapy in patients with smoldering MM is to delay the need for chemotherapy, a phase 3 randomized trial on the durability of response is needed before recommending this strategy for standard clinical practice.

1.2.6.5 Biclonal Gammopathy

Biclonal gammopathies are characterized by the presence of 2 different M proteins and occur in more than 5% of patients with monoclonal gammopathies. The 2 M proteins may be due to the proliferation of 2 different clones of plasma cells, each producing an unrelated monoclonal protein, or to 2 M proteins produced by a single clone of plasma cells.

Biclonal gammopathy of undetermined significance was found in 37 of 57 patients with a biclonal gammopathy. Their ages ranged from 39 to 93 years (median, 67 years). Twenty were women. The clinical findings of biclonal gammopathies are similar to those of monoclonal gammopathies (Kyle et al. 1981). The hemoglobin, leukocyte, and platelet values were normal. Electrophoresis on cellulose acetate showed 2 localized bands in only 18 cases; in the remainder, a 2nd M protein was recognized only with immunoelectrophoresis or immunofixation. Six of 22 patients had a monoclonal light chain in the urine. The bone marrow contained 1 to 7% plasma cells. In a patient with biclonal gammopathy (IgGκ and IgAκ) symptomatic MM developed 2 years later when the IgG value increased, but the IgA and IgM values were unchanged. In another patient, the biclonal gammopathy (IgGκ and IgMκ) disappeared without cause after 7 years' observation (Kyle et al. 1981).

Seven of the 37 patients died during a median follow-up of 31.5 months. The cause of death was acute granulocytic leukemia, metastatic prostatic carcinoma, malignant melanoma, alcoholic hepatitis, subdural hematoma, congestive heart failure, and undetermined cause (this patient was age 91 years) in 1 case each. Thirty-five percent of the 57 patients had MM, macroglobulinemia, or other malignant lymphoproliferative disorders (Kyle et al. 1981).

Almost one-half of 20 patients with biclonal gammopathy had biclonal gammopathy of undetermined significance. MM subsequently developed in 2 of them. Others reported that 2.5% of 1,135 patients with monoclonal gammopathy had a biclonal gammopathy. They postulated that complete class switching in a single plasma cell clone resulted in the production of 2 M proteins, whereas in other patients the M proteins arose from 2 separate plasma cell clones. Another group reported on a patient with IgAκ and IgGκ biclonal gammopathy in which the plasma cell clone simultaneously synthesized a, γ, and κ chains. They postulated that the plasma cell clone was "frozen" at the IgG to IgA switch. Sensorimotor peripheral neuropathy has been reported with biclonal gammopathy. Others described a patient with WM who had an IgM and an IgG M protein with the same λ light chain. Region 3 of the 2 γ and μ transcripts showed 100% homology, whereas immunofluorescence revealed that most cells stained with both IgG and IgM. This is an example of a single population of plasma cells producing 2 M proteins. Other authors emphasized the regulatory interactions between 2 monoclonal clones.

1.2.6.6 Triclonal Gammopathy

Triclonal gammopathy was reported in a patient with plasma cell dyscrasia in whom acquired immunodeficiency syndrome subsequently developed and in a patient with non-Hodgkin lymphoma. In a patient with triclonal gammopathy (IgMκ, IgGκ, and IgAκ) and a plasmacytoid lymphoma of the ileum and gastric wall, the tumor contained 3 different cell types that stained for IgG, IgA, and IgM. The authors believed that the 3 types of malignant cells, producing different classes of immunoglobulins, were derived from a single clone of plasma cells that had undergone a "class switch." They also reported that 11 of 15 patients reported in the literature with triclonal gammopathy had a malignant lymphoma or lymphoproliferative disorder.

Grosbois et al. (1997) also described a patient with a triclonal gammopathy (IgMκ, IgGκ, and IgAκ) and reviewed a group of cases with triclonal gammopathy from the literature. Sixteen cases were associated with a malignant immunolymphoproliferative disorder, 5 appeared in nonhematologic diseases, and 3 were of undetermined significance. Saito et al. (1998) described 2 patients with lymphoma who had a triclonal gammopathy (IgMλ, IgGκ, and IgGλ and IgMλ, IgMκ, and IgGκ). Using electron microscopy, they demonstrated that the immunoglobulins were synthesized at the same time in a single cell.

1.2.7 Benign Monoclonal Light Chain Idiopathic (Bence Jones) Proteinuria

Benign monoclonal gammopathy of the light chain type must be considered even though Bence Jones proteinuria is a recognized feature of MM, AL, WM, and other lymphoproliferative diseases. In 1 study, 2 patients with a stable serum M protein also excreted 0.8 g/day or more of Bence Jones protein for more than 17 years without progression. One of the patients had proteinuria documented 10 years before it was recognized as Bence Jones proteinuria, so proteinuria existed 27 years before the patient died of pneumonia. The second patient died of a hypernephroma 19 years after Bence Jones proteinuria was recognized. Neither patient developed symptomatic MM or amyloidosis.

Seven additional patients have been described who presented with Bence Jones proteinuria (more than 1 g/24 h) but in whom no M protein was found in the serum and who had no evidence of MM or a related disorder (Kyle and Greipp 1982). MM developed in 1 of the 7 patients after 20 years, and he died of a bleeding diathesis. He had no significant renal insufficiency despite having excreted more than 45 kg of λ light chain protein. His kidneys had "proved equal to the novel office assigned them" and had "discharged the task" without sustaining, on their part, the slightest danger. In the second patient, symptomatic MM developed 8.8 years after recognition of the Bence Jones proteinuria. Severe renal insufficiency developed in a 3rd patient after 2 episodes of acute renal failure. His renal failure was attributed to nephrosclerosis rather than to myeloma kidney or amyloidosis. A 4th patient probably had a slowly evolving MM during a 9-year period, but he died before symptomatic myeloma developed. Another patient developed symptoms of carpal tunnel syndrome after 14 years of Bence Jones proteinuria. He had systemic amyloidosis. The 6th patient produced 3 g/d of Bence Jones protein for 7.7 years and then developed an extensive squamous cell carcinoma involving the lungs and mediastinum. The 7th patient excreted up to 1.8 g/d of κ light chain for 30 years without developing symptomatic myeloma or a related disorder. Although idiopathic Bence Jones proteinuria may remain stable for years, MM or AL often results. These patients must be followed indefinitely.

1.2.7.1 IgD MGUS

The presence of an IgD M protein almost always indicates MM, AL, or plasma cell leukemia. However, IgD MGUS has been reported. A patient with an IgDλ protein of 0.5 g/dL was followed for more than 6 years without evidence of progressive disease. Another patient was described with metastatic thyroid medullary carcinoma and a serum IgDλ protein, without evidence of myeloma. Another patient with an IgDλ MGUS and axonal neuropathy was reported, but no follow-up information was given. We evaluated a patient with an IgDλ MGUS at Mayo Clinic who was followed for more than 8 years without development of MM or amyloidosis.

1.2.8 Association of Monoclonal Gammopathy With Other Diseases

Certain diseases are associated with MGUS, as would be expected in an older population. The association of 2 diseases depends on the frequency with which each occurs independently. In addition, an apparent association may occur because of differences in the referral practice or in other selected patient groups. One must use valid epidemiologic and statistical methods in evaluating these associations. The need for appropriate control populations cannot be overemphasized.

For example, the association of monoclonal gammopathy and hyperparathyroidism has been reported. Among 911 patients who met these criteria and who were age 50 years or older, immunoelectrophoresis demonstrated MGUS in 9 patients (1%), which is the expected number (Mundis and Kyle, 1982). This prevalence of MGUS is similar to the 1.25% to 1.7% found in studies of 3 normal populations (Axelsson et al. 1966; Kyle et al. 1972). In another report, 4 of 386 patients with primary hyperparathyroidism had MGUS. In a recent report, 20 of 101 patients with hyperparathyroidism but only 2 of 127 controls had an M protein (Arnulf et al. 2002). Thus, there is controversy concerning the association of hyperparathyroidism and MGUS.

An increased prevalence of monoclonal gammopathy in association with carcinoma of the colon has been reported on several occasions. However, in 2 large studies the prevalence of monoclonal gammopathies was no greater than that expected in a similar population. These studies also demonstrate the need for comparison with a satisfactory control population before it can be assumed that an association exists between monoclonal gammopathy and any disease.

1.2.8.1 Lymphoproliferative Disorders

In 1957, Azar et al. reported that malignant lymphoma and lymphatic leukemia were associated with a myeloma-type serum protein. In 1960, Kyle et al. described 6 patients with lymphoma who had serum or electrophoretic patterns consistent with that of MM. The presence of M proteins in patients with lymphoma was confirmed by others. Five patients were described with reticulum cell sarcoma and a serum M protein. IgM proteins may be increased in patients with malignant lymphoproliferative disorders.

Among 1,150 patients with lymphoma, M proteins were found in 49. M proteins were reported in 29 of 640 patients (4.5%) with a diffuse lymphoproliferative disease (chronic lymphocytic leukemia, lymphocytic lymphoma, or reticulum cell sarcoma) but in none of 292 with a nodular lymphoma. Another group reported that two-thirds of patients with an IgM protein had a diffuse histologic pattern, but only 13% had a follicular pattern. Others concluded that the association of nodular lymphoma and a serum M protein was rare. One group found an M protein in 20 of 108 patients with a well-differentiated lymphocytic lymphoma. More recently, IgM proteins were found with agarose gel electrophoresis and immunofixation in the serum of 12 of 21 patients with Burkitt lymphoma as well as in those with non-Burkitt types. These proteins disappeared after successful therapy but reappeared at relapse. In contrast, M proteins were rarely found in patients with Hodgkin disease.

We reviewed the medical records of 430 patients in whom a serum IgM monoclonal gammopathy had been identified between 1956 and 1978 at Mayo Clinic (Table 1.13). The patients were classified as follows: 1) WM: IgM spike of 3 g/dL or more in the serum protein electrophoretic pattern and an increase in lymphocytes or plasmacytoid lymphocytes in the bone marrow; 2) lymphoma: biopsy findings consistent with lymphoma in a lymph node or extranodal lymphoid tumor; 3) chronic lymphocytic leukemia: lymphocyte count of more than 9×10^9/L; 4) AL: biopsy specimen containing amyloid; 5) MGUS: IgM protein value less than 3 g/dL, absence of constitutional symptoms, hepatosplenomegaly, or lymphadenopathy and no anemia or other findings requiring therapy; and 6) malignant lymphoproliferative disease: could not be classified in the foregoing categories and characterized by IgM protein less than 3 g/dL, bone marrow infiltration with lymphocytes or plasmacytoid lymphocytes, and therapy required because of anemia or constitutional symptoms.

More than one-half of patients (56%) with an IgM protein had MGUS. During follow-up, 40 of the 242 (17%) with MGUS developed a malignant lymphoid disorder requiring therapy. In 22 patients, typical WM developed, 9 others had a malignant lymphoproliferative process requiring chemotherapy, and lymphoma developed in 6 others. The median duration from the detection of the IgM protein until the diagnosis of lymphoid disease was more than 4 years (range, 0.4–22 years). In addition, 10 patients with MGUS (4%) had an increase in serum M protein of more than 1 g/dL, and 9 others had an increase of 0.5 to 0.9 g/dL. None of these 19 patients developed symptomatic WM or other lymphoid disease requiring therapy.

Table 1.13. Classification of IgM monoclonal gammopathies among 430 patients (1956–1978)

Classification	Patients	
	No.	%
Monoclonal gammopathy of undetermined significance	242	56
Waldenström macroglobulinemia	71	17
Lymphoma	28	7
Chronic lymphocytic leukemia	21	5
Primary amyloidosis (AL)	6	1
Lymphoproliferative disease	62	14
Total	430	100

From Kyle and Garton (1987). By permission of Mayo Foundation.

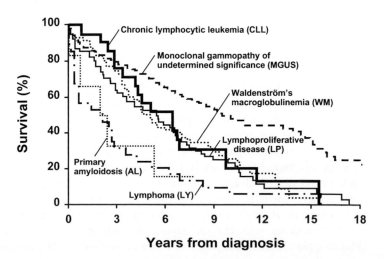

Fig. 1.21. Survival curves of patients with IgM monoclonal gammopathies. (From Kyle and Garton [1987]. By permission of Mayo Foundation.)

More than two-thirds of the 430 patients with IgM monoclonal gammopathy have died. The median survival of patients with WM and of those with a malignant lymphoproliferative disease requiring therapy was similar (5 and 5.5 years, respectively) (Fig. 1.21).

It is evident that patients with WM and lymphoproliferative disease who have lymphocytic proliferation of the marrow producing constitutional symptoms or anemia requiring chemotherapy are not different except for the occurrence of hyperviscosity syndrome. Consequently, no reason exists for differentiating patients with lymphoproliferative disease from those with WM. They can be included in future prospective studies of WM (Kyle and Garton 1987).

Approximately 2% of patients with angioimmunoblastic lymphadenopathy have a monoclonal gammopathy. Two groups reported the presence of M proteins in patients with angioimmunoblastic lymphadenopathy. A polyclonal increase in immunoglobulins is much more common in this disease. Castleman disease (angiofollicular lymph node hyperplasia) may be associated with a monoclonal gammopathy. Five of 10 Japanese patients with Sjögren syndrome had an IgA monoclonal protein. Two patients with Sjögren syndrome and an M protein subsequently developed a malignant lymphoma. Kaposi sarcoma has also been associated with a monoclonal gammopathy.

1.2.8.2 Leukemia

M proteins have been reported in the sera of patients with leukemia. We described 100 patients with chronic lymphocytic leukemia and an M protein in the serum or urine (Noel and Kyle 1987). IgM accounted for only 28% of cases, whereas IgG was found in 51%. The size of the M protein was modest, with a median concentration of 1 g/dL. No major differences were apparent in patients with chronic lymphocytic leukemia, regardless of monoclonal protein type (IgG or IgM). By use of immunoisoelectric focusing, an M protein was detected in 61% of 56 patients with chronic lymphocytic leukemia. Eighty-eight percent of the M proteins were IgM.

Monoclonal gammopathy has also been recognized in hairy cell leukemia and adult T-cell leukemia. Another group described a 14-year-old male with T-cell acute lymphoblastic leukemia with hairy cell features and a monoclonal κ light chain in the serum and urine.

Of 8 patients with chronic myelocytic leukemia (Philadelphia chromosome positive) and a monoclonal gammopathy, 7 had the λ isotype. Another patient who had Philadelphia positive chronic myelocytic leukemia developed a monocytic blast transformation associated with an IgGλ protein. We have also seen several patients with chronic myelocytic leukemia and an M protein in their serum, but it is not known whether an association exists between the 2 entities.

Transient M proteins have been reported with acute myelomonocytic leukemia. In a patient with acute myelomonocytic leukemia and an IgGκ monoclonal gammopathy, the leukemic cells were the most likely candidates for IgGκ monoclonal protein production. The patient also had eosinophilia. An IgGκ M protein was found in the serum and on the surface of the leukemic cells of a patient with acute promyelocytic leukemia. The blast cells did not appear to secrete the M protein. A patient was reported with an IgGκ (2.8 g/dL) M protein in whom plasma cell leukemia developed 5 months later. Data are inadequate to determine whether there is an increased incidence of M protein in patients with leukemia.

1.2.8.3 Other Hematologic Diseases

Acquired von Willebrand disease is an uncommon disorder but it is often associated with a monoclonal gammopathy (Federici et al. 1998). Treatment has been challenging. Federici et al. (1998) found that intravenous gamma globulin improved the laboratory abnormalities and bleeding in 8 patients with an IgG M protein, but it was ineffective in the 2 patients with an IgMκ monoclonal protein. Desmopressin has also been reported to be helpful. Severe bleeding may occur from binding of a monoclonal protein with thrombin.

Patients with monoclonal gammopathy and lupus anticoagulant activity have been reported. An increased incidence of antiphospholipid antibodies has been reported in patients with MGUS. A transient IgMκ monoclonal protein was detected in a patient with hydralazine-induced lupus erythematosus.

Monoclonal gammopathies have been reported with pernicious anemia. Three of 20 patients in a family with congenital dyserythropoietic anemia type III had a monoclonal IgGκ protein (1 had MM). Pure red cell aplasia and an M protein have been reported in 6 patients. Some thought that red cell aplasia was caused by a block in the maturation of the erythroid burst-forming unit that might be related to the M protein.

Polycythemia vera, myelofibrosis, and chronic myelocytic leukemia have been associated with monoclonal gammopathies. Three of 46 patients with idiopathic myelofibrosis had an M protein. An M protein was found in 6 of 52 patients with myelodysplastic syndrome.

An IgGκ monoclonal protein was found in 4 of 16 patients with Gaucher disease. Six others had a monoclonal increase in IgG. In another series, 2 of 23 had a monoclonal gammopathy, 6 had an oligoclonal gammopathy, and 10 had diffuse hypergammaglobulinemia. The IgGκ protein concentration decreased after splenectomy in a patient with Gaucher disease.

1.2.8.4 Connective Tissue Disorders

Rheumatoid arthritis and seronegative erosive arthritis have been reported with monoclonal gammopathies.

Lupus erythematosus and other connective tissue disorders have been described with M proteins. MGUS was reported in 4 of 120 patients with systemic lupus erythematosus. An M protein was found in 1.3% of 555 cases of ankylosing spondylitis, but this incidence is similar to that expected in a normal population.

Polymyalgia rheumatica has been noted with monoclonal gammopathy, but both conditions occur more often in an older population. The relationship is questionable. Polymyalgia rheumatica-like symptoms were reported in 4 patients with a monoclonal gammopathy and underlying lymphoreticular neoplasia. Three patients with polymyositis and an IgGκ M protein have been described. Relapsing polymyositis and IgG M protein have been reported. An M protein was found in 16 of 70 patients (23%) with inclusion body myositis. Eighty-one percent had an IgG M protein (Dalakas et al. 1997). In another report, immunoabsorption appeared to benefit a patient who had inclusion body myositis with an IgG M protein (Nakayama et al. 2000). Discoid lupus erythematosus that followed a benign course was reported in 8 patients with an M protein. The association of scleroderma with an IgGκ M protein and the subsequent development of MM has been reported. One case of monoclonal gammopathy with psoriatic arthritis has been described.

1.2.8.5 Osteosclerotic Myeloma (POEMS)

Osteosclerotic myeloma, or POEMS (polyneuropathy, organomegaly, endocrinopathy, M protein, and skin changes) syndrome, is characterized by a chronic sensorimotor polyneuropathy with predominating motor disability (Dispenzieri et al. 2003). Bardwick et al. (1980) suggested the acronym POEMS syndrome. Polyneuropathy of single or multiple osteosclerotic bone lesions is an important feature. The cranial nerves are not involved, except for papilledema. Hepatosplenomegaly and lymphadenopathy may occur. Hyperpigmentation, hypertrichosis, gynecomastia, and testicular atrophy may be seen. Polycythemia or thrombocytosis may be a prominent feature. Almost all patients have a monoclonal protein of the λ light chain class. The concentration of the M protein is modest and is almost always less than 3 g/dL. In contrast to MM, this syndrome is rarely associated with Bence Jones proteinuria, renal insufficiency, hypercalcemia, and skeletal fractures. The bone marrow aspirate and biopsy specimen usually contain less than 5% plasma cells.

The cause of osteosclerotic myeloma is unknown. Patients have higher values of IL-1β, tumor necrosis factor-a, and IL-6 than patients with MM. Increased levels of vascular endothelial growth factor are found frequently and often decrease with successful therapy. Single or multiple osteosclerotic lesions in a limited area should be treated with radiation therapy in tumoricidal doses of 40 to 50 cGy. More than half of patients have substantial improvement of the neuropathy. Improvement may be slow, and we have seen patients who continue to improve for 2 to 3 years after radiation therapy.

If the patient has widespread osteosclerotic lesions, systemic therapy is necessary. Five of 6 patients treated with melphalan and prednisone improved. Corticosteroids and plasma exchange generally have little benefit. Autologous stem cell transplantation after high-dose melphalan therapy is a consideration for younger patients with widespread osteosclerotic lesions (Dispenzieri et al. 2001b; Jaccard et al. 2002). The stem cells should be collected before the patient is exposed to alkylating agents, because these agents reduce the number of hematopoietic stem cells. The mortality rate associated with this procedure in MM is currently only 1%.

1.2.8.6 Dermatologic Diseases

Lichen myxedematosus (papular mucinosis, scleromyxedema) is a rare dermatologic condition frequently associated with a cathodal IgGλ protein. It is characterized by dermal papules, macules, and plaques that infiltrate the skin. Biopsy specimens exhibit an increased deposition of acid mucopolysaccharides. Scleredema (Buschke disease) has been noted with an M protein, but the role of the M protein is unknown. Cardiomyopathy and congestive heart failure from deposition of acid mucopolysaccharide have been reported in a patient with scleredema. Hyperpigmentation and hyperlipoproteinemia have also been seen in scleredema.

Pyoderma gangrenosum has been associated with M proteins (Duguid and Powell 1993). In a review of 67 patients, 7 patients had a benign M protein and 1 patient had multiple myeloma. Seven of the 8 patients had an IgA monoclonal gammopathy. Necrobiotic xanthogranuloma is frequently found with an IgG monoclonal protein (Mehregan and Winkelmann 1992; Nestle et al. 1999). Schnitzler syndrome is characterized by the presence of chronic urticaria and an IgM monoclonal gammopathy (Puddu et al. 1997). Monoclonal gammopathy has been noted in patients with diffuse plane xanthomatosis. M proteins have been reported with psoriasis, but it is doubtful that an association exists. Subcorneal pustular dermatosis has been associated with monoclonal gammopathy. An IgA M protein was found in 3 and IgG in 1 of 7 patients with subcorneal pustular dermatosis (Lutz et al. 1998). A comprehensive review of monoclonal gammopathies and skin disorders has been published (Daoud et al. 1999).

More than a dozen patients have been reported with an M protein and Sézary syndrome; only 2 had multiple myeloma (Venencie et al. 1984a). Five patients with mycosis fungoides and monoclonal gammopathy have been described (Venencie et al. 1984b). Thus, cutaneous T-cell lymphomas may be associated with monoclonal gammopathies. Several cases of Kaposi sarcoma and monoclonal gammopathy have been recognized (Strumia and Roveggio 1994). Erythema elevatum diutinum has been reported with monoclonal gammopathy.

1.2.8.7 Immunosuppression

M proteins were found in more than half of a series of patients with acquired immunodeficiency syndrome. In another series of 130 homosexual men, human immunodeficiency virus (HIV) antibody was found in 65. Four patients had an M protein: 2 with IgGκ and 2 with IgMκ. The appearance or disappearance of a monoclonal gammopathy in patients with HIV infection does not seem to have prognostic significance. Even when M proteins are identified in HIV-infected patients, the bone marrow plasma cells are atypical and present in aggregates, but they stain with both κ and λ light chains (polyclonal).

M proteins were detected in 18 of 141 patients (12.8%) who had undergone renal transplantation. In 7, the gammopathy was transient. In another series, 27 of 213 patients (12.7%) had a monoclonal or multiclonal gammopathy after renal transplantation. In 3 additional patients with persistent gammopathy, MM (2 patients) or solitary plasmacytoma (1 patient) subsequently developed. Others reported M proteins in 4 of 110 patients with renal transplants. A monoclonal gammopathy was found in 70 of 232 patients (30%) who were receiving immunosuppressive therapy after renal transplantation. The incidence was 10 times greater than that in a control group of 30 patients with chronic renal insufficiency who were receiving dialysis. In 74% of the 23 patients in whom a longitudinal study was available, the monoclonal gammopathy was transient. This finding suggests that immunosuppression leads to a temporary immunodeficiency state similar to that observed with aging of the immune system.

The presence of cytomegalovirus infection after renal transplantation in pediatric patients is associated with an increased incidence of M proteins. In a study of 80 pediatric patients who had kidney transplantation, 57% of patients with a cytomegalovirus infection had an M protein, whereas only 8% of those without a cytomegalovirus infection had an M protein. In another series of 182 renal transplantations, an M protein was found in 30% of patients. The authors concluded that the M protein was a reflection of the T-cell immune defect (Ducloux et al. 1999). A case of transient MM was reported after immunosuppression for renal transplantation. A biclonal gammopathy (IgGκ and IgGλ) developed, and the bone marrow contained 30% plasma cells. No lytic lesions were found. Immunosuppression was reduced, the M protein disappeared, and the bone marrow plasma cell content decreased to less than 5%.

Transient monoclonal gammopathies after bone marrow transplantation were found in 18 of 42 patients (43%); the gammopathy was most often of the IgGλ class. In another report, transient oligoclonal and monoclonal gammopathies were found in 31 of 60 patients (52%) who underwent allogeneic (57 cases) or syngeneic (3 cases) bone marrow transplantation. A monoclonal gammopathy was detected at an average of 3 months after transplantation and persisted for approximately 6 months. The development of graft-versus-host disease correlated strongly with the appearance of an M protein. Most of the Igs were IgG. M proteins appeared frequently and as early as 6 weeks after bone marrow transplantation in 40 children. IgM, IgG3, and IgG1 were the most common isotypes. In a report of 550 patients receiving autologous stem cell transplants, abnormal protein bands developed in 10%. Forty-eight additional patients had oligoclonal bands and 23 had an isotype switch. The authors concluded that the oligoclonal bands and isotype switching were due to recovery of immunoglobulin production rather than alteration in the biology of the malignant plasma cell clone (Zent et al. 1998). In 12 of 47 patients, an M protein developed after allogeneic bone marrow transplantation. Eleven of the 12 patients had had a cytomegalovirus infection.

In 57 of 201 patients (28%), an M protein developed after liver transplantation. Five of 7 in whom a posttransplantation lymphoproliferative disorder developed had an M protein, whereas only 52 of 194 (27%) without a posttransplantation lymphoproliferative disorder had an M protein (Badley et al. 1996). In another series, 26 of 86 liver transplant recipients had an M protein. There was a strong correlation between the occurrence of viral infections and the presence of an M protein (Pageaux et al. 1998). In a series of 88 patients receiving a liver transplant, there was no difference in the incidence of M proteins between cyclosporine and FK506 (tacrolimus) immunosuppression. Both monoclonal and oligoclonal Ig banding are common in recipients of heart transplants. The M proteins are small, transient, and of little clinical significance.

1.2.8.8 Miscellaneous Conditions

A patient with angioneurotic edema and acquired deficiency of C1 esterase inhibitor was described and the records were reviewed of 14 other patients reported in the literature, including 5 with a 7S IgM M protein. Others described 2 patients with acquired C1 esterase inhibitor deficiency, an IgGκ protein, and recurrent episodes of febrile panniculitis and hepatitis. Another group reported that 8 of 9 patients with systemic capillary leak syndrome had an M protein in the serum. In a review of the literature, all 21 patients with a capillary leak syndrome had a monoclonal serum protein (IgGκ, 12; IgGλ, 7; IgA, 1; IgG with an unspecified light chain, 1) (Droder et al. 1992).

Although polyclonal increases in immunoglobulin are most common in liver disease, M proteins have been noted in chronic active hepatitis. In a retrospective study of patients with an M protein or severe hypergammaglobulinemia, an M protein was found in 11 of 272 patients with chronic active hepatitis. These investigators found a higher incidence of M proteins (26%) in the sera of 50 randomly selected patients who had chronic active hepatitis. M proteins have also been recognized in patients with primary biliary cirrhosis. There is an association of hepatitis C virus (HCV) and monoclonal gammopathies. The incidence of HCV was 69% in 94 patients with mixed cryoglobulinemia and only 14% in 107 patients without cryoglobulinemia. In another series of 102 cases of MM, macroglobulinemia, or MGUS, HCV infection was found in 16% but in only 5% of controls. An M protein was found in 11% of 239 HCV-positive patients but in only 1% of 98 HCV-negative patients. Thus, the prevalence of M proteins is high in patients with HCV-related chronic liver diseases (Andreone et al. 1998).

Also reported in association with monoclonal gammopathies were Schönlein-Henoch purpura, bacterial endocarditis, Hashimoto thyroiditis, septic arthritis, purpura fulminans, idiopathic pulmonary fibrosis, pulmonary alveolar proteinosis, idiopathic pulmonary hemosiderosis, sarcoidosis, thymoma, hereditary spherocytosis, Doyne macular heredodystrophy, eosinophilic fibrohistiocytic lesions of the bone marrow, and hyperlipoproteinemia. The relationship of monoclonal gammopathy to these diseases is not clear and may be fortuitous.

Active glomerular lesions consisting of epithelial crescents and a rapidly progressive glomerulonephritis have been reported with monoclonal gammopathy. The association of proliferative glomerulonephritis with monoclonal gammopathy has been recognized in 25 cases, but the causal relationship is unknown. One of these patients had recurrence of the crescentic glomerulonephritis and deposition of IgGλ in a cadaveric renal transplant.

We are not aware of any well-documented instances in which surgical removal of a nonhematologic tumor resulted in the disappearance of the M protein. In 1 case an IgG M protein in the serum and urine disappeared 2 years after surgical removal of a carcinoma of the colon. However, the M protein in the serum and urine was first recognized 2 months after operation, indicating that the tumor did not produce the M protein.

1.2.8.9 M Proteins With Antibody Activity

Of 612 patients in whom monoclonal Igs were studied for their antibody activity against actin, tubulin, thyroglobulin, myosin, myoglobin, fetuin, albumin, transferrin, and double-stranded DNA, 36 (5.9%) possessed antibody activity. In 32 of the 36 patients, the antibody activity was directed mainly against actin. Most of these patients had a malignant lymphoplasmacytic disorder. Others reported the presence of an IgG3 M protein with antiactin activity in a patient who had 3 episodes of thrombotic thrombocytopenic purpura and who appeared to be developing a malignant lymphoproliferative process.

In some patients with MGUS, myeloma, or macroglobulinemia, the monoclonal Ig has exhibited unusual specificities to dextran, antistreptolysin O, antinuclear activity, smooth muscle, riboflavin, von Willebrand factor, thyroglobulin, insulin, double-stranded DNA, apolipoprotein, thyroxine, cephalin, lactate dehydrogenase, anti-HIV, and antibiotics.

In 1 patient, xanthoderma and xanthotrichia (yellow discoloration of the skin and hair) were caused by an IgGλ protein with antiriboflavin antibody activity. Xanthoderma disappeared when the IgG value decreased to < 2 g/dL after chemotherapy. Another patient with similar clinical and laboratory features has been reported.

One group described a patient with MM and a bleeding diathesis in whom an IgG1κ protein reacted with platelet glycoprotein IIIa. This produced a thrombasthenic-like state. An IgMκ M protein that agglutinated platelets and produced a pseudothrombocytopenia has been reported.

The binding of calcium by M protein may produce hypercalcemia without symptomatic or pathologic consequences. This situation must be recognized so that patients are not treated for hypercalcemia (Annesley et al. 1982). Copper-binding M protein has been found in 2 patients with MM. Hypercupremia was noted in a patient with a benign IgGλ M protein and carcinoma of the lung. Binding of an M protein with transferrin, producing a high serum iron level, has been reported.

One group described a patient with multiple thrombi from intravascular precipitation of an IgGλ monoclonal cryoglobulin with transferrin and fibrinogen. Others described a patient with an IgGκ protein that bound phosphate, producing a spurious elevation of the serum phosphorus value. Two other similar patients – one with MM and 1 with MGUS – have been described with hyperphosphatemia, presumably from binding of serum phosphorus by the M protein.

Transient M proteins with antibody activity have been recognized after infection. One report described a newborn with congenital toxoplasmosis who had an IgGλ protein. Such a protein was not found in the mother, and it did not display antibody activity.

Waldenström (1986) emphasized the antibody activity of M proteins. M proteins with antibody activity in plasma cell dyscrasias were reviewed by Merlini et al. (1986).

References

Andreone P, Zignego AL, Cursaro C, Gramenzi A, Gherlinzoni F, Fiorino S, Giannini C, Boni P, Sabattini E, Pileri S, Tura S, Bernardi M (1998) Prevalence of monoclonal gammopathies in patients with hepatitis C virus infection. Ann Intern Med 129:294–298

Annesley TM, Burritt MF, Kyle RA (1982) Artifactual hypercalcemia in multiple myeloma. Mayo Clin Proc 57:572–575

Arnulf B, Bengoufa D, Sarfati E, Toubert ME, Meignin V, Brouet JC, Fermand JP (2002) Prevalence of monoclonal gammopathy in patients with primary hyperparathyroidism: a prospective study. Arch Intern Med 162:464–467

Avet-Loiseau H, Facon T, Daviet A, Godon C, Rapp MJ, Harousseau JL, Grosbois B, Bataille R, Intergroupe Francophone du Myelome (1999 a) 14q32 translocations and monosomy 13 observed in monoclonal gammopathy of undetermined significance delineate a multistep process for the oncogenesis of multiple myeloma. Cancer Res 59:4546–4550

Avet-Loiseau H, Li JY, Morineau N, Facon T, Brigaudeau C, Harousseau JL, Grosbois B, Bataille R, Intergroupe Francophone du Myelome (1999 b) Monosomy 13 is associated with the transition of monoclonal gammopathy of undetermined significance to multiple myeloma. Blood 94:2583–2589

Axelsson U, Bachmann R, Hallen J (1966) Frequency of pathological proteins (M-components) in 6,995 sera from an adult population. Acta Med Scand 179:235–247

Azar HA, Hill WT, Osserman EF (1957) Malignant lymphoma and lymphatic leukemia associated with myeloma-type serum proteins. Am J Med 23:239–249

Badley AD, Portela DF, Patel R, Kyle RA, Habermann TM, Strickler JG, Ilstrup DM, Wiesner RH, de Groen P, Walker RC, Paya CV (1996) Development of monoclonal gammopathy precedes the development of Epstein-Barr virus-induced posttransplant lymphoproliferative disorder. Liver Transpl Surg 2:375–382

Baldini L, Guffanti A, Cesana BM, Colombi M, Chiorboli O, Damilano I, Maiolo AT (1996) Role of different hematologic variables in defining the risk of malignant transformation in monoclonal gammopathy. Blood 87:912–918

Bardwick PA, Zvaifler NJ, Gill GN, Newman D, Greenway GD, Resnick DL (1980) Plasma cell dyscrasia with polyneuropathy, organomegaly, endocrinopathy, M protein, and skin changes: the POEMS syndrome. Report on two cases and a review of the literature. Medicine (Baltimore) 59:311–322

Bataille R, Chappard D, Basle MF (1996) Quantifiable excess of bone resorption in monoclonal gammopathy is an early symptom of malignancy: a prospective study of 87 bone biopsies. Blood 87:4762–4769

Bellaiche L, Laredo JD, Liote F, Koeger AC, Hamze B, Ziza JM, Pertuiset E, Bardin T, Tubiana JM, the GRI Study Group (1997) Magnetic resonance appearance of monoclonal gammopathies of unknown significance and multiple myeloma. Spine 22:2551–2557

Bladé J, Lopez-Guillermo A, Rozman C, Cervantes F, Salgado C, Aguilar JL, Vives-Corrons JL, Montserrat E (1992) Malignant transformation and life expectancy in monoclonal gammopathy of undetermined significance. Br J Haematol 81:391–394

Cesana C, Klersy C, Barbarano L, Nosari AM, Crugnola M, Pungolino E, Gargantini L, Granata S, Valentini M, Morra E (2002) Prognostic factors for malignant transformation in monoclonal gammopathy of undetermined significance and smoldering multiple myeloma. J Clin Oncol 20:1625–1634

Cohen HJ, Crawford J, Rao MK, Pieper CF, Currie MS (1998) Racial differences in the prevalence of monoclonal gammopathy in a community-based sample of the elderly. Am J Med 104:439–444

Dalakas MC, Illa I, Gallardo E, Juarez C (1997) Inclusion body myositis and paraproteinemia: incidence and immunopathologic correlations. Ann Neurol 41:100–104

Daoud MS, Lust JA, Kyle RA, Pittelkow MR (1999) Monoclonal gammopathies and associated skin disorders. J Am Acad Dermatol 40:507–535

Dimopoulos MA, Moulopoulos LA, Maniatis A, Alexanian R (2000) Solitary plasmacytoma of bone and asymptomatic multiple myeloma. Blood 96:2037–2044

Dispenzieri A, Gertz MA, Therneau TM, Kyle RA (2001a) Retrospective cohort study of 148 patients with polyclonal gammopathy. Mayo Clin Proc 76:476–487

Dispenzieri A, Lacy MQ, Litzow MR, Tefferi A, Inwards DJ, Micallef IN, Gastineau DA, Ansell S, Rajkumar SV, Fonseca R, Witzig TE, Lust JA, Kyle RA, Greipp PR, Gertz MA (2001b) Peripheral blood stem cell transplant (PBSCT) in patients with POEMS syndrome (abstract). Blood 98 no. 11, Part 2:391 b

Dispenzieri A, Kyle RA, Lacy MQ, Rajkumar SV, Therneau TM, Lars DR, Greipp PR, Witzig TE, Basu R, Suarez GA, Fonseca R, Lust JA, Gertz MA (2003) POEMS syndrome: definitions and long-term outcome. Blood 101:2496–2506

Droder RM, Kyle RA, Greipp PR (1992) Control of systemic capillary leak syndrome with aminophylline and terbutaline. Am J Med 92:523–526

Ducloux D, Carron P, Racadot E, Rebibou JM, Bresson-Vautrin C, Hillier YS, Chalopin JM (1999) T-cell immune defect and B-cell activation in renal transplant recipients with monoclonal gammopathies. Transpl Int 12:250–253

Duguid CM, Powell FC (1993) Pyoderma gangrenosum. Clin Dermatol 11:129–133

Ellis TM, Le PT, DeVries G, Stubbs E, Fisher M, Bhoopalam N (2001) Alterations in CD30(+) T cells in monoclonal gammopathy of undetermined significance. Clin Immunol 98:301–307

Federici AB, Stabile F, Castaman G, Canciani MT, Mannucci PM (1998) Treatment of acquired von Willebrand syndrome in patients with monoclonal gammopathy of uncertain significance: comparison of three different therapeutic approaches. Blood 92:2707–2711

Fonseca R, Ahmann GJ, Jalal SM, Dewald GW, Larson DR, Therneau TM, Gertz MA, Kyle RA, Greipp PR (1998) Chromosomal abnormalities in systemic amyloidosis. Br J Haematol 103:704–710

Fonseca R, Aguayo P, Ahmann GJ, Jalal SM, Rajkumar SV, Kyle RA, Gertz MA, Dewald GW, Dispenzieri A, Lust JA, Lacy MQ, Witzig TE, Greipp PR (1999) Translocations at 14q32 are common in patients with the monoclonal gammopathy of undetermined significance (MGUS) and involve several partner chromosomes (abstract). Blood 94 Suppl 1:663 a

Greipp PR, Witzig TE, Gonchoroff NJ, Habermann TM, Katzmann JA, O'Fallon WM, Kyle RA (1987) Immunofluorescence labeling indices in myeloma and related monoclonal gammopathies. Mayo Clin Proc 62:969–977

Grignani G, Gobbi PG, Formisano R, Pieresca C, Ucci G, Brugnatelli S, Riccardi A, Ascari E (1996) A prognostic index for multiple myeloma. Br J Cancer 73:1101–1107

Grosbois B, Jego P, de Rosa H, Ruelland A, Lancien G, Gallou G, Leblay R (1997) Triclonal gammopathy and malignant immunoproliferative syndrome. [French] Rev Med Interne 18:470–473

Guillerm G, Gyan E, Wolowiec D, Facon T, Avet-Loiseau H, Kuliczkowski K, Bauters F, Fenaux P, Quesnel B (2001) p16(INK4a) and p15(INK4b) gene methylations in plasma cells from monoclonal gammopathy of undetermined significance. Blood 98:244–246

Hjorth M, Hellquist L, Holmberg E, Magnusson B, Rodjer S, Westin J, Myeloma Group of Western Sweden (1993) Initial versus deferred melphalan-prednisone therapy for asymptomatic multiple myeloma stage I – a randomized study. Eur J Haematol 50:95–102

Jaccard A, Royer B, Bordessoule D, Brouet JC, Fermand JP (2002) High-dose therapy and autologous blood stem cell transplantation in POEMS syndrome. Blood 99:3057–3059

Keren DF, Alexanian R, Goeken JA, Gorevic PD, Kyle RA, Tomar RH (1999) Guidelines for clinical and laboratory evaluation of patients with monoclonal gammopathies. Arch Pathol Lab Med 123:106–107

Kurihara Y, Shiba K, Fukumura Y, Kobayashi I, Kamei S (2000) Occurrence of serum M-protein species in Japanese patients older than 50 years based on relative mobility in cellulose acetate membrane electrophoresis. J Clin Lab Anal 14:64–69

Kyle RA (1993) "Benign" monoclonal gammopathy – after 20 to 35 years of follow-up. Mayo Clin Proc 68:26–36

Kyle RA (1999) Sequence of testing for monoclonal gammopathies. Arch Pathol Lab Med 123:114–118

Kyle RA, Garton JP (1987) The spectrum of IgM monoclonal gammopathy in 430 cases. Mayo Clin Proc 62:719–731

Kyle RA, Greipp PR (1980) Smoldering multiple myeloma. N Engl J Med 302:1347–1349

Kyle RA, Greipp PR (1982) "Idiopathic" Bence Jones proteinuria: long-term follow-up in seven patients. N Engl J Med 306:564–567

Kyle RA, Bayrd ED, McKenzie BF, Heck FJ (1960) Diagnostic criteria for electrophoretic patterns of serum and urinary proteins in multiple myeloma: study of one hundred and sixty-five multiple myeloma patients and of seventy-seven nonmyeloma patients with similar electrophoretic patterns. JAMA 174:245–251

Kyle RA, Finkelstein S, Elveback LR, Kurland LT (1972) Incidence of monoclonal proteins in a Minnesota community with a cluster of multiple myeloma. Blood 40:719–724

Kyle RA, Robinson RA, Katzmann JA (1981) The clinical aspects of bi-clonal gammopathies. Review of 57 cases. Am J Med 71:999–1008

Kyle RA, Linos A, Beard CM, Linke RP, Gertz MA, O'Fallon WM, Kurland LT (1992) Incidence and natural history of primary systemic amyloidosis in Olmsted County, Minnesota, 1950 through 1989. Blood 79:1817–1822

Kyle RA, Beard CM, O'Fallon WM, Kurland LT (1994) Incidence of multiple myeloma in Olmsted County, Minnesota: 1978 through 1990, with a review of the trend since 1945. J Clin Oncol 12:1577–1583

Kyle RA, Katzmann JA, Lust JA, Dispenzieri A (2002a) Immunochemical characterization of immunoglobulins. In: Rose NR, Hamilton RG, Detrick B (eds) Manual of clinical laboratory immunology, 6th edn. ASM Press, Washington, DC, pp 71–91

Kyle RA, Therneau TM, Rajkumar SV, Offord JR, Larson DR, Plevak MF, Melton LJ III (2002b) A long-term study of prognosis in monoclonal gammopathy of undetermined significance. N Engl J Med 346:564–569

Kyle RA, Gertz MA, Witzig TE, Lust JA, Lacy MQ, Dispenzieri A, Fonseca R, Rajkumar SV, Offord JR, Larson DR, Plevak MF, Therneau TM, Greipp PR (2003) Review of 1027 patients with newly diagnosed multiple myeloma. Mayo Clin Proc 78:21–33

Lacy MQ, Donovan KA, Heimbach JK, Ahmann GJ, Lust JA (1999) Comparison of interleukin-1 beta expression by in situ hybridization in monoclonal gammopathy of undetermined significance and multiple myeloma. Blood 93:300–305

Laroche M, Attal M, Dromer C (1996) Bone remodelling in monoclonal gammopathies of uncertain significance, symptomatic and non-symptomatic myeloma. Clin Rheumatol 15:347–352

Lutz ME, Daoud MS, McEvoy MT, Gibson LE (1998) Subcorneal pustular dermatosis: a clinical study of ten patients. Cutis 61:203–208

Mariette X, Zagdanski AM, Guermazi A, Bergot C, Arnould A, Frija J, Brouet JC, Fermand JP (1999) Prognostic value of vertebral lesions detected by magnetic resonance imaging in patients with stage I multiple myeloma. Br J Haematol 104:723–729

Mehregan DA, Winkelmann RK (1992) Necrobiotic xanthogranuloma. Arch Dermatol 128:94–100

Merlini G, Farhangi M, Osserman EF (1986) Monoclonal immunoglobulins with antibody activity in myeloma, macroglobulinemia and related plasma cell dyscrasias. Semin Oncol 13:350–365

Milla F, Oriol A, Aguilar J, Aventín A, Ayats R, Alonso E, Domingo A, Feliu E, Florensa L, López A, Pérez-Vila E, Rozman M, Sanchez C, Vallespi T, Woessner S (2001) Usefulness and reproducibility of cytomorphologic evaluations to differentiate myeloma from monoclonal gammopathies of unknown significance. Am J Clin Pathol 115:127–135

Mundis RJ, Kyle RA (1982) Primary hyperparathyroidism and monoclonal gammopathy of undetermined significance. Am J Clin Pathol 77:619–621

Nakayama T, Horiuchi E, Watanabe T, Murayama S, Nakase H (2000) A case of inclusion body myositis with benign monoclonal gammo-

pathy successfully responding to repeated immunoabsorption. J Neurol Neurosurg Psychiatry 68:230–233

Nestle FO, Hofbauer G, Burg G (1999) Necrobiotic xanthogranuloma with monoclonal gammopathy of the IgG lambda type. Dermatology 198:434–435

Noel P, Kyle RA (1987) Monoclonal proteins in chronic lymphocytic leukemia. Am J Clin Pathol 87:385–388

Ocqueteau M, Orfao A, Almeida J, Bladé J, Gonzalez M, Garcia-Sanz R, Lopez-Berges C, Moro MJ, Hernandez J, Escribano L, Caballero D, Rozman M, San Miguel JF (1998) Immunophenotypic characterization of plasma cells from monoclonal gammopathy of undetermined significance patients. Implications for the differential diagnosis between MGUS and multiple myeloma. Am J Pathol 152:1655–1665

Pageaux GP, Bonnardet A, Picot MC, Perrigault PF, Coste V, Navarro F, Fabre JM, Domergue J, Descomps B, Blanc P, Michel H, Larrey D (1998) Prevalence of monoclonal immunoglobulins after liver transplantation: relationship with posttransplant lymphoproliferative disorders. Transplantation 65:397–400

Pasqualetti P, Festuccia V, Collacciani A, Casale R (1997) The natural history of monoclonal gammopathy of undetermined significance. A 5- to 20-year follow-up of 263 cases. Acta Haematol 97:174–179

Puddu P, Cianchini G, Girardelli CR, Colonna L, Gatti S, de Pita O (1997) Schnitzler's syndrome: report of a new case and a review of the literature. Clin Exp Rheumatol 15:91–95

Rajkumar SV, Leong T, Roche PC, Fonseca R, Dispenzieri A, Lacy MQ, Lust JA, Witzig TE, Kyle RA, Gertz MA, Greipp PR (2000) Prognostic value of bone marrow angiogenesis in multiple myeloma. Clin Cancer Res 6:3111–3116

Riches PG, Sheldon J, Smith AM, Hobbs JR (1991) Overestimation of monoclonal immunoglobulin by immunochemical methods. Ann Clin Biochem 28:253–259

Saito N, Hirai K, Torimoto Y, Taya N, Kohgo Y, Takemori N, Tokuyasu Y, Miyokawa N (1998) Plural immunoglobulin synthesis in a single cell: an ultrastructural study of two cases with three M-proteins. Ultrastruct Pathol 22:421–429

Sala P, Tonutti E, Giuliano M, Fuccaro V, Bramezza M (1989) Laboratory screening of monoclonal gammopathies: incidence of serum monoclonal immunoglobulins during a five years survey in a general hospital. Boll Ist Sieroter Milan 68:224–227

Saleun JP, Vicariot M, Deroff P, Morin JF (1982) Monoclonal gammopathies in the adult population of Finistère, France. J Clin Pathol 35:63–68

Strumia R, Roveggio C (1994) Kaposi's sarcoma and monoclonal gammopathy. Dermatology 188:76–77

Vacca A, Ribatti D, Roncali L, Ranieri G, Serio G, Silvestris F, Dammacco F (1994) Bone marrow angiogenesis and progression in multiple myeloma. Br J Haematol 87:503–508

Vejlgaard T, Abildgaard N, Jans H, Nielsen JL, Heickendorff L (1997) Abnormal bone turnover in monoclonal gammopathy of undetermined significance: analysis of type I collagen telopeptide, osteocalcin, bone-specific alkaline phosphatase and propeptides of type I and type III procollagens. Eur J Haematol 58:104–108

Venencie PY, Winkelmann RK, Friedman SJ, Kyle RA, Puissant A (1984a) Monoclonal gammopathy and mycosis fungoides. Report of four cases and review of the literature. J Am Acad Dermatol 11:576–579

Venencie PY, Winkelmann RK, Puissant A, Kyle RA (1984 b) Monoclonal gammopathy in Sézary syndrome. Report of three cases and review of the literature. Arch Dermatol 120:605–608

Waldenström JG (1986) Antibody activity of monoclonal immunoglobulins in myeloma, macroglobulinemia and benign gammapathy. Med Oncol Tumor Pharmacother 3:135–140

Weber DM, Dimopoulos MA, Moulopoulos LA, Delasalle KB, Smith T, Alexanian R (1997) Prognostic features of asymptomatic multiple myeloma. Br J Haematol 97:810–814

Witzig TE, Gonchoroff NJ, Katzmann JA, Therneau TM, Kyle RA, Greipp PR (1988) Peripheral blood B cell labeling indices are a measure of disease activity in patients with monoclonal gammopathies. J Clin Oncol 6:1041–1046

Witzig TE, Kyle RA, O'Fallon WM, Greipp PR (1994) Detection of peripheral blood plasma cells as a predictor of disease course in patients with smouldering multiple myeloma. Br J Haematol 87:266–272

Xu D, Zheng C, Bergenbrant S, Holm G, Bjorkholm M, Yi Q, Gruber A (2001) Telomerase activity in plasma cell dyscrasias. Br J Cancer 84:621–615

Zent CS, Wilson CS, Tricot G, Jagannath S, Siegel D, Desikan KR, Munshi N, Bracy D, Barlogie B, Butch AW (1998) Oligoclonal protein bands and Ig isotype switching in multiple myeloma treated with high-dose therapy and hematopoietic cell transplantation. Blood 91:3518–3523

Neuropathy Associated With Plasma Cell Proliferative Disorders

S. Vincent Rajkumar, M.D., Robert A. Kyle, M.D., Guillermo A. Suarez, M.D.,
Angela Dispenzieri, M.D.*

2.1 Overview 36

2.2 Epidemiology 36
   2.2.1 Incidence 36
      2.2.1.1 MGUS Neuropathy 36
      2.2.1.2 Primary Amyloid Neuropathy 37
      2.2.1.3 POEMS Syndrome 37
   2.2.2 Mortality 37
   2.2.3 Sex Ratio 37
   2.2.4 Race Ratio 37
   2.2.5 Age Ratio 37

2.3 Etiology 37
   2.3.1 MGUS Neuropathy 38
   2.3.2 Primary Amyloid Neuropathy 39
   2.3.3 POEMS Syndrome 39

2.4 Screening and Prevention 39

2.5 Molecular Biology and Genetics 39

2.6 Clinical Presentation 39
   2.6.1 MGUS Neuropathy 39
   2.6.2 Neuropathy Associated With Multi-
      ple Myeloma and Solitary Plasma-
      cytoma 40
   2.6.3 Primary Amyloid Neuropathy 40
   2.6.4 POEMS Syndrome 41

2.7 Classification 42

2.8 Diagnosis 42
   2.8.1 Antibodies to MAG
      and Other Neural Antigens 43
   2.8.2 Radiographic Studies 43
   2.8.3 Electromyographic Studies 43
      2.8.3.1 MGUS Neuropathy 43
      2.8.3.2 Primary Amyloid Neuropathy 43
      2.8.3.3. POEMS Syndrome 44
   2.8.4 Cerebrospinal Fluid Examination . 44
   2.8.5 Pathologic Findings 44
      2.8.5.1 MGUS Neuropathy 44
      2.8.5.2 Primary Amyloid Neuropathy 44
      2.8.5.3 POEMS Syndrome 44

2.9 Differential Diagnosis 44

2.10 Therapy 46
   2.10.1 MGUS Neuropathy 46
   2.10.2 Primary Amyloid Neuropathy . . . 47
   2.10.3 POEMS Syndrome 47

2.11 Prognosis 48
   2.11.1 Primary Amyloid Neuropathy . . . 48
   2.11.2 POEMS Syndrome 48

References 49

* Supported in part by Grants CA 93842, CA 85818, CA 91561, and CA 62242, National Cancer Institute, Bethesda, MD, USA. Dr. Rajkumar is a Leukemia and Lymphoma Society of America Translational Research Awardee and is also supported by the Judith and George Goldman Foundation Fighting Catastrophic Diseases, Deerfield, IL, USA, and by the Multiple Myeloma Research Foundation.

2.1 Overview

The association of peripheral neuropathy with monoclonal plasma cell proliferative disorders (monoclonal gammopathies) is well recognized (Kyle and Dyck 1993b). This includes distinct clinical and pathophysiologic entities such as peripheral neuropathy associated with monoclonal gammopathy of undetermined significance (MGUS), primary amyloid neuropathy, and neuropathy associated with osteosclerotic myeloma (POEMS syndrome) (Table 2.1) (Kyle and Dyck 1993 a, b, c). Each of these clinical entities differs in presentation, natural history, management, and prognosis. This chapter describes the epidemiology, etiology, classification, diagnosis, treatment, and prognosis of these disorders.

Patients with neuropathy associated with the monoclonal gammopathies should be distinguished from patients with MGUS (or other plasma cell disorder) who incidentally have neuropathic symptoms due to other unrelated factors or systemic disorders in which the causal relationship between the monoclonal (M) protein and neurologic syndrome is unclear. Therefore, before

making a diagnosis of neuropathy related to MGUS or other plasma cell proliferative disorders, it is important to consider other causes of neuropathy such as diabetes mellitus and alcoholism by evaluating the pattern of nerve damage, clinical course, electrophysiologic features, and cerebrospinal fluid findings.

2.2 Epidemiology

2.2.1 Incidence

2.2.1.1 MGUS Neuropathy

Kahn and colleagues (1980) detected 58 cases of monoclonal gammopathy without evidence of myeloma or Waldenström macroglobulinemia in 14,000 serum samples (0.4%) obtained from patients admitted to a neurologic tertiary care center. Sixteen of the 58 patients had peripheral neuropathy. In another series, of 132 patients with monoclonal gammopathy, 4 (3%) had peripheral neuropathy (Johansen and Leegaard 1985).

Kelly and colleagues (1981) studied 692 patients with a clinical peripheral neuropathy identified in an electromyography laboratory at Mayo Clinic over a 1-year period. The cause of neuropathy was apparent in 358 patients and included diseases such as diabetes, alcoholism, and connective tissue disorders. In the remaining 334 patients, no obvious etiology was apparent for the neuropathy. Two hundred seventy-nine of these patients had serum protein electrophoresis done, and 28 (10%) had an M protein. The associated diseases were MGUS (16 patients), primary amyloidosis (7 patients), macroglobulinemia (1 patient), and gamma heavy chain disease (1 patient).

In another study, Isobe and Osserman (1971) found M proteins in 5.4% of patients presenting with peripheral neuropathy or myopathy. Other studies have found a statistically significant increase in the prevalence of M proteins in patients with peripheral neuropathy compared with the prevalence in normal populations in Minnesota, France, and Sweden (Kelly et al. 1981).

It appears that MGUS may be associated with (or account for) about 3% to 5% of all cases of peripheral neuropathy, especially in patients referred to tertiary care centers with such symptoms. Among patients with peripheral neuropathy in whom no cause is apparent, the association may be as high as 10%. Because MGUS prevalence is 2% to 3% of the normal adult population

---

Table 2.1. Classification of neuropathies associated with plasma cell disorders

MGUS neuropathy

   IgM related

   Non-IgM related

Neuropathy due to primary systemic amyloidosis (primary amyloid neuropathy)

   Polyneuropathy

   Carpal tunnel syndrome (compressive or infiltrative neuropathy)

POEMS syndrome

Neuropathy related to multiple myeloma

   Compressive neuropathy or radiculopathy

   Neuropathy of the MGUS type[a]

Neuropathy related to Waldenström macroglobulinemia[b]

MGUS, monoclonal gammopathy of undetermined significance; POEMS, polyneuropathy, organomegaly, endocrinopathy, M proteins, and skin changes.

[a] Similar to non-IgM MGUS neuropathy.

[b] Similar to IgM MGUS neuropathy.

older than 50 years (Kyle et al. 2002), and although some associations are pathophysiologically related, some are likely coincidental.

2.2.1.2 Primary Amyloid Neuropathy

Of patients with primary amyloidosis, 15% to 20% have peripheral neuropathy. Among patients with primary amyloid neuropathy, only 25% have neuropathy as the presenting manifestation of the disease (Duston et al. 1989). Neuropathy is rarely the dominant manifestation of the disease. In one study, neuropathy was the dominant symptom in only 26 of 1,282 patients (2%) with primary systemic amyloidosis referred to a tertiary care center (Rajkumar et al. 1998). Carpal tunnel syndrome may coexist with polyneuropathy or may be the sole neurologic manifestation of primary amyloidosis (Kyle and Dyck 1993 a). Overall, approximately 25% of patients with primary amyloidosis have carpal tunnel syndrome at presentation.

2.2.1.3 POEMS Syndrome

In 1980 Bardwick et al. coined the acronym POEMS to represent polyneuropathy (P), organomegaly (O), endocrinopathy (E), M proteins (M), and skin changes (S). POEMS syndrome (also called osteosclerotic myeloma, Takatsuki syndrome, or Crow-Fukase syndrome) is associated with polyneuropathy. Primary osteosclerotic lesions occur in less than 3% of multiple myeloma patients. Dispenzieri et al. (2003), in a comprehensive study of 99 patients, confirmed the presence of osteosclerotic bone lesions in more than 80% of patients with POEMS syndrome and set forth criteria for the diagnosis of this paraneoplastic syndrome. These figures contrast significantly with the 1% to 8% incidence of neuropathy in patients with classic multiple myeloma. Moreover, of patients with myeloma and peripheral neuropathy, half have osteosclerotic lesions (Kelly et al. 1983).

2.2.2 Mortality

The natural history of neuropathies associated with the monoclonal gammopathies differs depending on the distinct clinical entities (see section on prognosis) (Kyle and Dyck 1993b). The precise mortality from neuropathy in patients with MGUS neuropathy is unclear. For pa-

tients with primary systemic amyloidosis who present with dominant neuropathy, the median survival is 2 to 3 years (Rajkumar et al. 1998). Patients with POEMS syndrome have a more indolent course, and in one study the mortality was 23% at 5-year follow-up and the median survival was more than 13 years (Dispenzieri et al. 2003).

2.2.3 Sex Ratio

There is a slightly increased incidence of plasma cell proliferative disorders, including MGUS, in males (Kyle et al. 2002). Similarly, there is a male predominance in neuropathy associated with plasma cell disorders. In fact, two-thirds of all patients with MGUS neuropathy, primary systemic amyloidosis, and POEMS syndrome are men (Dispenzieri et al. 2003; Gertz and Rajkumar 2002; Kyle and Dyck 1993 a, b, c).

2.2.4 Race Ratio

There are no population-based studies of race ratio for patients with peripheral neuropathy associated with plasma cell proliferative disorders. However, in general there is a higher incidence of plasma cell dyscrasias among blacks than whites. It was initially believed that the POEMS syndrome was more common in Japanese than in whites from the US or Europe, but this likely represented a higher awareness of the syndrome in Japan in the 1980s.

2.2.5 Age Ratio

The median age at diagnosis of patients with MGUS is approximately 72 years (Kyle et al. 2002). Monoclonal gammopathies are rare in patients younger than 40 years. MGUS neuropathy occurs typically in the 6th and 7th decades of life. The median age for primary amyloidosis is about 62 years (Gertz and Rajkumar 2002). The median age at diagnosis of POEMS syndrome is considerably younger (in the early 50s) (Dispenzieri et al. 2003).

2.3 Etiology

The cause of peripheral neuropathy in patients with monoclonal gammopathy is unknown. The pathogenesis of neuropathy varies in the specific disease entities listed in Table 2.1. In primary amyloidosis, the basic mechanism responsible for the neuropathy is not entirely known, but probably involves a combination of nerve infiltration, nerve compression, and ischemia caused by the amyloid deposition. In contrast, patients with IgM monoclonal gammopathies often have demonstrable anti-myelin-associated glycoprotein (MAG), which is probably causally related. POEMS syndrome is a paraneoplastic syndrome that is likely due to proinflammatory cytokines; data suggest that vascular-derived endothelial growth factor is implicated in this disorder (Hashiguchi et al. 2000; Soubrier et al. 1999).

2.3.1 MGUS Neuropathy

The pathogenesis of MGUS neuropathy (especially IgM) is probably related to the reactivity of the monoclonal immunoglobulins to specific antigens expressed on peripheral nerves such as MAG, gangliosides, and chondroitin sulfate and sulfatide. In preclinical studies, mice injected daily with purified monoclonal IgG or just monoclonal Fab fragments from patients with polyneuropathy associated with myeloma or monoclonal gammopathy developed a demyelinating peripheral neuropathy with slowed nerve conduction velocities (Besinger et al. 1981).

The most convincing pathogenic relationship is between IgM MGUS neuropathy and MAG antibodies, although there is still some controversy. In 1980, Latov et al. described a patient with sensorimotor peripheral neuropathy and a monoclonal IgM protein. The M protein was directed against peripheral nerve myelin; this was documented by complement fixation and immunoabsorption. MAG has a molecular weight of approximately 100,000 and consists of 30% carbohydrate. The monoclonal IgM protein binds to a carbohydrate moiety in MAG (Nobile-Orazio et al. 1984). The IgM proteins do not bind to *de*glycosylated MAG, which is consistent with this hypothesis that the reactive determinants contain carbohydrate moieties (Shy et al. 1984). It has also been shown that *de*glycosylation of MAG abolishes the recognition of MAG by the patient's IgM protein (Frail et al. 1984).

Direct electron microscopic immunochemical studies with colloidal gold revealed deposition of anti-MAG IgM antibodies within the myelin and extending throughout the compact myelin in large and small mye-

linated fibers (Dellagi et al. 1983). A pathogenetic role for anti-MAG antibodies in IgM MGUS neuropathy is also supported by a study showing demyelination of the sciatic nerve in cats after intraneural injection of these antibodies obtained from 3 patients. In this study, there was evidence of an M protein and complement on the surface of the myelin sheaths, suggesting that the M protein reacted with an epitope of myelin (Dalakas et al. 1983). Binding of the IgM protein to MAG is specific because it can be completely blocked by MAG isolated from human myelin (Steck et al. 1983).

Two experimental animal studies have reproduced the pathologic features of human IgM MGUS neuropathy. Tatum (1993) systemically injected purified anti-MAG antibodies into chicks and produced demyelination with widening of the myelin lamella, similar to the changes observed in nerve biopsy specimens of patients. Similar histopathologic findings were obtained by intraneural injection of anti-MAG antibodies into rabbits (Monaco et al. 1995). However, the development of an in vivo animal model of the disease has not been successful. Quarles and Weiss (1999) comprehensively reviewed autoantibodies associated with peripheral neuropathy.

Approximately one-half of patients with peripheral neuropathy and an IgM M protein have anti-MAG antibodies (Latov et al. 1988). The anti-MAG IgM titers in 16 patients with peripheral neuropathy and an IgM M protein reacting with MAG ranged from 1:12,800 to 1:100,000. Low antibody titers to MAG (1:400 or less) were found in 8 of 24 patients with an IgM M protein without neuropathy. Very low titers (1:200 or less) were found in 17% of normal control patients without monoclonal gammopathy (Nobile-Orazio et al. 1989), suggesting that these antibodies may be part of the normal human antibody spectrum.

In addition to MAG determinants, other antigens such as glycolipids have been implicated (Kusunoki et al. 1987). Antiglycolipid antibodies have been associated with IgM neuropathies, Guillain-Barré syndrome, and multifocal neuropathies (Fredman 1998). Gangliosides represent other target antigens. Ilyas et al. (1984) reported that a monoclonal IgM protein in 3 patients with peripheral neuropathy bound to the carbohydrate portion of MAG and also to a single ganglioside of sciatic nerve.

The IgM protein may react with chondroitin sulfate and produce axonal rather than myelin damage. In one patient, clusters were seen of thinly myelinated fibers consistent with regeneration after axonal degeneration. Others have reported binding of the IgM protein to chondroitin sulfate C (Sherman et al. 1983; Yee et al. 1989). A predominantly sensory neuropathy has been described in association with monoclonal or polyclonal IgM antibodies directed against sulfatide. Ilyas et al. (1985) reported reaction with antibody to GD_{1b} or disialosyl gangliosides. Motor neuropathy with anti-GM_{1b} associated with motor neuropathy has also been reported.

Ischemia may play a role in MGUS neuropathy, but mechanisms are unclear. Endothelial proliferation causing thickened vessel walls can be seen in the vasa nervorum, and these microvascular changes may produce ischemia and loss of axons.

In contrast to studies supporting an association between demyelinating forms of neuropathy and MGUS, injections of serum from patients with M proteins and chronic sensorimotor polyneuropathy into rat sciatic nerves resulted in no abnormalities (Bosch et al. 1982).

In summary, there is considerable evidence of the pathogenetic role of anti-MAG antibodies in IgM MGUS neuropathy but much remains to be clarified, such as the cause of the monoclonal expansion that reacts with peripheral nerve antibodies, the mechanism of nerve injury, and the usefulness of measurements of these antibodies in clinical practice.

2.3.2 Primary Amyloid Neuropathy

The neuropathy associated with primary amyloidosis is thought to be a result of direct nerve infiltration with amyloid, nerve compression, or ischemia (Rajkumar et al. 1998). In primary amyloid neuropathy, amyloid deposits are found surrounding the endoneurial capillaries or in the epineurium on sural nerve biopsy studies. Other findings include a marked decrease in myelin fiber density and axonal degeneration on examination of teased fibers.

2.3.3 POEMS Syndrome

The etiology of POEMS syndrome is unknown. Patients with POEMS syndrome have higher concentrations of interleukin-1β, tumor necrosis factor alpha, vascular endothelial growth factor, and interleukin-6 than patients with typical multiple myeloma, and these cytokines may have a significant role in the pathogenesis of peripheral

neuropathy. Interleukin-6 and vascular endothelial growth factor values decrease after therapy. The precise mechanism by which these cytokines lead to nerve damage is not clear.

Human herpesvirus type 8 DNA has been reported in POEMS syndrome and multicentric Castleman disease. Antibodies to human herpesvirus type 8 were found in 78% of patients with POEMS syndrome and Castleman disease and 22% of those with POEMS syndrome without multicentric Castleman disease (Bélec et al. 1999). This association and its relationship to neuropathy need further study.

Another possible mechanism may involve the reactivity of the secreted monoclonal λ immunoglobulin to specific epitopes on the peripheral nerves, although light chains are not typically observed in pathologic specimens.

2.4 Screening and Prevention

Screening for neuropathies or other neurologic syndromes is not recommended for patients with MGUS or related plasma cell disorders. Patients with neurologic symptoms, however, need further evaluation. There are no preventive therapies known for neuropathy associated with MGUS or other plasma cell proliferative disorders.

2.5 Molecular Biology and Genetics

A genetic effect may have a role in some cases of neuropathy associated with monoclonal gammopathies. Busis and colleagues (1985) reported on a mother and son with IgM MGUS neuropathy. In another report, a brother and sister had an IgM M protein and a demyelinating peripheral neuropathy (Jønsson et al. 1988). Familial reports of MGUS and myeloma do exist, but there is no indication that neuropathy is more frequent in familial cases of MGUS and myeloma than in sporadic cases.

2.6 Clinical Presentation

2.6.1 MGUS Neuropathy

The diagnosis of MGUS neuropathy is made after excluding other known causes of neuropathy (Kyle and

Dyck 1993 b). Features of primary systemic amyloidosis, POEMS syndrome (osteosclerotic myeloma), and related disorders are absent. The typical presentation is a symmetric sensorimotor polyradiculopathy or neuropathy that usually begins insidiously in the toes and extends to the feet and legs. Paresthesias, ataxia, and pain may be prominent, and cranial nerves are not involved. Sensory symptoms usually precede motor involvement. The lower extremities are involved in 90% of patients, and the deep tendon reflexes are decreased or absent. Occasionally, unilateral symptoms initiate the process. MGUS neuropathy most frequently involves the IgM immunoglobulin class, followed by IgG and IgA classes.

In IgM MGUS neuropathy, sensory symptoms and ataxia overshadow the motor deficits. Several large studies (Chassande et al. 1998; Gosselin et al. 1991; Simovic et al. 1998; Suarez and Kelly 1993), including our experience, have analyzed the IgM MGUS vs. non-IgM MGUS neuropathies. In general, IgM MGUS neuropathy is more frequent and has a more progressive course than IgG or IgA neuropathy, with more sensory symptoms and deficits. IgM MGUS is associated with antibodies against peripheral nerve antigens (eg, anti-MAG antibodies) whereas non-IgM MGUS neuropathy only occasionally has anti-nerve antibody activity. Non-IgM MGUS neuropathies are more heterogeneous in their clinical presentation, with motor or sensory deficits and mixed varieties.

The peripheral neuropathy in Waldenström macroglobulinemia and IgM-associated chronic lymphocytic leukemia does not differ from that occurring in patients with MGUS of the IgM type.

2.6.2 Neuropathy Associated With Multiple Myeloma and Solitary Plasmacytoma

Neurologic involvement in myeloma is most often due to compression of the nerve roots, spinal cord, or cauda equina by myeloma arising in the marrow cavity of a vertebral body and extending to the extradural space. It occurs in about 5% of patients and causes severe back pain with radicular features, weakness or paralysis of the lower extremities, and bowel or bladder incontinence.

Polyneuropathy is not commonly associated with multiple myeloma or solitary plasmacytoma. In a series of 23 patients with multiple myeloma, 3 had clinical neuropathy and 6 had electrophysiologic evidence of peripheral neuropathy (Walsh 1971). If neuropathy is present, consideration must be given first to the presence of coexistent primary amyloidosis. Silverstein and Doniger (1963) found peripheral neuropathy in 10 of 277 hospitalized patients (3.6%) with multiple myeloma. Three of the 10 patients had amyloidosis. In the remaining patients in whom neuropathy was present in association with myeloma or solitary plasmacytoma, the etiology and course were similar to mild sensorimotor non-IgM MGUS neuropathy if features of the POEMS syndrome were not present.

Occasionally other presentations occur. Davison and Balser (1937) described a patient with peripheral neuritis of the upper extremities and multiple myeloma. Demyelination was found at autopsy, but there was no evidence of myelomatous invasion of the nerves. Delauche et al. (1981) described 3 patients with multiple myeloma and progressive demyelinating sensorimotor polyneuropathy. The demyelinating neuropathy did not respond to melphalan and prednisone. Borges and Busis (1985) reported the presence of a λ light chain within the neurons of a patient with multiple myeloma.

Solitary plasmacytoma of bone may be associated with peripheral neuropathy. In one report, a sacral plasmacytoma produced a severe peripheral neuropathy. Surgical removal and irradiation were associated with improvement of the peripheral neuropathy (Davidson 1972). Read and Warlow (1978) reported on 3 patients with solitary myeloma and peripheral neuropathy and reviewed 13 previous cases from the literature.

2.6.3 Primary Amyloid Neuropathy

Peripheral nerve involvement in amyloidosis is well recognized. In most patients, neuropathy is an incidental finding and not the major cause of morbidity (Kelly et al. 1979). Involvement of other organs such as the heart or kidney usually dominates the clinical picture.

There are 2 distinct patterns of presentation: polyneuropathy and carpal tunnel syndrome (Kyle and Dyck 1993 a). Patients with amyloid polyneuropathy usually present with undiagnosed neuropathy or with neuropathy, and serum or urine M protein is detected on workup. Alternatively, neuropathy may be identified at presentation or may develop in patients with known systemic amyloidosis involving the heart, liver, kidney, or other organs. Sensory symptoms are more common than motor dysfunction, and lower extremities are affected before upper extremities. Numbness, paresthesias, dysesthesias, and pain are common symptoms. This may be followed by progressive muscle weakness. Postural hypotension, syncope, and other autonomic symptoms can occur and may cause significant distress in patients with advanced disease. Significant weight loss is common.

In a series of 1,282 patients with primary amyloidosis, there were 26 patients in whom neuropathy was the presenting symptom and the dominant manifestation of their illness (Rajkumar et al. 1998). In this study, the median duration of symptoms before diagnosis was 29 months. Paresthesias, muscle weakness, and numbness were the most common symptoms. The lower extremities were involved first in 88% of patients. Symptoms of autonomic neuropathy were present in 65%. Although neuropathy was the dominant symptom in these patients, most had amyloid involvement of other tissues at diagnosis or during the course of their illness. In this group of patients, neuropathy progressed relentlessly and most patients became markedly immobile or bedridden.

The diagnosis of amyloid neuropathy is often delayed, with a median time to diagnosis from the onset of symptoms of 1 to 2 years (Duston et al. 1989; Kyle et al. 1986; Rajkumar et al. 1998). The possible reasons for the delay in diagnosis include patient delays in seeking care, physicians not recognizing the clinical picture, and failure to initiate the appropriate diagnostic work-up. Serum and urine protein electrophoresis and immunofixation should be considered for symptomatic patients. Electromyography reveals evidence of axonal neuropathy for which a cause is not readily apparent. If an M protein is detected, stains for amyloid should be performed on biopsy specimens, including nerve, bone marrow, and fat aspirate. The diagnosis should also be suspected if other organ involvement, such as the heart or kidney, is detected in a patient with undiagnosed neuropathy. Primary amyloid neuropathy must be distinguished from neuropathy associated with other monoclonal gammopathies, including MGUS and POEMS syndrome.

Although polyneuropathy as a dominant manifestation of the disease is rare in primary amyloidosis, carpal tunnel syndrome is a frequent finding at presentation (Gertz and Kyle 1989). In most of the cases of carpal tunnel syndrome where amyloid deposits are found,

the deposition is localized and seldom leads to systemic amyloidosis if not already present. In a study of 152 patients with carpal tunnel syndrome and associated amyloid deposits, 124 patients (82%) had localized amyloidosis, 25 (16%) had primary systemic amyloidosis, 3 (2%) had secondary amyloidosis, and 1 had familial amyloidosis (Kyle et al. 1989). Of the 124 patients with localized amyloidosis, systemic amyloidosis developed in only 2 patients. In fact, in most cases the amyloid localized to the carpal ligament is not the light chain type (primary amyloidosis) but rather the unmutated transthyretin (TTR) type. It must be emphasized that amyloidosis is a rare cause of carpal tunnel syndrome, and amyloid deposits are found in only about 2% of cases. Specimen staining or work-up for amyloidosis is not recommended for patients seen with isolated carpal tunnel syndrome, unless there are other indications that suggest systemic amyloidosis.

Cranial nerve involvement is rare (Rajkumar et al. 1998).

2.6.4 POEMS Syndrome

POEMS syndrome is characterized by polyneuropathy, organomegaly, endocrinopathy, M protein, and skin changes (Kyle and Dyck 1993c). Solitary or multiple osteosclerotic lesions on radiographs are found in more than 90% of patients.

Patients with POEMS syndrome are about a decade younger than typical multiple myeloma patients. Symptoms of peripheral neuropathy usually dominate the clinical picture. The duration of symptoms is usually 1 to 2 years before diagnosis, but it may be longer. Symptoms begin in the feet and consist of tingling, pins and needles, and coldness. Motor involvement follows the sensory symptoms. The neuropathy is symmetrical and ascending, with either an insidious or rapidly progressing onset. Patients often describe numbness and dysesthesias, followed by progressive ascending weakness. The sensory impairment is overshadowed by progressive motor impairment for the majority. As the neuropathy ascends, upper extremity involvement is not uncommon. Severe weakness occurs in more than one-half of the patients and results in inability to climb stairs, arise from a chair, or grip objects firmly with their hands. The course is usually slowly progressive, and patients may be confined to a wheelchair. Autonomic symptoms are not a feature, but impotence is common. In contrast to multiple myeloma, bone pain and fractures rarely occur.

Physical examination reveals asymmetric sensorimotor neuropathy involving the extremities. Neuropathy is worse distally and, in contrast to MGUS neuropathy, motor loss is more marked than sensory loss. More than one-half of patients have severe muscle weakness with areflexia. Touch-pressure, vibratory, and joint position senses are usually involved. Loss of temperature discrimination and nociception is less frequent. Cranial nerves are not involved except for papilledema.

Endocrine abnormalities are defining features of the syndrome. POEMS has been associated with primary and secondary hypothyroidism, hypogonadism, adrenocortical insufficiency, parathyroid abnormalities, and diabetes mellitus (Dispenzieri et al. 2003). Typically, endocrine glands appear normal histologically. Diabetes mellitus and gonadal dysfunction are the most common endocrinopathies. The diabetes is often mild. Gonadal dysfunction is usually associated with increased concentrations of serum luteinizing hormone and follicle-stimulating hormone, indicative of primary failure. Hyperprolactinemia may account for hypogonadism or galactorrhea. The cause of hyperprolactinemia is not apparent. Gynecomastia is common and probably related to increased concentrations of estrogen in the majority of cases. Hypothyroidism is not uncommon but is usually mild. It is associated with low thyroxine values and increased thyroid-stimulating hormone values.

Hepatomegaly occurs in almost one-half of patients; splenomegaly and lymphadenopathy are found in 25% to 50%.

Numerous cutaneous pathologic findings have been described, including hyperpigmentation, hemangioma, skin thickening or scleroderma-like changes, hypertrichosis, opacity of fingernails, and Terry nails. Hyperpigmentation is the most common skin change in POEMS syndrome. In some instances, it may be due to excessive melanocyte-stimulating hormone from the pituitary. Thickening of the skin has been seen. Raynaud phenomenon and clubbing have been reported. Angiomas of the skin may be prominent.

Papilledema is observed in 30% to 55% of patients and may be asymptomatic or cause headache, transient obscurations of vision, scotoma, enlarged blind spots, and progressive constriction of the visual field.

Clubbing may be seen in more than 10% of patients. It is unclear whether the clubbing observed in association with POEMS syndrome is a function of undiagnosed pulmonary hypertension associated with POEMS syndrome.

Hypertrichosis is characterized by development of stiff, coarse black hair on the extremities. Gynecomastia and testicular atrophy may be seen. Pitting edema of the lower extremities is common. Occasionally, ascites and pleural effusions occur.

Castleman disease (giant lymph node hyperplasia, angiofollicular lymph node hyperplasia) often is associated with POEMS syndrome (Dispenzieri et al. 2003).

The diagnosis of POEMS syndrome depends on the demonstration of increased numbers of abnormal monoclonal plasma cells in a biopsy specimen from the osteosclerotic lesion. A metastatic bone survey is done to detect osteosclerotic lesions. These lesions can be subtle and easily confused with benign fibrous dysplasia or a vertebral hemangioma. An M protein is found in the serum in almost 90% of patients. The size of the M protein is small (rarely more than 3 g/dL). The M protein is usually IgG or IgA and almost always of the λ type (Dispenzieri et al. 2003). Bence Jones proteinuria is infrequent. The M protein in the serum and urine may be small and may easily be overlooked unless immunofixation is done.

In contrast to multiple myeloma, anemia is not a feature of POEMS syndrome. The hemoglobin concentration may be increased and POEMS syndrome may be confused with polycythemia. Thrombocytosis is found in more than one-half of patients (Kelly et al. 1983). In contrast to multiple myeloma, hypercalcemia and renal insufficiency are rarely present. The bone marrow usually contains fewer than 5% plasma cells

2.7   Classification

The classification of neuropathies associated with plasma cell disorders (the monoclonal gammopathies) is arbitrary and evolving. Table 2.1 provides a suggested classification.

2.8   Diagnosis

The initial evaluation should include a careful clinical examination to confirm and characterize the peripheral neuropathy, followed by appropriate laboratory studies as discussed below.

2.8.1 Antibodies to MAG and Other Neural Antigens

Although anti-MAG antibodies are important in the pathogenesis of the IgM MGUS neuropathy, their role in clinical practice has not been established definitively (Kyle and Dyck 1993b). Reasons may include 1) method of analysis is not standardized and varies among laboratories, 2) potential cross-reactivity with other antigens, 3) controversy on the correlation with response to treatment and outcome, and 4) financial issues. Commercial autoantibody testing can be expensive and sometimes heavily promoted and bundled in groups of "autoantibody profiles" containing several individual profiles. An in-depth review of the clinical use of anti-MAG and other autoantibodies in peripheral neuropathy was published recently (Wolfe and Nations 2001).

In some patients with IgM MGUS and demyelinating neuropathy, testing for anti-MAG antibodies may indicate the presence of an immune-mediated neuropathy. In a review of 40 patients with polyneuropathy associated with an IgM gammopathy, all but 1 had symmetrical polyneuropathy. It was predominantly sensory in 13 and purely sensory in 17 others. Electrophysiologic studies revealed demyelination in 83% and axonal degeneration in 15%. Anti-MAG antibodies were found in 65% and were associated with only demyelinating polyneuropathies (Chassande et al. 1998).

In a series of 52 patients with IgM monoclonal gammopathy, symptomatic neuropathy was present in 3 of 4 patients with a high anti-MAG titer compared with 3 of 21 with a low anti-MAG titer (Meucci et al. 1999). This suggests that anti-MAG activity correlates with peripheral neuropathy.

The patient who most likely benefits from anti-MAG testing will have a chronic, predominantly sensory neuropathy with evidence of demyelination on electrophysiologic studies and an IgM MGUS.

2.8.2 Radiographic Studies

A bone survey should be considered in any patient with an unexplained peripheral neuropathy. By definition, patients with MGUS do not have bone disease such as lytic lesions, fractures, or osteoporosis related to their plasma cell dyscrasia. However, such lesions are the hallmark of multiple myeloma. In solitary plasmacytoma, there is a single bone lesion, but no significant bone marrow involvement.

Osteosclerotic lesions are present in more than 90% of patients with POEMS syndrome. Almost half have a solitary sclerotic lesion and about a third have multiple sclerotic lesions. The lesions are often modest in size and may be misinterpreted as benign bony sclerosis. On the other hand, they may produce a striking ivory (sclerotic) vertebral body. Often both osteosclerotic and osteolytic lesions are found. One can easily overlook a small sclerotic rim surrounding a large lytic lesion. Computed tomography or tomography may help identify the lesions. The pelvis, spine, ribs, and proximal extremities are most often involved.

2.8.3 Electromyographic Studies

2.8.3.1 MGUS Neuropathy

Nerve conduction is characteristically abnormal in motor and sensory fibers in the upper and lower extremities (Kyle and Dyck 1993b). In one study, conduction velocity of motor fibers decreased below the normal range by approximately 20% in IgM MGUS neuropathy (Smith et al. 1983). The amplitude of the compound muscle action potential is severely decreased in the lower limb nerves. Frequently, responses cannot be elicited from the sensory fibers of the upper and lower limb nerves. Needle electromyography reveals denervation in 80% of patients. Both demyelination and denervation may be present (Kelly et al. 1983). The electrophysiologic features of the IgM MGUS neuropathy are, in general, more homogeneous and resemble demyelination. Slow conduction velocities and prolonged distal latencies out of proportion to the proximal slowing suggest distal demyelination. This finding may help separate this neuropathy from other acquired and inherited demyelinating neuropathies.

2.8.3.2 Primary Amyloid Neuropathy

In most cases of amyloid polyneuropathy, motor nerve conduction velocities are affected minimally, and compound muscle action potentials are decreased or absent (Kyle and Dyck 1993a). Sensory nerve action potentials are decreased or absent and affected to a greater degree than compound muscle action potentials. Needle electromyographic examination reveals fibrillation potentials (Rajkumar et al. 1998). These findings are characteristic of an axonal sensorimotor peripheral neuropathy. Occasionally, a predominant demyelinating neuro-pathy is seen (Rajkumar et al. 1998). Electromyographic studies in patients with primary amyloidosis may reveal evidence of clinically asymptomatic carpal tunnel syndrome. Autonomic function testing in patients with primary amyloid neuropathy usually reveals decreased sweating, orthostatic hypotension, and cardiovagal impairment indicative of generalized autonomic failure.

2.8.3.3 POEMS Syndrome

The neuropathy in POEMS syndrome is usually a chronic, distal, large-fiber sensorimotor neuropathy (Kyle and Dyck 1993 c). Nerve conduction studies reveal moderate slowing of the conduction velocity with prolonged distal latencies. The slowing of motor conduction is proportionately greater than the reduction in the compound muscle action potential amplitude. On electromyographic examination, distal fibrillation potentials and enlarged, polyphasic voluntary motor unit action potentials with decreased recruitment are found (Kelly et al. 1983). The results suggest a polyneuropathy with prominent demyelination and features of axonal degeneration.

2.8.4 Cerebrospinal Fluid Examination

Protein levels in the cerebrospinal fluid are increased in virtually all patients with POEMS syndrome (Dispenzieri et al. 2003). Over one-half of our patients have a protein value of more than 100 mg/dL. The cell count is almost always normal. Plasma cells are not present in the cerebrospinal fluid.

In a study of patients with primary amyloid neuropathy, increased concentration of protein in cerebrospinal fluid was noted in 3 of 9 patients who underwent the procedure (Rajkumar et al. 1998).

2.8.5 Pathologic Findings

2.8.5.1 MGUS Neuropathy

Histopathologic studies of sural nerves of patients with IgM MGUS neuropathy have demonstrated segmental demyelination with remyelination and axonal degeneration on teased-fiber preparations (Kyle and Dyck 1993 b). There was a reduction in the number of myelinated fi-

bers on semithin sections without evidence of significant inflammatory infiltrates, vasculitis, or amyloid deposits. Electron micrographs showed a typical widening of the outer myelin lamella. This feature is found in the majority of patients with anti-MAG antibodies.

2.8.5.2 Primary Amyloid Neuropathy

When histologic evidence of primary systemic amyloidosis has already been established by fat aspirate, bone marrow examination, or biopsy of other involved organs, it is usually not necessary to subject the patient to a sural nerve biopsy unless the findings are atypical. However, at times biopsy of the sural nerve is required to make the diagnosis. Histologic examination reveals Congo red-positive amyloid deposits surrounding the endoneurial capillaries or in the epineurium. Other findings include a marked decrease in myelin fiber density and axonal degeneration on examination of teased fibers (Rajkumar et al. 1998).

2.8.5.3 POEMS Syndrome

Biopsy of the sural nerve usually shows axonal degeneration and demyelination (Kyle and Dyck 1993 c). Findings include a polymorphous and mononuclear cell infiltration around the epineurium, usually in a perivascular location; a decrease in number of myelinated axons of all sizes with segmental demyelination and remyelination; and an active demyelination process in spinal roots. Severe endoneurial edema may also be seen, and uncompacted myelin lamellae are observed frequently. In most cases, monoclonal immunoglobulin is not associated with the nerve specimens. Amyloid deposits are also not found.

2.9 Differential Diagnosis

Table 2.2 summarizes the clinical features of and differences among MGUS neuropathy, POEMS syndrome, and primary amyloid neuropathy. MGUS neuropathy must be distinguished from inherited neuropathies and acquired neuropathies such as chronic inflammatory demyelinating polyneuropathy (CIDP), amyloidosis, osteosclerotic myeloma (POEMS syndrome) and multiple myeloma, T-cell and B-cell lymphomatosis involvement, paraneoplastic neuropathies, and metabolic and toxic neuropathies.

Table 2.2. Clinical features and differential diagnosis of plasma cell disorders

Feature	MGUS	Multiple myeloma	Primary amyloidosis	POEMS syndrome
Symptoms	Asymptomatic	Bone pain, fatigue, infections	Edema, fatigue, paresthesias	Paresthesias
Peripheral neuropathy	Present in 3–5%	Rare	15–20%	100%
Bone marrow plasma cells	<10%	>10%	<20%	<10%
Hemoglobin	Normal	<12 g/dL in 65%	Normal	Normal or increased
Serum creatinine	Normal	>2 mg/dL in 20%	>2 mg/dL in 20%	Normal
Nephrotic syndrome	No	No	Present in 30%	No
Skeletal radiographs	Normal	Lytic lesions or fracture	Normal	Sclerotic
Diagnosis	M protein <3 g/dL, BMPC <10%, AND no other features of myeloma	BMPC ≥10%, M protein in serum or urine in 97% of patients, AND lytic lesions, renal failure, anemia, or hypercalcemia*	Positive amyloid in tissue stain AND evidence of monoclonal plasma cell proliferative disorder (M protein, monoclonal plasma cells in bone marrow, or positive staining of amyloid tissue for light chains)	Biopsy of sclerotic lesion reveals monoclonal plasma cells

BMPC, bone marrow plasma cells; MGUS, monoclonal gammopathy of undetermined significance.

* Patients who have ≥10% bone marrow plasma cells or M protein ≥3 g/dL but no evidence of lytic lesions, anemia, renal failure, or hypercalcemia are considered to have smoldering (asymptomatic) myeloma.

CIDP may occur at any age. In a comparison of 45 patients with CIDP and 15 with MGUS-associated neuropathy, the latter had less severe weakness; greater imbalance, ataxia, and vibration loss in the hands; and absent median and ulnar sensory potentials (Gorson et al. 1997). In another study, the clinical course was progressive in most patients with MGUS, whereas those with CIDP were more likely to have a relapsing course. Impairment appeared to develop more slowly in the MGUS patients, and they also had less severe functional impairment and a lesser degree of weakness and sensory changes (Simmons et al. 1995). In contrast, Maisonobe et al. (1996) noted no significant clinical or electrophysiologic differences between patients with CIDP and those with CIDP and a monoclonal gammopathy. They reported that patients with anti-MAG antibody had more pronounced slowing of the peroneal motor nerve conduction velocity, a lower frequency of conduction block, and a distal accentuation of conduction slowing. In CIDP, motor symptoms dominate sensory symptoms and there is a greater tendency for the course to be relapsing.

MGUS neuropathy differs from primary amyloid neuropathy in that the lower limbs are preferentially affected in MGUS neuropathy, whereas upper and lower limbs tend to be affected in amyloidosis. In addition, the course of neuropathy in amyloidosis is slowly progressive compared to MGUS neuropathy, which may remain stable for long periods. Finally, autonomic features (postural hypotension, sphincter dysfunction, and anhidrosis) and organ (heart or kidney) failure are seen often in primary amyloidosis but are rare in MGUS neuropathy.

Primary amyloid neuropathy must be differentiated from familial amyloid polyneuropathy, which is an autosomal dominant, inherited multisystem disorder that is characterized by a progressive peripheral neuropathy and autonomic neuropathy. The most common variety is type 1. This is of Portuguese origin, and the amyloid protein is a mutated form of TTR (TTR MET 30), in which methionine is substituted for valine at position 30 of the *TTR* gene. TTR is produced mainly by the liver and in small amounts by the choroid plexus. Symptoms of familial amyloid neuropathy usually start in the 3rd or 4th decade of life, and patients usually die within 10 to 15 years. The major therapeutic option is liver transplantation, which stops the production of TTR MET 30.

POEMS syndrome should be differentiated from MGUS neuropathy. Not all 5 components are required for the diagnosis of POEMS syndrome. When MGUS neuropathy is associated with features such as sclerotic bone lesions, Castleman disease, papilledema, pleural effusion, edema, ascites, and thrombocytosis (Dispenzieri et al. 2003), the possibility of POEMS must be considered. Minimal criteria for diagnosis include a sensorimotor peripheral neuropathy, evidence of a monoclonal plasma cell proliferative disorder, and at least one other paraneoplastic feature.

POEMS syndrome should also be differentiated from multiple myeloma. Patients with POEMS syndrome are at least a decade younger than those with multiple myeloma. Patients with multiple myeloma often present with bone pain, weakness, or fatigue, whereas peripheral neuropathy is a cardinal feature of osteosclerotic myeloma. In contrast, peripheral neuropathy is rarely seen in multiple myeloma and, when it does occur, it is usually due to amyloidosis. The infrequency of anemia, hypercalcemia, renal insufficiency, and bone pain; the rarity of fractures; the low values of M protein in the serum and urine; and the small number of plasma cells in the bone marrow of patients with osteosclerotic myeloma (POEMS syndrome) differentiate them. In addition, the clinical features of POEMS syndrome such as sensorimotor peripheral neuropathy, osteosclerotic bone lesions, endocrine features, hepatosplenomegaly, and skin changes help to distinguish the 2 entities. Unlike myeloma, patients with POEMS syndrome do not develop renal insufficiency or multiple fractures and rarely if ever die of typical multiple myeloma.

2.10   Therapy

2.10.1   MGUS Neuropathy

Treatment of patients with MGUS neuropathy is suboptimal. In general, IgM MGUS neuropathy is less responsive to treatment than the non-IgM MGUS group. Plasma exchange has been tried with mixed results. Plasma exchange produced improvement of neuropathy in 6 of 10 patients with polyneuropathy and a monoclonal gammopathy. Three others had stabilization of their neuropathy. With cessation of plasma exchange, the neuropathy progressed (Sherman et al. 1984). In a randomized trial, 39 patients with MGUS neuropathy were assigned to receive either plasma exchange twice weekly or sham plasma exchange in a double-blind fashion. Patients who initially underwent sham plasma exchange subsequently underwent plasma exchange in an open trial. The average neuropathy disability score improved by 2 points in the sham exchange group and by 12 points in the plasma exchange group. In the open trial in which patients who initially underwent sham exchange were treated with plasma exchange, the neuropathy disability score, weakness score, and summed compound muscle action potentials improved more with plasma exchange than with sham exchange. In both the double-blind and open trials, patients who had IgG or IgA gammopathy responded better to plasma exchange than those with IgM gammopathy (Dyck et al. 1991). In another study, 8 of 13 patients with monoclonal gammopathy and peripheral neuropathy benefited from plasma exchange (Mazzi et al. 1999).

A second option for therapy is the use of alkylating agents. In a study of 16 patients with monoclonal gammopathy (IgM 11 patients, IgG 5 patients) and sensorimotor peripheral neuropathy, the use of cyclophosphamide plus prednisone produced improvement in 8 and stabilization of the neuropathy in 6 others (Notermans et al. 1996). We have used chlorambucil for patients with IgM monoclonal gammopathy and melphalan for those with IgG and IgA monoclonal gammopathies and peripheral neuropathy. Some of these patients have had gratifying responses to therapy. Kelly et al. (1988) reported that 9 of 10 patients with peripheral neuropathy and an IgM M protein responded to prednisone, cyclophosphamide, chlorambucil, azathioprine, or plasmapheresis. In another study, chlorambucil alone was compared with chlorambucil in combination with plasma exchange in patients with IgM monoclonal polyneuropathy. Forty-four patients were randomized prospectively in this comparative trial. At the end of the study 15 patients, 8 from the chlorambucil group and 7 from the chlorambucil plus plasma exchange group, reported clinical improvement. A similar number reported clinical worsening. In this study, no advantage was observed with the addition of plasma exchange to chlorambucil therapy in IgM polyneuropathy (Oksenhendler et al. 1995). In patients with IgM polyneuropathy in association with chronic lymphocytic leukemia or Waldenström macroglobulinemia, treatment of the malignancy often decreases the number of anti-MAG–secreting malignant cells. But most patients do not respond in terms of neuropathy.

The use of intravenous gamma globulin (IVIG) has been beneficial in some patients with CIDP but has been disappointing for patients with peripheral neuropathy associated with a monoclonal gammopathy. A randomized study of 11 patients in which IVIG was compared with placebo, followed by a crossover, revealed improved strength in 2 patients and improved sensory neuropathy in 1 other. Antibody titers to MAG or gangliosides did not change. Thus, less than 20% had any benefit (Dalakas et al. 1996). The mechanism of IVIG in the treatment of IgM monoclonal neuropathy is unclear. Anti-idiotypic antibodies contained in the IVIG may neutralize anti-MAG antibodies. IVIG may also contain antibodies against the CD5-bearing subset of B cells that produce the anti-MAG antibody. Theoretically, it may also down-regulate anti-MAG antibody production.

Mariette and colleagues (1997) conducted a randomized, multicenter clinical trial that compared interferon-α and IVIG in polyneuropathy associated with IgM monoclonal neuropathy. Interferon-α was administered at 3 million units/m^2 subcutaneously 3 times per week. IVIG was administered at a dose of 2.0 g/kg and then 1.0 g/kg every 3 weeks. Twenty patients were studied. Interferon-α was effective in decreasing the clinical neuropathy disability score in 8 of 10 patients at 6 months. In contrast, IVIG did not improve symptoms of IgM polyneuropathy. Nevertheless, at the end of treatment all patients continued to have anti-MAG antibody in their sera.

Newer options for therapy include the use of purine nucleoside analogs and rituximab, but data are limited. Fludarabine, a purine analog, produced clinical and neurophysiologic improvement in 3 of 4 patients with an IgM M protein and peripheral neuropathy (Wilson et al. 1999). In addition, another study reported that 7 of 10 patients with an IgM M protein and neuropathy responded to fludarabine. Rituximab produced improvement in all 5 patients with neuropathy and IgM antibody to MAG or GM1 ganglioside. All 5 patients had been treated successfully with plasma exchange and cyclophosphamide but had relapsed (Levine and Pestronk 1999).

2.10.2 Primary Amyloid Neuropathy

No therapy seems to greatly improve neuropathy. Chemotherapy may have benefit. In one study, patients receiving chemotherapy seemed to have significantly better survival than those receiving other forms of therapy or no treatment (median survival, 38 vs. 18.5 months) (Rajkumar et al. 1998). Chemotherapy consisted of melphalan and prednisone in 15 patients (melphalan 0.15 mg/kg days 1–7 and prednisone 60 mg days 1–7, repeated every 6 weeks) and 1 patient received vincristine, BCNU, melphalan, cyclophosphamide, and prednisone (VBMCP). Ten of 16 patients (63%) who received chemotherapy had a decrease in their M protein value, but only 2 patients had stabilization of neuropathy. The median duration of chemotherapy was 15 months (range, 1–36 months).

Agents such as colchicine, tocopherol, and interferon-α have not shown benefit. The role of autologous stem cell transplantation for eligible candidates remains to be determined. Because the best treatment for this group of patients, similar to other patients with primary amyloidosis, is yet to be determined, we recommend continued enrollment of these patients in clinical trials.

2.10.3 POEMS Syndrome

Single or multiple osteosclerotic lesions in a limited area can be treated with radiation in a tumoricidal dosage of 40 to 50 cGy. More than half of patients show substantial improvement of the neuropathy (Dispenzieri et al. 2003). This improvement may be slow and not apparent for the first 6 months. Patients can continue to improve for 2 to 3 years after radiation therapy. Response of systemic symptoms and skin changes tend to precede those of the neuropathy, with the former beginning to respond within a month and the latter within 3 to 6 months.

In addition to radiation, a multitude of strategies have been used, including plasmapheresis, IVIG, interferon-a, corticosteroids, alkylators, azathioprine, autologous stem cell transplantation, tamoxifen, and transretinoic acid. Because slow responders are not uncommon, systemic therapies should be reserved for only those patients who demonstrate progression after radiation therapy. If the patient has widespread osteosclerotic lesions, systemic therapy is necessary. Kuwabara et al. (1997) reported that 5 of 6 patients treated with melphalan and prednisone showed various degrees of improvement of their neuropathy and other symptoms. The schedule we use is melphalan (0.15 mg/kg daily) plus prednisone (20 mg 3 times daily) for 7 days every 6 weeks. The leukocyte and platelet counts should be determined every 3 weeks, and the dosage of melphalan altered so that there is some cytopenia at midcycle. We usually treat patients for 1 year and then discontinue treatment if they are stable. There is some risk of myelodysplasia or acute leukemia with continued therapy. Others have also noted benefit from melphalan and prednisone (Donofrio et al. 1984; Parra et al. 1987).

Autologous stem cell transplantation after high-dose melphalan is a consideration for younger patients with widespread osteosclerotic lesions. The mortality from the procedure is currently only 2%. We and others have had success in performing autologous stem cell transplantation in small groups of patients (Dispenzieri et al. 2001; Hogan et al. 2001; Jaccard et al. 2002; Rovira et al. 2001). For patients being considered for this approach, stem cells should be collected before the patient is exposed to alkylating agents.

Although corticosteroids may occasionally produce a response, they are generally ineffective in the long run (Tobin and Fitzgerald 1982). From our experience and review of the literature, plasmapheresis is also not considered an effective treatment of this disorder (Silberstein et al. 1985). IVIG also cannot be recommended for the same reason.

2.11   Prognosis

2.11.1   Primary Amyloid Neuropathy

Rajkumar and colleagues (1998) studied patients with primary amyloidosis and neuropathy as the dominant manifestation. In general, neuropathy was chronic and showed relentless progression. The median survival

was 25 months. On multivariate analysis, serum albumin was a predictor of survival as a continuous variable and as a discrete variable. Survival was significantly better in patients with a serum albumin concentration greater than 3 g/dL (median, 31 months) than in those with a serum albumin value less than 3 g/dL (median, 18 months).

Duston and colleagues (1989) reported a median survival of 35 months and a 3-year survival rate of 50% in patients with amyloid neuropathy. Previous studies of amyloid neuropathy from Mayo Clinic indicated a median survival of approximately 30 months and a 5-year survival rate of approximately 25% (Kyle and Dyck 1993 a, b; Rajkumar et al. 1998). These reports suggested that patients with amyloid neuropathy have a better prognosis than others with primary amyloidosis. The median survival of patients who have primary amyloidosis with dominant neuropathy (25–30 months) is better than survival of patients who have primary amyloidosis with dominant cardiomyopathy (6 months), hepatic amyloid (11 months), or nephrotic syndrome (17 months) (Rajkumar et al. 1998).

Studies are ongoing to determine the role of autologous stem cell transplantation for patients with primary systemic amyloidosis (Comenzo and Gertz 2002).

2.11.2   POEMS Syndrome

The prognosis of patients who have POEMS was considered initially to be poor, with estimated median survivals of 12 to 33 months. However, more recent data indicate that the disease runs a chronic course, and the median survival in a large Mayo Clinic study was 13.8 years (Dispenzieri et al. 2003). In a French study, at least 7 of 15 patients were alive for more than 5 years, with the longest survivor alive at 25 years. Survival does not seem to be affected by the number of POEMS features. In the Mayo Clinic series of 99 patients, 35 died during follow-up (Dispenzieri et al. 2003). Even those patients with multiple bone lesions or those with more than 10% plasma cells do not progress to classic multiple myeloma.

The cause of death in POEMS syndrome is not the excessive proliferation of plasma cells and a large tumor mass. The natural history is one of progressive peripheral neuropathy until the patient is bedridden. Death usually results from inanition or a terminal bronchopneumonia. Progressive capillary leak – effusions, ascites, and resultant renal failure – may also contribute to a patient's death. Stroke and myocardial infarction, which may or may not be related to the POEMS syndrome, are also observed causes of death.

References

Bardwick PA, Zvaifler NJ, Gill GN, Newman D, Greenway GD, Resnick DL (1980) Plasma cell dyscrasia with polyneuropathy, organomegaly, endocrinopathy, M protein, and skin changes: the POEMS syndrome: report on two cases and a review of the literature. Medicine (Baltimore) 59:311–322

Bélec L, Mohamed AS, Authier FJ, Hallouin MC, Soe AM, Cotigny S, Gaulard P, Gherardi RK (1999) Human herpesvirus 8 infection in patients with POEMS syndrome-associated multicentric Castleman's disease. Blood 93:3643–3653

Besinger UA, Toyka KV, Anzil AP, Fateh-Mognadam A, Rouscher R, Heininger K (1981) Myeloma neuropathy: passive transfer from man to mouse. Science 213:1027–1030

Borges LF, Busis NA (1985) Intraneuronal accumulation of myeloma proteins. Arch Neurol 42:690–694

Bosch EP, Ansbacher LE, Goeken JA, Cancilla PA (1982) Peripheral neuropathy associated with monoclonal gammopathy: studies of intraneural injections of monoclonal immunoglobulin sera. J Neuropathol Exp Neurol 41:446–459

Busis NA, Halperin JJ, Stefansson K, Kwiatkowski DJ, Sagar SM, Schiff SR, Logigian EL (1985) Peripheral neuropathy, high serum IgM, and paraproteinemia in mother and son. Neurology 35:679–683

Chassande B, Leger JM, Younes-Chennoufi AB, Bengoufa D, Maisonobe T, Bouche P, Baumann N (1998) Peripheral neuropathy associated with IgM monoclonal gammopathy: correlations between M-protein antibody activity and clinical/electrophysiological features in 40 cases. Muscle Nerve 21:55–62

Comenzo RL, Gertz MA (2002) Autologous stem cell transplantation for primary systemic amyloidosis. Blood 99:4276–4282

Dalakas MC, Flaum MA, Rick M, Engel WK, Gralnick HR (1983) Treatment of polyneuropathy in Waldenström's macroglobulinemia: role of paraproteinemia and immunologic studies. Neurology 33:1406–1410

Dalakas MC, Quarles RH, Farrer RG, Dambrosia J, Soueidan S, Stein DP, Cupler E, Sekul EA, Otero C (1996) A controlled study of intravenous immunoglobulin in demyelinating neuropathy with IgM gammopathy. Ann Neurol 40:792–795

Davidson S (1972) Solitary myeloma with peripheral polyneuropathy – recovery after treatment. Calif Med 116:68–71

Davison C, Balser BH (1937) Myeloma and its neural complications. Arch Surg 35:913–936

Delauche MC, Clauvel JP, Seligmann M (1981) Peripheral neuropathy and plasma cell neoplasias: a report of 10 cases. Br J Haematol 48:383–392

Dellagi K, Dupouey P, Brouet JC, Billecocq A, Gomez D, Clauvel JP, Seligmann M (1983) Waldenström's macroglobulinemia and peripheral neuropathy: a clinical and immunologic study of 25 patients. Blood 62:280–285

Dispenzieri A, Lacy MQ, Litzow MR, Tefferi A, Inwards DJ, Micallef IN, Gastineau DA, Ansell SM, Rajkumar SV, Fonseca R, Witzig TE, Lust JA, Kyle RA, Greipp PR, Gertz MA (2001) Peripheral blood stem cell transplant (PBSCT) in patients with POEMS syndrome (abstract). Blood 98:391b

Dispenzieri A, Kyle RA, Lacy MQ, Rajkumar SV, Therneau TM, Lars DR, Greipp PR, Witzig TE, Basu R, Suarez GA, Fonseca R, Lust JA, Gertz MA (2003) POEMS syndrome: definitions and long-term outcome. Blood 101:2496–2506

Donofrio PD, Albers JW, Greenberg HS, Mitchell BS (1984) Peripheral neuropathy in osteosclerotic myeloma: clinical and electrodiagnostic improvement with chemotherapy. Muscle Nerve 7:137–141

Duston MA, Skinner M, Anderson J, Cohen AS (1989) Peripheral neuropathy as an early marker of AL amyloidosis. Arch Intern Med 149:358–360

Dyck PJ, Low PA, Windebank AJ, Jaradeh SS, Gosselin S, Bourque P, Smith BE, Kratz KM, Karnes JL, Evans BA, Pineda AA, O'Brien PC, Kyle RA (1991) Plasma exchange in polyneuropathy associated with monoclonal gammopathy of undetermined significance. N Engl J Med 325:1482–1486

Frail DE, Edwards AM, Braun PE (1984) Molecular characteristics of the epitope in myelin-associated glycoprotein that is recognized by a monoclonal IgM in human neuropathy patients. Mol Immunol 21:721–725

Fredman P (1998) The role of antiglycolipid antibodies in neurological disorders. Ann N Y Acad Sci 845:341–352

Gertz MA, Kyle RA (1989) Primary systemic amyloidosis – a diagnostic primer. Mayo Clin Proc 64:1505–1519

Gertz MA, Rajkumar SV (2002) Primary systemic amyloidosis. Curr Treat Options Oncol 3:261–271

Gorson KC, Allam G, Ropper AH (1997) Chronic inflammatory demyelinating polyneuropathy: clinical features and response to treatment in 67 consecutive patients with and without a monoclonal gammopathy. Neurology 48:321–328

Gosselin S, Kyle RA, Dyck PJ (1991) Neuropathy associated with monoclonal gammopathies of undetermined significance. Ann Neurol 30:54–61

Hashiguchi T, Arimura K, Matsumuro K, Otsuka R, Watanabe O, Jonosono M, Maruyama Y, Maruyama I, Osame M (2000) Highly concentrated vascular endothelial growth factor in platelets in Crow-Fukase syndrome. Muscle Nerve 23:1051–1056

Hogan WJ, Lacy MQ, Wiseman GA, Fealey RD, Dispenzieri A, Gertz MA (2001) Successful treatment of POEMS syndrome with autologous hematopoietic progenitor cell transplantation. Bone Marrow Transplant 28:305–309

Ilyas AA, Quarles RH, MacIntosh TD, Dobersen MJ, Trapp BD, Dalakas MC, Brady RO (1984) IgM in a human neuropathy related to paraproteinemia binds to a carbohydrate determinant in the myelin-associated glycoprotein and to a ganglioside. Proc Natl Acad Sci U S A 81:1225–1229

Ilyas AA, Quarles RH, Dalakas MC, Fishman PH, Brady RO (1985) Monoclonal IgM in a patient with paraproteinemic polyneuropathy binds to gangliosides containing disialosyl groups. Ann Neurol 18:655–659

Isobe T, Osserman EF (1971) Pathologic conditions associated with plasma cell dyscrasias: a study of 806 cases. Ann N Y Acad Sci 190:507–518

Jaccard A, Royer B, Bordessoule D, Brouet JC, Fermand JP (2002) High-dose therapy and autologous blood stem cell transplantation in POEMS syndrome. Blood 99:3057–3059

Johansen P, Leegaard OF (1985) Peripheral neuropathy and paraproteinemia: an immunohistochemical and serologic study. Clin Neuropathol 4:99–104

Jønsson V, Schroder HD, Staehelin Jensen T, Nolsoe C, Stigsby B, Trojaborg W, Svejgaard A, Hippe E (1988) Autoimmunity related to IgM monoclonal gammopathy of undetermined significance: peripheral neuropathy and connective tissue sensibilization caused by IgM M-proteins. Acta Med Scand 223:255–261

Kahn SN, Riches PG, Kohn J (1980) Paraproteinaemia in neurological disease: incidence, associations, and classification of monoclonal immunoglobulins. J Clin Pathol 33:617–621

Kelly JJ Jr, Kyle RA, O'Brien PC, Dyck PJ (1979) The natural history of peripheral neuropathy in primary systemic amyloidosis. Ann Neurol 6:1–7

Kelly JJ Jr, Kyle RA, Miles JM, O'Brien PC, Dyck PJ (1981) The spectrum of peripheral neuropathy in myeloma. Neurology 31:24–31

Kelly JJ Jr, Kyle RA, Miles JM, Dyck PJ (1983) Osteosclerotic myeloma and peripheral neuropathy. Neurology 33:202–210

Kelly JJ, Adelman LS, Berkman E, Bhan I (1988) Polyneuropathies associated with IgM monoclonal gammopathies. Arch Neurol 45:1355–1359

Kusunoki S, Kohriyama T, Pachner AR, Latov N, Yu RK (1987) Neuropathy and IgM paraproteinemia: differential binding of IgM M-proteins to peripheral nerve glycolipids. Neurology 37:1795–1797

Kuwabara S, Hattori T, Shimoe Y, Kamitsukasa I (1997) Long term melphalan-prednisolone chemotherapy for POEMS syndrome. J Neurol Neurosurg Psychiatry 63:385–387

Kyle RA, Dyck PJ (1993 a) Amyloidosis and neuropathy. In: Dyck PJ, Thomas PK, Griffin JW, Low PA, Poduslo JF (eds) Peripheral neuropathy, 3rd edn, vol 2. WB Saunders Company, Philadelphia, pp 1294–1309

Kyle RA, Dyck PJ (1993 b) Neuropathy associated with the monoclonal gammopathies. In: Dyck PJ, Thomas PK, Griffin JW, Low PA, Poduslo JF (eds) Peripheral neuropathy, 3rd edn, vol 2. WB Saunders Company, Philadelphia, pp 1275–1287

Kyle RA, Dyck PJ (1993 c) Osteosclerotic myeloma (POEMS syndrome). In: Dyck PJ, Thomas PK, Griffin JW, Low PA, Poduslo JF (eds) Peripheral neuropathy, 3rd edn, vol 2. WB Saunders Company, Philadelphia, pp 1288–1293

Kyle RA, Greipp PR, O'Fallon WM (1986) Primary systemic amyloidosis: multivariate analysis for prognostic factors in 168 cases. Blood 68:220–224

Kyle RA, Eilers SG, Linscheid RL, Gaffey TA (1989) Amyloid localized to tenosynovium at carpal tunnel release: natural history of 124 cases. Am J Clin Pathol 91:393–397

Kyle RA, Therneau TM, Rajkumar SV, Offord JR, Larson DR, Plevak MF, Melton LJ III (2002) A long-term study of prognosis in monoclonal gammopathy of undetermined significance. N Engl J Med 346:564–569

Latov N, Sherman WH, Nemni R, Galassi G, Shyong JS, Penn AS, Chess L, Olarte MR, Rowland LP, Osserman EF (1980) Plasma-cell dyscrasia and peripheral neuropathy with a monoclonal antibody to peripheral-nerve myelin. N Engl J Med 303:618–621

Latov N, Hays AP, Sherman WH (1988) Peripheral neuropathy and anti-MAG antibodies. Crit Rev Neurobiol 3:301–332

Levine TD, Pestronk A (1999) IgM antibody-related polyneuropathies: B-cell depletion chemotherapy using Rituximab. Neurology 52:1701–1704

Maisonobe T, Chassande B, Verin M, Jouni M, Leger JM, Bouche P (1996) Chronic dysimmune demyelinating polyneuropathy: a clinical and electrophysiological study of 93 patients. J Neurol Neurosurg Psychiatry 61:36–42

Mariette X, Chastang C, Clavelou P, Louboutin JP, Leger JM, Brouet JC (1997) A randomised clinical trial comparing interferon-alpha and intravenous immunoglobulin in polyneuropathy associated with monoclonal IgM. The IgM-associated Polyneuropathy Study Group. J Neurol Neurosurg Psychiatry 63:28–34

Mazzi G, Raineri A, Zucco M, Passadore P, Pomes A, Orazi BM (1999) Plasma-exchange in chronic peripheral neurological disorders. Int J Artif Organs 22:40–46

Meucci N, Baldini L, Cappellari A, Di Troia A, Allaria S, Scarlato G, Nobile-Orazio E (1999) Anti-myelin-associated glycoprotein antibodies predict the development of neuropathy in asymptomatic patients with IgM monoclonal gammopathy. Ann Neurol 46:119–122

Monaco S, Ferrari S, Bonetti B, Moretto G, Kirshfink M, Nardelli E, Nobile-Orazio E, Zanusso G, Rizzuto N, Tedesco F (1995) Experimental induction of myelin changes by anti-MAG antibodies and terminal complement complex. J Neuropathol Exp Neurol 54:96–104

Nobile-Orazio E, Hays AP, Latov N, Perman G, Golier J, Shy ME, Freddo L (1984) Specificity of mouse and human monoclonal antibodies to myelin-associated glycoprotein. Neurology 34:1336–1342

Nobile-Orazio E, Francomano E, Daverio R, Barbieri S, Marmiroli P, Manfredini E, Carpo M, Moggio M, Legname G, Baldini L, Scarlato G (1989) Anti-myelin-associated glycoprotein IgM antibody titers in neuropathy associated with macroglobulinemia. Ann Neurol 26:543–550

Notermans NC, Lokhorst HM, Franssen H, Van der Graaf Y, Teunissen LL, Jennekens FG, Van den Berg LH, Wokke JH (1996) Intermittent cyclophosphamide and prednisone treatment of polyneuropathy associated with monoclonal gammopathy of undetermined significance. Neurology 47:1227–1233

Oksenhendler E, Chevret S, Leger JM, Louboutin JP, Bussel A, Brouet JC (1995) Plasma exchange and chlorambucil in polyneuropathy associated with monoclonal IgM gammopathy. IgM-associated Polyneuropathy Study Group. J Neurol Neurosurg Psychiatry 59:243–247

Parra R, Fernandez JM, Garcia-Bragado F, Bueno J, Biosca M (1987) Successful treatment of peripheral neuropathy with chemotherapy in osteosclerotic myeloma. J Neurol 234:261–263

Quarles RH, Weiss MD (1999) Autoantibodies associated with peripheral neuropathy. Muscle Nerve 22:800–822

Rajkumar SV, Gertz MA, Kyle RA (1998) Prognosis of patients with primary systemic amyloidosis who present with dominant neuropathy. Am J Med 104:232–237

Read D, Warlow C (1978) Peripheral neuropathy and solitary plasmacytoma. J Neurol Neurosurg Psychiatry 41:177–184

Rovira M, Carreras E, Bladé J, Graus F, Valls J, Fernandez-Aviles F, Montserrat E (2001) Dramatic improvement of POEMS syndrome following autologous haematopoietic cell transplantation. Br J Haematol 115:373–375

Sherman WH, Latov N, Hays AP, Takatsu M, Nemni R, Galassi G, Osserman EF (1983) Monoclonal IgM kappa antibody precipitating with chondroitin sulfate C from patients with axonal polyneuropathy and epidermolysis. Neurology 33:192–201

Sherman WH, Olarte MR, McKiernan G, Sweeney K, Latov N, Hays AP (1984) Plasma exchange treatment of peripheral neuropathy associated with plasma cell dyscrasia. J Neurol Neurosurg Psychiatry 47:813–819

Shy ME, Vietorisz T, Nobile-Orazio E, Latov N (1984) Specificity of human IgM M-proteins that bind to myelin-associated glycoprotein: peptide mapping, deglycosylation, and competitive binding studies. J Immunol 133:2509–2512

Silberstein LE, Duggan D, Berkman EM (1985) Therapeutic trial of plasma exchange in osteosclerotic myeloma associated with the POEMS syndrome. J Clin Apheresis 2:253–257

Silverstein A, Doniger DE (1963) Neurologic complications of myelomatosis. Arch Neurol 147:534–544

Simmons Z, Albers JW, Bromberg MB, Feldman EL (1995) Long-term follow-up of patients with chronic inflammatory demyelinating polyradiculoneuropathy, without and with monoclonal gammopathy. Brain 118:359–368

Simovic D, Gorson KC, Ropper AH (1998) Comparison of IgM-MGUS and IgG-MGUS polyneuropathy. Acta Neurol Scand 97:194–200

Smith IS, Kahn SN, Lacey BW, King RH, Eames RA, Whybrew DJ, Thomas PK (1983) Chronic demyelinating neuropathy associated with benign IgM paraproteinaemia. Brain 106:169–195

Soubrier M, Sauron C, Souweine B, Larroche C, Wechsler B, Guillevin L, Piette JC, Rousset H, Deteix P (1999) Growth factors and proinflammatory cytokines in the renal involvement of POEMS syndrome. Am J Kidney Dis 34:633–638

Steck AJ, Murray N, Meier C, Page N, Perruisseau G (1983) Demyelinating neuropathy and monoclonal IgM antibody to myelin-associated glycoprotein. Neurology 33:19–23

Suarez GA, Kelly JJ Jr (1993) Polyneuropathy associated with monoclonal gammopathy of undetermined significance: further evidence that IgM-MGUS neuropathies are different than IgG-MGUS. Neurology 43:1304–1308

Tatum AH (1993) Experimental paraprotein neuropathy, demyelination by passive transfer of human IgM anti-myelin-associated glycoprotein. Ann Neurol 33:502–506

Tobin MJ, Fitzgerald MX (1982) The Japanese plasma cell dyscrasia syndrome: case report and theory of pathogenesis. Postgrad Med J 58:786–789

Walsh JC (1971) The neuropathy of multiple myeloma. An electrophysiological and histological study. Arch Neurol 25:404–414

Wilson HC, Lunn MP, Schey S, Hughes RA (1999) Successful treatment of IgM paraproteinaemic neuropathy with fludarabine. J Neurol Neurosurg Psychiatry 66:575–580

Wolfe GI, Nations SP (2001) Guide to autoantibody testing in peripheral neuropathies. Neurologist 7:195–207

Yee WC, Hahn AF, Hearn SA, Rupar AR (1989) Neuropathy in IgM lambda paraproteinemia. Immunoreactivity to neural proteins and chondroitin sulfate. Acta Neuropathol 78:57–64

Multiple Myeloma

Angela Dispenzieri, M.D., Martha Q. Lacy, M.D., Philip R. Greipp, M.D.*

Contents

3.1 Introduction 54

3.2 History 55
   3.2.1 The Earliest Diagnoses
      and Diagnostic Methods 55
   3.2.2 The Earliest Treatments
      for Multiple Myeloma 55

3.3 Incidence and Epidemiology 56
   3.3.1 Epidemiology of Myeloma 56
   3.3.2 Etiologic Factors 57
      3.3.2.1 Radiation Exposures 57
      3.2.2.2 Workplace Exposures ... 57
      3.3.2.3 Lifestyle Factors 57
      3.3.2.4 Precursor Medical
         Conditions 57

3.4 Pathogenesis and Pathophysiology ... 57
   3.4.1 Cytokines and Cell Signaling 58
   3.4.2 Bone Marrow Microenvironment .. 59
   3.4.3 Cell Cycle 59

3.5 Clinical Manifestations 59
   3.5.1 Anemia 60
   3.5.2 Monoclonal Proteins 60
   3.5.3 Bone Disease 60
   3.5.4 Hypercalcemia 61
   3.5.5 Renal Insufficiency 61
   3.5.6 Infection 63
   3.5.7 Bone Marrow Pathologic Features . 63
   3.5.8 Hemostasis in Myeloma 64

3.5.9 "Acute Terminal Phase of Plasma Cell
      Myeloma" and Cause
      of Death 65
3.5.10 Special Cases of Myeloma 65
      3.5.10.1 Nonsecretory Multiple
         Myeloma 65
      3.5.10.2 Immunoglobulin D
         Myeloma 65
      3.5.10.3 Immunoglobulin E
         Myeloma 66

3.6 Diagnosis 66

3.7 Differential Diagnosis 67
   3.7.1 Reactive Plasmacytosis and Poly-
      clonal Hypergammaglobulinemia . 67
   3.7.2 MGUS 68
   3.7.3 Primary Systemic Amyloidosis ... 68
   3.7.4 Waldenström Macroglobulinemia . 68
   3.7.5 Light Chain Deposition Disease .. 68
   3.7.6 Acquired Fanconi Syndrome 69
   3.7.7 POEMS Syndrome
      (Osteosclerotic Myeloma) 69

3.8 Treatment for Multiple Myeloma 70
   3.8.1 Systemic Therapy 70
      3.8.1.1 General Comments 70
      3.8.1.2 Interpreting Study
         Response and Survival
         Data 71
      3.8.1.3 Efficacy of Single
         Chemotherapeutic
         Agents 74
      3.8.1.4 Induction Chemotherapy
         Regimens 77

* This work was supported in part by grant CA 91561-01.

3.8.2   Hematopoietic Stem Cell
         Transplantation   84
         3.8.2.1   Autologous Transplant . .   84
         3.8.2.2   Allogeneic Transplant . . .   87
         3.8.2.3   Donor Lymphocyte
                    Infusions   88
         3.8.2.4   Nonmyeloablative
                    Allogeneic Transplant . . .   88
3.8.3   Radiation   95
3.8.4   Sequential Half-body (Hemibody)
         Irradiation   95

3.9   **Staging and Prognosis**   96
3.9.1   Individual Prognostic Markers With
         Standard Intensity Chemotherapy   97
         3.9.1.1 β_2-Microglobulin   97
         3.9.1.2   C-reactive Protein   97
         3.9.1.3   Lactate Dehydrogenase .   97
         3.9.1.4   Bone Marrow Plasma
                    Cell Number and
                    Morphology   97
         3.9.1.5   Plasma Cell Labeling
                    Index   99
         3.9.1.6   Cytogenetics, Fluorescence
                    In Situ Hybridization,
                    and Other Genetic
                    Abnormalities   99
         3.9.1.7   Angiogenesis   100
         3.9.1.8   Lymphocyte Subsets . . .   100
         3.9.1.9   Other Prognostic Factors   101

3.9.1.10 Drug Resistance   101
3.9.2   Significance of the Extent
         of Response After Therapy   101
         3.9.2.1   Significance of Response
                    After Standard Intensity
                    Chemotherapy   101
         3.9.2.2   Significance of a Complete
                    Response After High-Dose
                    Therapy   101
3.9.3   New Staging Systems   102

3.10 **Treatment of Complications
      and Supportive Care**   102
3.10.1 Treatment of Myeloma Bone
        Disease   102
3.10.2 Spinal Cord Compression   103
3.10.3 Hypercalcemia   103
3.10.4 Hematologic Complications
        Including Anemia, Secondary
        Leukemia, Hyperviscosity,
        and Cryoglobulinemia   104
        3.10.4.1 Anemia   104
        3.10.4.2 Secondary Myelodysplasia
                  and Acute Leukemia   104
        3.10.4.3 Cryoglobulinemia   104
        3.10.4.4 Hyperviscosity   104
3.10.5 Renal Failure   104
3.10.6 Infection Management   105

References   105

3.1   Introduction

Multiple myeloma is a neoplastic plasma cell dyscrasia (PCD) characterized by a clinical pentad: 1) anemia, 2) a monoclonal protein in the serum or urine or both, 3) abnormal bone radiographs and bone pain, 4) hypercalcemia, and 5) renal insufficiency or failure. With the exception of monoclonal gammopathy of undetermined significance (MGUS), it is the most common PCD, with an incidence of about 4.5 per 100,000 per year in the United States. Solitary plasmacytoma and plasma cell leukemia (PCL) are recognized as separate entities and are much less prevalent. The underlying pathogenesis of the plasma cell malignancies is not well understood but is an area of active investigation. At present, according to WHO (World Health Organization) and REAL (Revised European-American Lymphoma) classification systems, there is only 1 category for multiple myeloma. Results of clinical trials are confounded by this underclassification. Emerging information about the disease, however, will likely change this underclassification.

The interactions among the plasma cells, their antibody product, the local bone and bone marrow environment, and other organs are complex. There is no cure for multiple myeloma, but there are many effective treatments that prolong and improve the quality of life in patients with the disease.

3.2 History

3.2.1 The Earliest Diagnoses and Diagnostic Methods

Samuel Solley reported the first well-documented case of myeloma in Sarah Newbury in 1844 (mollities ossium) (Kyle 2000). Several years later, William MacIntyre described and recorded the properties of the disease we now call multiple myeloma in Thomas Alexander McBean. Both Drs. MacIntyre and Bence Jones noted and described some of the peculiar urine properties of this same patient. On heating, the urine was found to "abound in animal matter," which dissolved on the addition of nitric acid but reappeared after cooling. These urinary proteins became known as Bence Jones proteins. MacIntyre and Dalrymple described the postmortem examination of Mr. McBean's bones. The former described the affected bones as softened and fragile, with their interiors replaced with a soft "gelatinform" blood-red substance. Dalrymple suggested that the disease began in the cancellous bone and extended through the periosteum. The nucleated cells, which formed the bulk of the gelatinous material, were heterogeneous in size and shape, but the majority were round to oval. Many of the larger and more irregular cells frequently contained 2 and often 3 nuclei. The term "multiple myeloma" was coined in 1873 by von Rustizky who independently described a similar patient to emphasize the multiple bone tumors that were present.

In 1889, Professor Otto Kahler described a case involving a 46-year-old physician with multiple myeloma and executed a major review of the disease. He described the skeletal pain, albuminuria, pallor, anemia, a precipitable urinary protein, and the findings on necroscopy and linked these findings as part of a clinical syndrome, which bears his name (multiple myeloma is also known as Kahler disease).

In 1898 Weber postulated that bone marrow was the site of production of the Bence Jones protein. Wright emphasized that multiple myeloma arose specifically from plasma cells of the marrow in 1933. In 1917 and 1921, respectively, Jacobson and Walters recognized Bence Jones proteins in the bloodstream and concluded that the Bence Jones protein was probably derived from blood proteins through the action of the abnormal cells in the bone marrow.

In 1922 Bayne-Jones and Wilson identified 2 similar but distinct groups of Bence Jones proteins by immuniz-ing rabbits with Bence Jones proteins from patients. Using the Ouchterlony test, Korngold and Lipari showed that antisera to Bence Jones protein also reacted with myeloma proteins. The 2 classes of Bence Jones proteins have been designated kappa and lambda as a tribute to these 2 men. In 1962, Edelman and Gally showed that the light chains prepared from an IgG monoclonal protein and the Bence Jones protein from the same patient's urine were identical. Longsworth et al. applied electrophoresis to the study of multiple myeloma and described the tall narrow-based "church spire" peak. Paper electrophoresis was supplanted by filter paper in 1957. Most recently, high-resolution electrophoresis on agarose gel is used in most laboratories. Immunoelectrophoresis and immunofixation or direct immunoelectrophoresis make it possible to detect small monoclonal light chains not recognizable on electrophoresis.

In 1928, Geschickter and Copeland reported on the largest case series of multiple myeloma – 13 cases – and reviewed the 412 cases reported in the literature since 1848. They documented a higher incidence in men than women and an overall survival of about 2 years. They emphasized 6 features: 1) involvement by the tumor of the skeletal trunk, 2) pathologic fractures of the ribs, 3) Bence Jones proteinuria in 65% of cases, 4) backache with early paraplegia, 5) anemia in 77% of cases, and 6) chronic renal disease. They did not note abnormalities of blood protein or increased erythrocyte sedimentation rate (Kyle 2000). In 1931, Magnus-Levy described amyloidosis as a complication of multiple myeloma. Salmon, Durie, and Smith developed methods to quantitate the total body burden of tumor cells and to stage patients (Durie and Salmon 1975) in the 1970s.

3.2.2 The Earliest Treatments for Multiple Myeloma

In 1947 Snapper reported that stilbamidine along with a low animal protein diet relieved myeloma pain in 14 of 15 patients (Kyle 2000). Subsequent studies did not confirm a benefit. Urethane was believed to be effective until 1966. It was first used in the treatment of multiple myeloma by Alwall in 1947 and then by Loge and Rundles in 1949. Their early observations were encouraging, and the use became widespread. Toxic effects included severe anorexia, nausea, vomiting, cytopenias, and hepatic damage. In 1966, however, Holland et al. published

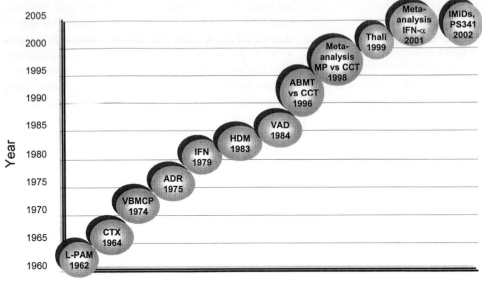

Fig. 3.1. Landmark therapeutic innovations. *ABMT*, autologous bone marrow transplant; *ADR*, doxorubicin; *CCT*, conventional chemotherapy; *CTX*, cyclophosphamide; *HDM*, high-dose melphalan; *IFN-α*, interferon-α; *IMiDs*, immunomodulatory derivatives of thalidomide; *L-PAM*, melphalan; *MP*, melphalan and prednisone; *PS341*, proteosome inhibitor; *Thali*, thalidomide; *VAD*, vincristine, doxorubicin, and dexamethasone; *VBMCP*, vincristine, BCNU, melphalan, cyclophosphamide, and prednisone (M-2 regimen).

the results of a randomized controlled trial of urethane versus placebo in 83 patients with symptomatic multiple myeloma. The median overall survival was higher in the placebo group: previously untreated patients had a median survival of 12 or 5 months depending on whether they received placebo or urethane.

In 1950, Thorn et al. reported the first observations on the beneficial effects of adrenocorticotropic hormone on myeloma. During that decade, it was recognized that adrenocorticotropic hormone, cortisone, and prednisone were all useful agents in patients with multiple myeloma. Corticosteroids decreased bone pain, improved hypercalcemia, increased hemoglobin values, and decreased abnormal serum and urine globulin concentrations.

In 1958 Blokhin et al. reported benefits in 3 of 6 patients with multiple myeloma who were treated with sarcolysin (a racemic mixture of the *d*- and *l*-isomers of phenylalanine mustard). Subsequently, the *d*- and *l*-isomers were tested separately, and the anti-myeloma activity was found to reside in the *l*-isomer, melphalan. In 1962, Bergsagel et al. reported significant improvement in 14 of 24 patients with multiple myeloma with the use of melphalan; this activity was quickly substan-

tiated by others (Bergsagel et al. 1967). Similar activity was noted with cyclophosphamide. Subsequently, interferon-α, doxorubicin, carmustine, and thalidomide have each been reported to have activity as a single agent in myeloma (Alberts et al. 1976; Myeloma Trialists' Collaborative Group 2001) (Fig. 3.1).

3.3 Incidence and Epidemiology

3.3.1 Epidemiology of Myeloma

There are approximately 14,400 new cases of multiple myeloma diagnosed each year and 11,200 deaths. SEER (Surveillance, Epidemiology, and End Results) data incidence age-adjusted rates from 1992 through 1998 show an overall incidence of 4.5 per 100,000 per year, with the incidence among whites at 4.2 per 100,000 per year and among blacks at 9.3 per 100,000 per year. Male-to-female ratio is 1.4 to 1. The median age at diagnosis of myeloma is 71 years. Mortality rates are consistently higher among men than women and among blacks than whites in each age group. Myeloma accounts for 1% of all malignancies and 10% of all hematologic malignancies in whites and 20% in African Americans. International mortality data reveal that the highest rates of myeloma occur in Northern Europe, North America, Australia, and New Zealand and the lowest rates are in Japan, Yugoslavia, and Greece.

3.3.2 Etiologic Factors

3.3.2.1 Radiation Exposures

Reports of increased myeloma incidence and mortality among Japanese atomic bomb survivors have suggested an association between ionizing radiation and multiple myeloma. Evaluations of cancer incidence and mortality among Japanese atomic bomb survivors demonstrated an increased risk of multiple myeloma with increasing radiation dose. However, with an additional 12 years of follow-up from the previous comprehensive report, the findings of an increased myeloma risk associated with atomic bomb irradiation were refuted.

An excess of myeloma deaths was reported among American radiologists more than 40 years ago, but subsequent reports have been contradictory. For example, increases in multiple myeloma incidence and mortality have been observed among British military men who participated in atmospheric nuclear weapons testing but not among New Zealand military who participated in similar nuclear weapons testing.

Diagnostic x-ray exposure has not been linked clearly with multiple myeloma, and most epidemiologic studies have reported no association with diagnostic x-rays. Studies of the effects of therapeutic irradiation on myeloma risk have shown conflicting results.

3.3.2.2 Workplace Exposures

Several epidemiologic studies have evaluated the risk of myeloma among agricultural workers, with positive associations reported by many but not all of the studies. Workers in various metal occupations and industries have been reported to have an increased myeloma risk. There is no evidence of a link between benzene exposure and myeloma.

3.3.2.3 Lifestyle Factors

There is no evidence of a link between cigarette smoking or alcohol consumption and the development of multiple myeloma. There may be a higher risk among people whose diets contain large quantities of liver and butter and a lower risk among people who consume large amounts of cruciferous vegetables, fish, and vitamin C supplements. Obesity, lower socioeconomic status, and personal use of dark hair dyes appear to be risk factors for multiple myeloma.

3.3.2.4 Precursor Medical Conditions

MGUS is considered a potential precursor condition for multiple myeloma. In a long-term study of prognosis in MGUS, Kyle and colleagues (2002) identified 1,384 patients in southeastern Minnesota in whom MGUS was diagnosed. During 11,009 person-years of follow-up, 115 of the 1,384 MGUS patients progressed to multiple myeloma, IgM lymphoma, primary amyloidosis, macroglobulinemia, chronic lymphocytic leukemia, or plasmacytoma. The risk of progression of MGUS to multiple myeloma-related disorders is thus about 1% per year.

Repeated or chronic antigenic stimulation of the immune system may lead to myeloma. Several case-control studies have suggested that myeloma risk is associated with past history of inflammatory conditions, connective tissue disorders, autoimmune illnesses, and allergy-related disorders, but other studies of individuals with these conditions have not been confirmatory.

Patients with human immunodeficiency virus may have an increased likelihood of developing myeloma. In addition, myeloma and hepatitis C may be associated. Human herpesvirus 8 has been suggested as a possible etiologic agent (Rettig et al. 1997), but it has not been confirmed.

Familial clusters of myeloma among first-degree relatives have been documented. Epidemiologic studies have reported higher frequencies of myeloma among cases compared with controls.

3.4 Pathogenesis and Pathophysiology

To date no single molecular defect can account for the pathogenesis of multiple myeloma. Malignant plasma cells are long-lived cells, typically with low proliferative rates and labeling indices. A postgerminal cell origin is indicated by their somatically hypermutated rearranged immunoglobulin genes. Abnormalities of signaling pathways, apoptotic mechanisms, bone marrow microenvironment, and cell cycle have been identified. Factors including level of gene expression, protein expression, and gene product phosphorylation status of cell cycle molecules may all be relevant for propagation of the malignant plasma cells. Extracellular signaling alterations include changes in stromal cell, osteoblast, osteoclast, vessel endothelial cell, and immune cell interactions. These changes may in turn result in activation, adhesion, and cytokine production that fuel myeloma cell proliferation and survival.

3.4.1 Cytokines and Cell Signaling

Interleukin (IL)-6 is among the most important proliferation and survival factors in myeloma. Predominantly produced by the bone marrow stromal cells – macrophages, fibroblasts, osteoblasts, osteoclasts, and monocytes (Fig. 3.2) – it serves both as a growth factor and as an antiapoptotic factor. In the majority of cases, myeloma cells and cell lines are capable of producing IL-6 and the IL-6 receptor, resulting in autocrine stimulation. IL-6 transmits messages intracellularly through the signal-transducing protein gp130, which can activate 2 pathways: the JAK-STAT pathway and the Ras-MAP kinase pathway (Hallek et al. 1998). Through the former pathway, which includes JAK-2 and STAT3, the antiapoptotic proteins Mcl-1 and Bcl-X_L are up-regulated; through the latter pathway, transcription factors such

as ELK-1, AP-1, and NF-IL-6 are up-regulated. NF-kappaB and IL-6 may also mediate increases in the antiapoptotic proteins Bcl-2, Mcl-1, and Bcl-X_L. The overall effect of these pathways is prevention of apoptosis and enhancement of multiple myeloma proliferation. In addition, the constitutive activation of STAT3 may also be important in the pathogenesis of multiple myeloma, independent of IL-6. Finally, CD40 activation of myeloma cells can alter cell surface phenotype, triggering autocrine IL-6 secretion regulating myeloma cell cycle in a *p53*-dependent fashion.

Other cytokines and growth factors produced by myeloma and stromal cells that maintain myeloma growth include IL-1β (Lacy et al. 1999), vascular-derived endothelial growth factor (VEGF), insulin-like growth factor (IGF), and tumor necrosis factor-α (Dalton et al. 2001). Aberrant expression of IL-1β may be a critical step in the transition of MGUS to multiple myeloma. IL-1β up-regulates production of IL-6, changes expression of cell adhesion molecules, and has been shown to have osteoclast-activating factor activity. Myeloma cells are capable of expressing and secreting VEGF and responding to the cytokine in an autocrine fashion. Moreover, stromal and microvascular endothelial cell exposure to VEGF induces an increase in IL-6 secretion, which then further stimulates myeloma cells. IGF, which is believed to signal through the phosphatidylinositol-3′-kinase (PI-3K) pathway, is capable of directly stimulating myeloma cell growth and enhancing myeloma cell respon-

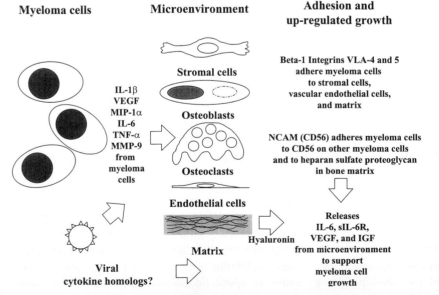

Fig. 3.2. Paracrine myeloma cell growth model. Putative pathogenic mechanisms in myeloma. *IGF*, insulin-like growth factor; *IL*, interleukin; *MIP*, macrophage inflammatory factor; *MMP*, metalloproteinase; *NCAM*, neural cell adhesion molecule; *TNF*, tumor necrosis factor; *VEGF*, vascular-derived endothelial growth factor; *VLA*, very late antigen.

siveness to IL-6 through mitogen-activated protein (MAP) kinase and also inhibiting apoptosis by increasing expression of BAD.

3.4.2 Bone Marrow Microenvironment

There is a synergistic, pathologic relationship between myeloma cells and the cells comprising the bone marrow microenvironment, including fibroblasts, osteoblasts, and osteoclasts. High levels of IL-6 are produced in vitro by the stromal cells of the marrow of myeloma patients. The IL-6 serves as a growth and survival factor for benign and malignant plasma cells, which thereby produce IL-1β, VEGF, and macrophage inflammatory protein-1a (MIP-1a). In turn, IL-1β and MIP-1a regulate and activate osteoclasts.

A cell adhesion molecule belonging to the immunoglobulin superfamily, CD56 (N-CAM), is strongly expressed in most plasma cells of myeloma patients and is believed to play a role in myeloma homing and cell adhesion to the marrow. In a majority of patients, increased levels of the adhesion molecules lymphocyte function-associated antigen (LFA)-3, LFA-1 (CD11a), and very late antigen-4 (VLA-4) are expressed on myeloma cells. VLA-4 may act to bind myeloma cells to fibronectin in bone marrow, which under appropriate conditions can significantly increase IL-6 production by stroma (Dalton et al. 2001). Cell-cell contact between marrow stromal cells and myeloma cells via VCAM-1 and $a_4\beta_1$-integrin enhances production of osteoclast-stimulating activity.

The endothelial microvascular environment has also been shown to be important in multiple myeloma biology. VEGF plays an important role in angiogenesis by acting as a potent inducer of vascular permeability as well as serving as a specific endothelial cell mitogen. Plasma cells in the bone marrow from multiple myeloma patients express VEGF, which can thereby interact with the Flt-1 and KDR high-affinity VEGF receptors highly expressed on bone marrow myeloid and monocytic cells surrounding the tumor.

3.4.3 Cell Cycle

Regulatory signals underlying proliferation of myeloma cells include increased cyclin D1 expression, hypermethylation of the cyclin-dependent kinase (CDK) pathway regulatory gene p16, mutations of the *ras* oncogene, and loss of *p53* (Hallek et al. 1998).

Approximately one-third of myeloma patients have up-regulation of cyclin D1 by immunohistochemistry; these same patients' plasma cells tend to have higher proliferative rate (Rajkumar and Greipp 1999). Peculiarly, the t(11;14)(q13;q32) translocation, which juxtaposes the immunoglobulin heavy chain promoter and the cyclin D1 gene, is seen in approximately 25% of multiple myeloma patients but is not typically associated with a worse prognosis.

Both p15 and p16 are important cell cycle inhibitors that suppress cell proliferation through inhibition of CDK4 or CDK6 or both, thereby preventing the phosphorylation of the retinoblastoma gene (*RB*). Although large deletions of *p15* and *p16* are rare in myeloma, selective methylation of these genes, a form of transcriptional inactivation, occurs in as many as 67% and 75% of cases, respectively. Most data suggest that hypermethylation of *p15* or *p16* is associated with disease progression.

K- and N-*ras* mutations have been described in 25% to 100% of newly diagnosed multiple myeloma patients, depending on the technique used for detection. A *p53* tumor suppressor gene deletion is present in less than one-third of plasma cells from newly diagnosed myeloma patients and mutations are even less common. Dysregulation of c-*myc* appears to be caused principally by complex genomic rearrangements that occur during late stages of multiple myeloma progression. The c-*myc* protein and c-*myc* RNA are overexpressed in about 25% of multiple myeloma patients. Rearrangements of the c-*myc* gene are present in about 15% of patients with multiple myeloma or primary PCL.

3.5 Clinical Manifestations

The symptoms of multiple myeloma may be nonspecific (Table 3.1). They may include fatigue, bone pain, easy bruisability and bleeding, and recurrent infections, which may be manifestations of underlying anemia, hypercalcemia, lytic bone lesions, hyperviscosity, thrombocytopenia, and hypogammaglobulinemia. Weakness, infection, bleeding, and weight loss are reported in as many as 82%, 13%, 13%, and 24% of patients, respectively (Kapadia 1980; Kyle et al. 2003). Hypercalcemia is present in 18% to 30% of patients. One- to two-thirds

Table 3.1. Symptoms and signs of multiple myeloma at presentation

Symptom or sign	Patients, %
Spontaneous bone pain	66
Fatigue	32
Weight loss (>20 pounds)	12
Infection and bleeding	<15
Paresthesia	5
"Tumor fever"	<1
M protein in serum or urine	97
Lytic lesions, osteoporosis, or fracture on plain radiograph	79
Hemoglobin <12 g/dL	73
Creatinine >2 mg/dL	19
Calcium >11 mg/dL	13
Viscosity >4 cP	<7

Data from Kyle et al. (2003).

of patients present with spontaneous bone pain. "Tumor fever" is present in less than 1% of presenting patients.

3.5.1 Anemia

The most common clinical feature of multiple myeloma is anemia. A hemoglobin concentration of less than 12 g/dL occurs in 40% to 72% of patients at presentation (Kyle et al. 2003). The anemia is normochromic, normocytic in most patients, but macrocytosis may also be observed. In the presence of high concentrations of serum immunoglobulin, rouleau formation may be observed on peripheral blood smear (Fig. 3.3). The combination of anemia and hyperproteinemia leads to marked increase of the erythrocyte sedimentation rate in more than 90% of cases.

The anemia is related partially to direct infiltration and replacement of the bone marrow. Hemoglobin concentration is also correlated with the percentage of myeloma cells in S phase, suggesting that the bone marrow cytokine milieu permissive for myeloma cell proliferation is not conducive to efficient erythropoiesis. Cytokines, like tumor necrosis factor-a and IL-1, may inhibit erythropoiesis. Fas ligand-mediated erythroid apoptosis is also increased in patients with myeloma. Finally, rel-

ative erythropoietin deficiency from myeloma-induced renal insufficiency also contributes to the observed anemia.

3.5.2 Monoclonal Proteins

The M protein (M component, myeloma protein, or M spike) is a hallmark of the disease in that 97% of myeloma patients have either an intact immunoglobulin or a free light chain that can be detected by protein electrophoresis, immunoelectrophoresis, or immunofixation studies of the serum or urine (Fig. 3.4) (Kyle et al. 2003). Monoclonal proteins are used to calculate myeloma tumor burden and kinetics, to stage myeloma patients, and to document their response to treatment.

An M protein represents overproduction of a homogeneous immunoglobulin or immunoglobulin fragment. In a series of 1,027 newly diagnosed cases of myeloma, the immunoglobulin type was IgG, IgA, IgD, and free light chain only (Bence Jones myeloma) in 52%, 20%, 2%, and 16% of cases, respectively (Kyle et al. 2003). Less than 1% of myeloma cases are IgM; most IgM cases are MGUS, lymphoma, Waldenström macroglobulinemia, or primary systemic amyloidosis. Ninety-three percent of patients have a monoclonal protein detected in their serum. About 70% have a monoclonal protein – or fragment thereof – detected in the urine.

3.5.3 Bone Disease

Approximately one-third to two-thirds of patients present with bone pain (Kapadia 1980; Kyle et al. 2003). Myeloma bone disease is a major source of morbidity in patients and may present as an area of persistent pain or as a vague migratory bone pain, often in the lower back and pelvis. The type, location, and duration of the pain are not characteristic. It may be sudden in onset, especially when associated with a pathologic fracture. Persistent localized pain or tenderness of sudden onset is usually referable to a pathologic fracture.

A myelomatous lesion may extend through the cortex of a vertebral body and cause either nerve root or spinal cord compression. More commonly, the myeloma disturbs the mechanical integrity of a vertebral body, resulting in compression fracture and pain (Fig. 3.5 D). Occasionally, there may be retropulsion of either plasmacytoma or bony fragments into the spinal canal, again causing neurologic deficit.

Because myelomatous bone lesions are characteristically lytic, conventional radiography is superior to technetium-99m bone scanning. About twice as many myelomatous bone lesions are detected by radiograph as by bone scan; an exception to this general finding is at the lumbar spine and the rib cage, where the 2 methods are equally reliable. The role of fluorodeoxyglucose positron emission tomography is yet to be defined.

Computed tomography and magnetic resonance imaging (MRI) are more sensitive than conventional radiography. Both reveal specific lesions in 40% of stage I myeloma patients. The presence of lacunae larger than 5 mm with trabecular disruption on computed tomography appears to be sensitive and specific for myeloma. This information may be useful in distinguishing between senile and myelomatous osteoporosis and compression fracture.

The finding of diffusely decreased signal intensity and a multinodular appearance on MRI may also be useful for the same indication. Among asymptomatic multiple myeloma patients with normal radiographs, 50% have tumor-related abnormalities on MRI of the lower spine. MRI is superior to radiographs for lesion detection in the pelvis and the spine, but overall it is inferior for detecting overall bone involvement. Given the expense of MRI, it cannot be recommended for routine clinical use in all symptomatic patients.

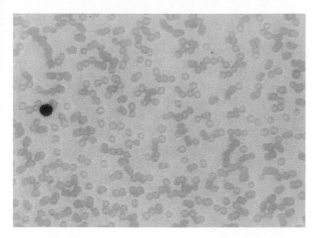

Fig. 3.3. Rouleaux

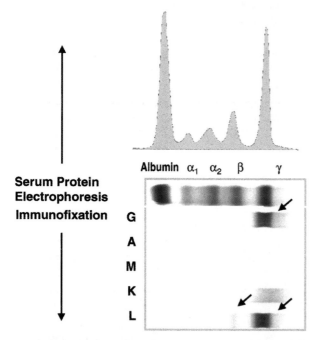

Fig. 3.4. Serum protein electrophoresis patterns and immunofixation patterns

3.5.4 Hypercalcemia

Rates of hypercalcemia at presentation have been decreasing in the last few decades, suggesting earlier diagnosis (Kapadia 1980; Kyle et al. 2003). Incidence rates of hypercalcemia at diagnosis are 18% to 30%, and about 13% have concentrations greater than 11 mg/dL. Patients may complain of fatigue, constipation, nausea, or confusion. Hypercalcemia can precipitate and aggravate renal insufficiency. The inorganic phosphorus is rarely decreased, except in cases of acquired Fanconi syndrome.

3.5.5 Renal Insufficiency

Approximately 25% of myeloma patients have a serum creatinine value greater than 2 mg/dL at diagnosis. Another 25% have a mildly elevated creatinine value (Kapadia 1980; Kyle et al. 2003). Contributing factors to renal insufficiency include hypercalcemia, free light chain

Approximately 75% of patients have punched-out lytic lesions, osteoporosis, or fractures on conventional radiography. The vertebrae, skull, ribs, sternum, proximal humeri, and femora are involved most frequently (Kapadia 1980; Kyle et al. 2003) (Fig. 3.5). A small subset of patients have de novo osteosclerotic lesions (Dispenzieri et al. 2003), but in general osteosclerosis is seen after therapy in a minority of patients and may serve as a marker of healing.

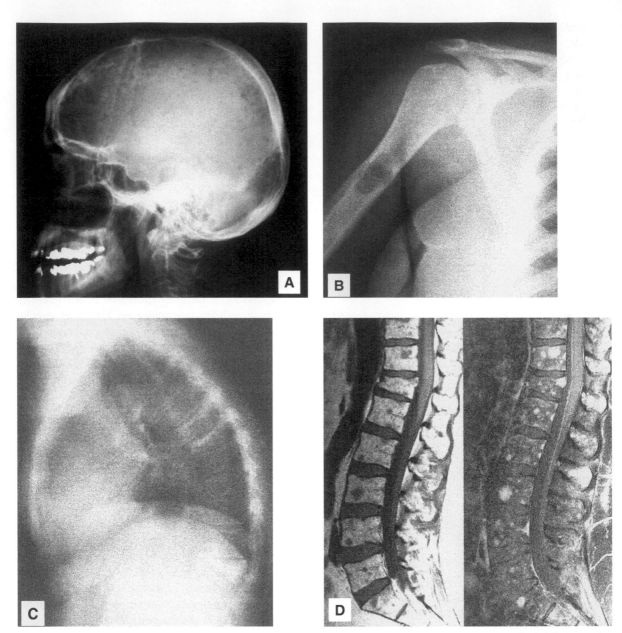

Fig. 3.5 A. *Skull, punched-out lesions* . **B–D.** *B*, Humerus, lytic lesion. *C*, Compression fractures, osteopenia, and kyphosis. *D*, MRI, bone marrow infiltration, compression fracture, and extradural extension extending from thoracic levels T6-T9 (T1 with gadolinium and T2 images)

proteinuria, dehydration, hyperuricemia, and nephrotoxic drugs (MRC Working Party on Leukaemia in Adults 1984).

The pathologic lesion of myeloma kidney is the presence of monoclonal light chains in the tubules in the form of dense, often laminated, tubular casts. These casts contain albumin and Tamm-Horsfall protein. Light chains are normally passed through the glomeruli and reabsorbed and catabolized in the nephron's proximal tubules. It is postulated that these systems become overwhelmed, and casts result. The most common abnormal renal findings on autopsy of 60 patients with myeloma were tubular atrophy and fibrosis (77%), tubular hyaline casts (62%), tubular epithelial giant cell reaction (48%), and nephrocalcinosis (42%). Acute and chronic pyelonephritis were observed in 20% and 23% of cases, respectively. Plasma cell infiltrates and amyloid may be observed in 10% and 5% of cases, respectively (Kapadia 1980). Rarely, myeloma may be associated with acquired Fanconi syndrome.

An important feature of myeloma kidney is that it is primarily a tubular, rather than a glomerular, disease. Glomerular function is preserved initially, and there is a predominance of immunoglobulin light chain protein in the urine instead of the nonspecific protein loss observed in glomerular disease. This feature helps predict the renal lesion: a free light chain predominance is consistent with myeloma kidney, whereas nonspecific protein loss (ie, mostly albumin) is more compatible with primary systemic amyloidosis, light chain deposition disease of the kidney, or proteinuria unrelated to the plasma cell dyscrasia.

3.5.6 Infection

Patients with multiple myeloma are at high risk for bacterial infections and for dying of overwhelming bacteremia. During the first 2 months after initiating chemotherapy the infection incidence is as high as 4.68 infections per patient-year but decreases to 0.44 to 0.49 per patient-year in those reaching plateau phase. Serum creatinine value greater than or equal to 2 mg/dL is a risk factor for infection.

At disease onset, infections with encapsulated organisms like *Streptococcus pneumoniae* and *Haemophilus influenzae* are most common. After diagnosis, the proportion of infections due to gram-negative bacilli and *Staphyloccocus aureus* increases markedly, and they

are responsible for more than 90% of deaths from infection.

3.5.7 Bone Marrow Pathologic Features

There is a complex interaction among the malignant clone, its surrounding stromal cells, and the remaining immune cells within the bone marrow. The morphologic and immunologic phenotypes of myeloma cells can vary, and they often resemble normal plasma cells. Plasma cells are at least 2 to 3 times the size of peripheral lymphocytes and are round to oval, with one or more eccentrically placed nuclei (Fig. 3.6). The nucleus, which contains either diffuse or clumped chromatin, is displaced from the center by an abundance of rough-surfaced endoplasmic reticulum – the site of specialized immunoglobulin synthesis. There is a perinuclear clear zone that is the site of the Golgi apparatus. Intranuclear and cytoplasmic inclusions are not uncommon. Derangements of immunoglobulin secretion are responsible for an assortment of cytologic aberrations, including flaming cells, Mott cells, Russell bodies, and Gaucher-like cells. Flaming cells are plasma cells that have intensely eosinophilic cytoplasm with a magenta or carmine coloring of their margins, which is caused by plugging of peripheral secretory channels by precipitated immunoglobulin or immunoglobulin fragments. These cells are most commonly seen in IgA myeloma. Thesaurocytes are large flaming cells with a pyknotic nucleus that is pushed to the side. Mott cells (grape cells or morula forms) are plasma cells filled with dense spherical immunoglobulin inclusions; these inclusions are colorless, pink, or blue. Other inclusions are Russell bodies and their intranuclear counterparts (intranuclear dense bodies); these appear cherry red and can be as large as several microns in diameter. Gaucher-like cells are not uncommon in myeloma infiltrates; these cells are macrophages laden with sphingolipids released by the dying plasma cells. None of these inclusions are specific for malignancy nor do they have prognostic value.

In myeloma, there is often discordance between the nucleus and cytoplasm, the former appearing immature and the latter highly differentiated. About 20% of myeloma cases have plasmablastic morphology: a diffuse chromatin pattern, nucleus >10 mm or nucleolus >2 mm, relatively less abundant cytoplasm, and a concentrically placed nucleus with little or no hof (Rajku-

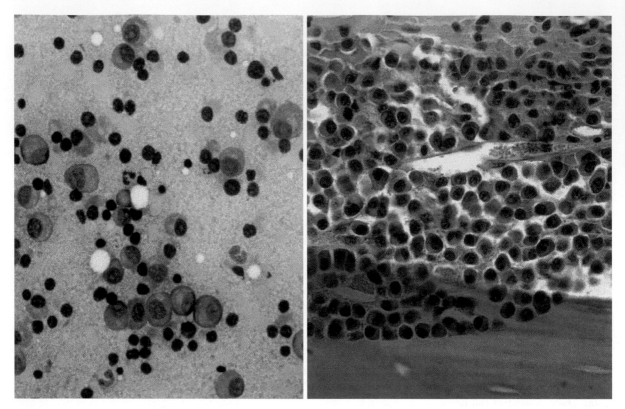

Fig. 3.6. Bone marrow: normal plasma cells and sheets

mar and Greipp 1999). Both diffuse and nodular infiltration patterns can be observed, although the former is more common. Myeloma cells are commonly present in cords around bone marrow microvessels. Mild marrow fibrosis may be observed in as many as 27% of cases; extensive fibrosis is rare. Less than 1% of cases have an extensive idiopathic granulomatous reaction.

The immunophenotype of myeloma cells is complex. In general, myeloma cells are CD45 negative and CD38 and CD138 positive. CD19 and CD20 are earlier B-cell antigens that are variably expressed on myeloma cells. CD56 is strongly positive in as many as three-quarters of myeloma cases, and CD56-negative myeloma cells tend to be present in more aggressive disease, such as end-stage myeloma or PCL. Other surface antigens like CD10 (CALLA), CD28, *c-kit*, and CD20 are present on a minority of patients' myeloma cells.

The labeling index of bone marrow plasma cells can be useful to identify plasma cell clonality and rate of division. This assay has some value in differentiating

MGUS from myeloma and indolent myeloma from active myeloma. In general, myeloma is a low growth fraction tumor with only a small percentage of myeloma cells in the S phase of the cell cycle at any given time.

3.5.8 Hemostasis in Myeloma

Multiple myeloma can be associated with hemostatic abnormalities, more often bleeding than thrombosis. Bleeding as a complication of myeloma may be present in as many as one-third of patients and is related to thrombocytopenia, uremia, hyperviscosity, and interference with coagulation factors. The association with thrombosis is less clear because coexisting old age and immobility confound interpretation of thrombosis rates.

Fewer than 7% of myeloma patients have a viscosity greater than 4 (Kyle et al. 2003). Symptoms of hyperviscosity include bleeding (particularly of the oronasal areas), purpura, dyspnea, decrease in visual acuity from retinopathy, neurologic symptoms, expanded plasma volume, and congestive heart failure. Most patients become symptomatic when the serum viscosity is 6 or 7 centipoise (normal is less than or equal to 1.8 centipoise).

Myeloma proteins may also interact with coagulation proteins. The immunoglobulin may interfere with fibrin monomer aggregation or serve as a specific inhibitor of thrombin, von Willebrand factor, or factor VIII. Nonspecific inhibitors may also be present, but unlike the specific inhibitors they do not correlate with clinical bleeding. Depression of clotting factors II, V, VII, VIII, X, and fibrinogen has been described.

At the opposite hemostatic extreme, thrombosis risk may be increased in myeloma patients. Individual cases of aberrance have been reported. Paraproteins have been shown to be responsible for lupus anticoagulants, acquired protein S deficiency, acquired activated protein C resistance, and inhibition of tissue plasminogen activator.

3.5.9 "Acute Terminal Phase of Plasma Cell Myeloma" and Cause of Death

Bergsagel and Pruzanski described the "acute terminal phase" of patients with myeloma, which they observed in about one-third of their preterminal patients. This syndrome is characterized as rapidly progressive disease with an unexplained temperature and pancytopenia with a hypercellular marrow. Extramedullary plasmacytomas may also occur. As disease progresses, and at autopsy, cutaneous, visceral, and even meningeal involvement is possible. Besides "progressive disease," the most frequent causes of death are infection in 24% to 52% and renal failure in about 20%. Acute leukemia, myelodysplastic syndrome, and hemorrhage are the cause of death in a minority of patients (Kapadia 1980). In one autopsy series, 85% of patients had evidence of either bacterial or fungal infection and myelomatous involvement was found in the spleen, liver, lymph nodes, and kidneys in 45%, 28%, 27%, and 10% of patients, respectively. Other less frequent areas of myelomatous involvement were the lung, pleura, adrenal glands, pancreas, and testis (Kapadia 1980).

3.5.10 Special Cases of Myeloma

3.5.10.1 Nonsecretory Multiple Myeloma

Nonsecretory multiple myeloma accounts for 1% to 5% of myeloma cases (Bladé and Kyle 1999). More than 85% of cases have a cytoplasmic monoclonal protein when immunoperoxidase or immunofluorescence studies are performed; in the remainder, no monoclonal protein can be detected in the cytoplasm. Individuals in this latter group are "nonproducers." From a clinical standpoint, both are referred to as "nonsecretory." With more sensitive testing like immunofixation and free light chain assay (Drayson et al. 2001), many of these "nonsecretory" patients are found to be low secretors or oligosecretory.

At presentation, hypercalcemia and anemia may be present (Bladé and Kyle 1999). A reduction in background immunoglobulins is common. There is minimal to no risk of myeloma kidney. Lytic bone disease is present in most patients. Median survival of these patients is at least as good as for those with secretory myeloma. Response is difficult to document, but with the new serum assays, quantitation of free light chain is possible in about two-thirds of these patients (Drayson et al. 2001).

3.5.10.2 Immunoglobulin D Myeloma

IgD myeloma accounts for about 2% of all cases of myeloma. The presence of a monoclonal IgD in the serum usually indicates myeloma, but there have been 3 cases of IgD MGUS documented (Bladé and Kyle 1999). Patients with IgD myeloma generally present with a small band or no evident M spike on serum protein electrophoresis. Their clinical presentation is most similar to that of patients with Bence Jones myeloma (light chain myeloma) in that they both have higher incidences of renal insufficiency and coincident amyloidosis as well as a higher degree of proteinuria than in IgG or IgA myeloma. With an incidence of 19% to 27%, extramedullary involvement is more prevalent in patients with IgD myeloma. Though initial reports suggested that survival with IgD myeloma was inferior to that with other forms of myeloma, in the Mayo Clinic series in patients diagnosed after 1980, this was not the case.

3.5.10.3 Immunoglobulin E Myeloma

IgE myeloma is a rare form of myeloma. A disproportionate number of cases are PCL, although the sample size is small, with only about 40 cases of IgE myeloma reported in the literature.

3.6   Diagnosis

The definition of multiple myeloma has unfortunately not been a static one. In 1973, the Chronic Leukemia-Myeloma Task Force set forth guidelines for the diagnosis of myeloma (Table 3.2). These criteria, which by today's standards are not stringent, have been replaced by a more modern definition (Table 3.2) (Kyle and Greipp 1980). In the last 3 decades, the terms and definitions of MGUS, smoldering myeloma, indolent myeloma, and symptomatic multiple myeloma (Alexanian 1980; Kyle and Greipp 1980) have evolved and will be replaced by the following expressions: MGUS, inactive (smoldering) myeloma, and active (or symptomatic) myeloma (Kyle et al. 2003) (Fig. 3.7).

This internationally accepted diagnostic classification schema is derived from more than 4 decades of ex-

Table 3.2. Chronic Leukemia-Myeloma Task Force definition of multiple myeloma 1973

If M protein present in serum or urine, 1 or more of the following must be present:

Marrow plasmacytosis >5% in absence of underlying reactive process

Tissue biopsy demonstrating replacement and distortion of normal tissue by plasma cells

More than 500 plasma cells/mm^3 in peripheral blood

Osteolytic lesion unexplained by other causes

If M protein absent in serum and urine, there must be radiologic evidence of osteolytic lesions or palpable tumors and 1 or more of the following must be present:

Marrow plasmacytosis of >20% from 2 sites in absence of reactive process

Tissue biopsy demonstrating replacement and distortion of normal tissue by plasma cells

Data from Committee of the Chronic Leukemia-Myeloma Task Force, National Cancer Institute (1973).

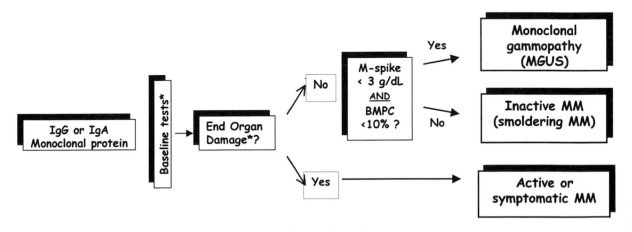

* End organ damage without other explanation
- **Bone marrow: hemoglobin, more than 2 g/dl below normal**
- **Bones:**
    - **Lytic lesions or osteoporosis with compression fracture**
    - **Serum calcium, more than 1 mg/dl above normal**
- **Kidneys: serum creatinine, more than 1 mg/dl above normal**

Fig. 3.7. Diagnostic criteria. *BMPC*, bone marrow plasma cells; *MGUS*, monoclonal gammopathy of undetermined significance; *MM*, multiple myeloma. Personal communication from Dr. R. A. Kyle

perience of treating and studying multiple myeloma patients. Because multiple myeloma includes a spectrum of biologic and clinical features, treatment should not commence based on a single threshold value. The diagnosis of active myeloma is not a straightforward pathologic one; rather, it is a clinical diagnosis that requires thoughtful synthesis of multiple variables. Those patients with Durie-Salmon stage I disease, who also meet the criteria for inactive, smoldering, or asymptomatic myeloma, should be managed expectantly. Median progression-free survival in asymptomatic stage I patients, observed without any therapy, is 12 to more than 48 months (Facon et al. 1995; Hjorth et al. 1993; Peest et al. 1995; Riccardi et al. 2000); for similar stage II patients, progression-free survival is 12 months (Peest et al. 1995). No survival advantage has been demonstrated by treating asymptomatic myeloma patients (Alexanian 1980; Hjorth et al. 1993; Riccardi et al. 2000).

3.7   Differential Diagnosis

The diagnosis of multiple myeloma is made from a constellation of findings, including anemia, monoclonal proteins, bone lesions, renal complications, hypercalcemia, and bone marrow plasmacytosis. Often the diagnosis is straightforward, but other disease entities associated with hypergammaglobulinemia or monoclonal bone marrow plasma cells must also be considered. These include reactive plasmacytosis, MGUS, primary systemic amyloidosis, Waldenström macroglobulinemia, light chain deposition disease, Fanconi syndrome,

Table 3.3. Differential diagnosis of multiple myeloma

Reactive plasmacytosis and polyclonal hypergamma-globulinemia

Monoclonal gammopathy of undetermined significance

Primary systemic amyloidosis

Plasma cell leukemia

POEMS syndrome (osteosclerotic myeloma)

Solitary plasmacytoma

Waldenström macroglobulinemia

Light chain deposition disease

Acquired Fanconi syndrome

Table 3.4. Criteria for diagnosis of MGUS, SMM, and MM according to Kyle and Greipp

MGUS[a]

  Serum monoclonal protein (<3 g/dL)

  No anemia, renal failure, or hypercalcemia

  Bone lesions absent on radiographic bone survey[b]

  Bone marrow <10% plasma cells

SMM[a]

  Serum monoclonal protein (≥3 g/dL) and/or ≥10% marrow plasma cells or aggregates on biopsy

  No anemia, renal failure, or hypercalcemia attributable to myeloma

MM

  Monoclonal protein present in serum or urine

  ≥10% marrow plasma cells on biopsy or histologic evidence of plasmacytoma

  Plus one or more of the following

    Anemia

    Lytic lesions or osteoporosis and ≥30% plasma cells in marrow

    Bone marrow plasma cell labeling index >1%

    Renal insufficiency

    Hypercalcemia

MM, multiple myeloma; MGUS, monoclonal gammopathy of undetermined significance; SMM, smoldering multiple myeloma.
[a] Patients with MGUS and SMM must not have solitary plasmacytoma, amyloidosis, or light-chain deposition disease.
[b] Computed tomography or magnetic resonance imaging may be needed to rule out skeletal lesions.
Data from Kyle and Greipp (1980).

solitary plasmacytoma, osteosclerotic myeloma or POEMS syndrome, and plasma cell leukemia (Table 3.3).

3.7.1   Reactive Plasmacytosis and Polyclonal Hypergammaglobulinemia

Reactive plasmacytosis and polyclonal hypergammaglobulinemia must be distinguished from a clonal process. Patients with liver disease, chronic infections including human immunodeficiency virus, connective tissue diseases, other lymphoproliferative disorders, and carcinoma can have increased bone marrow plasmacytosis (polyclonal) and hypergammaglobulinemia (polyclonal). These conditions should not be confused with multiple myeloma or MGUS, which are clonal processes.

3.7.2 MGUS

Two percent of patients older than age 50 years have MGUS, which is a benign counterpart or precursor lesion of multiple myeloma (Kyle et al. 2002). It is characterized by an M protein in the serum or urine, without evidence of multiple myeloma or other serious gammopathy-related disorder. MGUS patients do not have bone marrow suppression, lytic bone lesions, hypercalcemia, renal failure, or increased susceptibility to infection. Standard clinical features do not accurately predict which patients will remain stable, and multiple myeloma develops in approximately 1% of MGUS patients per year. The clinical distinction between MGUS and asymptomatic multiple myeloma has been derived from an arbitrary definition (Table 3.4 and Fig. 3.7), although the underlying biologic conditions should prove to be distinct.

The greatest challenges in differentiating MGUS from myeloma occur in patients who have MGUS and 1) senile osteoporosis, 2) renal insufficiency from another cause, or 3) hypercalcemia due to hyperparathyroidism. Approximately 50% of women older than age 60 years have osteoporosis, and a fraction of these even have a vertebral compression fracture. Computed tomographic scan of the spine may help distinguish between senile osteoporosis and myelomatous bone disease. Similarly, renal insufficiency due to long-standing diabetes, hypertension, or nonsteroidal drug use is not uncommon. In such cases, a patient may still have MGUS (or asymptomatic myeloma, for that matter) and "end-organ damage." The key is whether the damage is attributable to the plasmaproliferative disorder or another cause. In some instances, renal biopsy may be required to clarify this issue.

3.7.3 Primary Systemic Amyloidosis

Primary systemic amyloidosis is a rare disorder that is characterized by the deposition of amyloid fibrils. These fibrils are composed of immunoglobulin light chain fragments in a β-pleated sheet conformation. It should be suspected when a patient with a monoclonal protein in the serum or urine presents with nephrotic-range proteinuria (primarily albumin) with or without renal insufficiency, cardiomyopathy, hepatomegaly, or peripheral neuropathy. Patients usually present with weight loss or fatigue. Anemia is rare at presentation. Symptoms related to the affected organ are also seen. Median percentage of clonal plasma cells in these patients is only 5%. A histologic diagnosis is made by demonstrating the amyloid fibrils – green birefringence under polarized light by using a Congo red stain or 8- to 10-nm nonbranching fibrils by electron microscopy. Nearly 90% of patients with amyloid have a bone marrow or fat aspirate specimen positive for amyloid. In the remaining 10%, a biopsy specimen of the affected organ is positive.

3.7.4 Waldenström Macroglobulinemia

Waldenström macroglobulinemia should not be confused with IgM myeloma, which comprises only about 1% of myeloma cases (Kyle et al. 2003). Patients with Waldenström macroglobulinemia may have anemia, hyperviscosity, B symptoms, bleeding, and neurologic symptoms. Significant lymphadenopathy or splenomegaly may also be present. Lytic bone disease would be exceptional; if present, IgM myeloma should be considered. In Waldenström macroglobulinemia, bone marrow biopsy typically reveals infiltration with clonal lymphoplasmacytic cells which are CD20 positive. The natural history and treatment options for Waldenström macroglobulinemia are different from those of multiple myeloma.

3.7.5 Light Chain Deposition Disease

The nonamyloidogenic light chain deposition diseases (LCDD) are due to pathologic protein deposition in various tissues and organs. Unlike the light chain deposits observed in patients with primary systemic amyloidosis, these infiltrates are not congophilic by light microscopy, and by electron microscopy nonbranching fibrils are not observed. Instead, amorphous nodular deposits are observed.

LCDD may occur with or without coexistent multiple myeloma. Renal involvement is most common, followed distantly by cardiac and hepatic. Clinically, LCDD can be differentiated from multiple myeloma and primary systemic amyloidosis by the following findings.

As in primary systemic amyloidosis, early in the disease course the light chain deposits have a predilection for the renal glomeruli rather than the tubules. This results in nonselective proteinuria, that is, a predominance of albuminuria, which is not usual in multiple myeloma. It is impossible clinically to distinguish the nephropathy, cardiomyopathy, or hepatopathy from primary systemic amyloidosis without tissue biopsy. The underlying clone is more commonly monoclonal κ than λ in LCDD.

The prognosis of patients who have this disorder depends on whether there is underlying multiple myeloma. In one retrospective study of 19 patients with LCDD, 5-year actuarial patient survival and survival free of end-stage renal disease were 70% and 37%, respectively.

3.7.6 Acquired Fanconi Syndrome

Fanconi syndrome is a rare complication of plasma cell dyscrasias characterized by diffuse failure in reabsorption at the level of the proximal renal tubule and resulting in glycosuria, generalized aminoaciduria, and hypophosphatemia. Acquired Fanconi syndrome is usually associated with MGUS. Overt hematologic malignancies may occur, such as multiple myeloma, Waldenström macroglobulinemia, or other lymphoproliferative disorders. The prognosis for survival is good in the absence of overt malignant disease. Clinical manifestations include slowly progressive renal failure and bone pain due to osteomalacia. The diagnosis of Fanconi syndrome can be made when a patient with a monoclonal plasma cell disorder presents with hypophosphatemia, hypouricemia, aminoaciduria, phosphaturia, and glycosuria. Bence Jones proteinuria is usually present and is almost always of the κ type. Rare patients have been reported with Fanconi syndrome associated with λ Bence Jones proteinuria.

Treatment consists of supplementation with phosphorus, calcium, and vitamin D. Chemotherapy may benefit patients with rapidly progressive renal failure or symptomatic malignancy.

3.7.7 POEMS Syndrome (Osteosclerotic Myeloma)

Osteosclerotic myeloma is a rare variant of myeloma ($\leq 3.3\%$ of cases). There is a straight osteosclerotic variant that is similar to multiple myeloma in that anemia, significant bone marrow plasmacytosis, hypercalcemia, and renal insufficiency occur. Survival in these patients is comparable to that of classic multiple myeloma patients. There is, however, a more interesting form, which is known as Crow-Fukase syndrome, Takatsuki syndrome, and POEMS syndrome (*p*olyneuropathy, *o*rganomegaly, *e*ndocrinopathy, *M* protein, and *s*kin changes) (Dispenzieri et al. 2003). This variant is associated with multiple paraneoplastic phenomena, and its natural history is not similar to that of classic multiple myeloma. The acronym POEMS captures several of the dominant features of the syndrome, but it omits the sclerotic bone lesions, Castleman disease, papilledema, peripheral edema, ascites, polycythemia, thrombocytosis, fatigue, and clubbing commonly observed in the disorder. Not all features are required to make the diagnosis; at a minimum, however, a patient must have: 1) peripheral neuropathy, 2) osteosclerotic myeloma (i.e., a clonal plasma cell dyscrasia and at least 1 sclerotic bone lesion) or Castleman disease, and 3) at least 1 of the other features mentioned. The peak incidence of POEMS syndrome is in the 5th and 6th decades of life, and there is a male predominance.

Although the precise mechanism of POEMS syndrome is unknown, VEGF appears to be a driving factor in this disorder. Despite the presence of osteosclerotic bone lesions that microscopically contain clonal plasma cell infiltrates, bone marrow aspirate and biopsy of the iliac crest typically yield only about 5% monoclonal lambda plasma cells.

Treatment for this disorder is not standardized. For an isolated plasmacytoma, external beam irradiation is the preferred first-line treatment. It produces substantial improvement of the neuropathy in more than half of the patients who have a single lesion or multiple lesions in a limited area. If there are widespread lesions, chemotherapy and, potentially, peripheral blood stem cell transplantation should be considered. Responses of systemic symptoms and skin changes tend to precede those of the neuropathy, with the former beginning to respond within a month and the latter within 3 to 6 months. The most common causes of death are cardiorespiratory failure, progressive inanition, infection, capillary leak–like syndrome, and renal failure. The neuropathy may be unrelenting and contribute to progressive inanition and eventual cardiorespiratory failure and pneumonia. Patients do not die of classic myeloma (ie, progressive bone marrow failure or hypercalcemia).

3.8   Treatment for Multiple Myeloma

Before starting therapy for multiple myeloma, a distinction must be made between inactive (smoldering, indolent, asymptomatic) myeloma and active myeloma, which requires therapy (Fig. 3.7) (International Myeloma Working Group, 2003). Approximately 20% of patients with multiple myeloma are recognized by chance without significant symptoms; such patients can be carefully monitored without instituting therapy. Risk factors for progression include serum M protein >3 g/dL, IgA isotype, and Bence Jones protein excretion >50 mg per day. Patients with 2 or more of these features required treatment at a median of 17 months, whereas the absence of any adverse variable was associated with prolonged stability (median, 95 months) ($P<0.01$) (Weber et al. 1997). Patients with one or more lytic bone lesions or circulating plasma cells on peripheral blood labeling index are also at higher risk for early progression.

Once the decision has been made to institute therapy for symptomatic disease, a long-term plan for managing the disease should be formulated before instituting therapy. Figure 3.8 outlines a possible treatment algorithm. Because high-dose therapy with hematopoietic stem cell support has been accepted as an important treatment modality for patients younger than age 65 years, alkylator-based therapy should be avoided before hematopoietic stem cell collection in patients considered candidates for high-dose therapy.

3.8.1   Systemic Therapy

3.8.1.1   General Comments

Historically, the bifunctional alkylating agents, like melphalan and cyclophosphamide, have been the foundation of standard therapy for multiple myeloma (Fig. 3.1). Myeloma cells tend to be slowly proliferating,

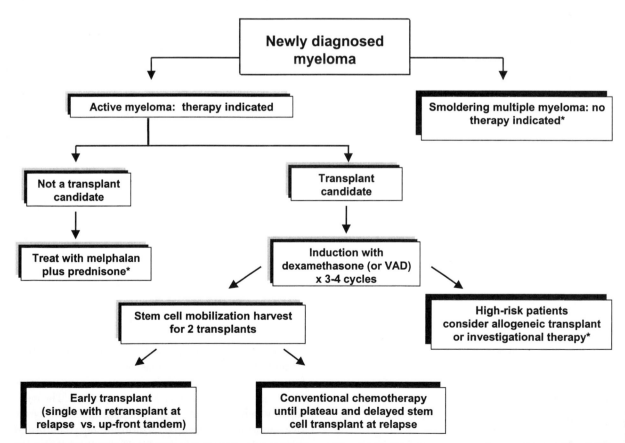

Fig. 3.8. Possible treatment algorithm. *At any point in the disease, consider clinical trial or investigational therapy directed at particular phase of disease. *VAD*, vincristine, doxorubicin, and dexamethasone

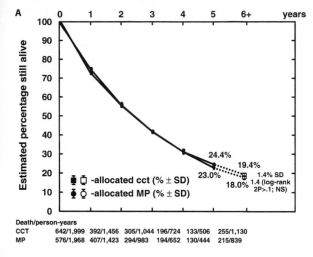

Death/person-years
CCT	642/1,999	392/1,456	305/1,044	196/724	133/506	255/1,130
MP	576/1,968	407/1,423	294/983	194/652	130/444	215/839

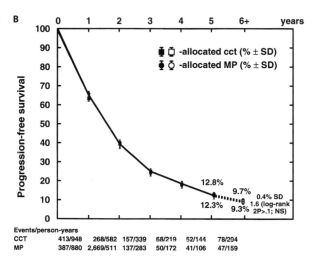

Events/person-years
CCT	413/948	268/582	157/339	68/219	52/144	78/294
MP	387/880	2,669/511	137/283	50/172	41/106	47/159

Fig. 3.9. Melphalan and prednisone (*MP*) versus combined chemotherapy (*cct*) as induction. Results from 6,633 patients from 27 randomized trials. *A,* Overall survival. *B,* Response duration. (From the Myeloma Trialists' Collaborative Group [1998]. By permission of the American Society of Clinical Oncology.)

and alkylators, which do not rely heavily on cell division and DNA replication, are useful. Before the recognition of thalidomide's activity in myeloma, the bifunctional alkylators, nitrosoureas, doxorubicin, and glucocorticoids were the primary agents shown to have single agent activity against multiple myeloma in vivo. These drugs and vincristine, either singly or in combination, have been the mainstay of chemotherapy for myeloma from the early 1960s to the present. Even though vincristine has not been shown to have significant single agent in vivo activity or to clearly improve overall sur-

vival (MacLennan et al. 1992; Tribalto et al. 1985), it is included in multiple therapeutic regimens. Decades of study suggest that although response rates are higher with regimens that combine multiple active agents as part of initial therapy, these regimens do not improve overall survival rates (Myeloma Trialists' Collaborative Group 1998).

Interferon-α has been incorporated into both induction and maintenance protocols with modest benefit since the 1980s because of its single agent activity (Myeloma Trialists' Collaborative Group 2001). Both autologous and allogeneic stem cell transplantation have received considerable attention since McElwain and Powles' description in 1983 of the benefit of dose intensification of melphalan in patients with multiple myeloma. With the recognition of thalidomide as a new agent with activity against multiple myeloma in 1999 and exciting new agents like the IMiDs and proteosome inhibitors, there is hope that the next 4 decades of myeloma treatment will be even more promising than the last (Fig. 3.1).

Before discussing induction (Fig. 3.9), transplantation, maintenance, and salvage therapies, 2 general concepts will be reviewed: interpretation of study response data and the efficacy of single chemotherapeutic agents commonly used to treat myeloma. Table 3.5 serves as a reference for commonly cited regimens.

3.8.1.2 Interpreting Study Response and Survival Data

Four points are emphasized regarding the interpretation and comparisons of the myeloma treatment literature. First, definitions of response vary. Second, definitions of evaluable patients may be different. Third, concurrent corticosteroid therapy, either as part of the regimen or for other indications, may confound interpretation of efficacy. Finally, patient population risk and prognosis may differ substantially. Lead-time bias and inappropriate incorporation of patients with MGUS or inactive myeloma can significantly distort survival estimates, as can effective salvage regimens.

The measurement of myeloma disease burden, and therefore response, is complex, and different investigators have used different methods to determine response (Table 3.6). The 4 most common response criteria are those of the Chronic Leukemia-Myeloma Task Force (CLMTF) (1973), Southwest Oncology Group (SWOG)

Table 3.5. Commonly cited regimens and their dosage schedules

Drug regimen	VCR	Mel	CTX	BCNU	ADR	Gluco
MP	–	9 mg/m^2 per d d 1–4 q 4 wk or 0.15 mg/kg per d d 1–7 q 6 wk	–	–	–	Pred 100 mg/d d 1–4 q 4 wk or Pred 60 mg/d d 1–7 q wk
CP[a]	–	–	250 mg/m^2 per d d 1–4 or 1,000 mg/m^2 IV	–	–	Pred 100 mg/d d 1–4 or Pred 50 mg qod
VMCP[b]	1 mg d 1	6 mg/m^2 per d d 1–4	125 mg/m^2 per d d 1–4	–	–	Pred 60 mg/m^2 per d d 1–4
VBAP[b]	1 mg d 1	–	–	30 mg/m^2 IV d 1	30 mg/m^2 IV d 1	Pred 60 mg/m^2 per d d 1–4
ABCM[c] (MacLennan et al. 1992)	–	6 mg/m^2 per d d 1–4	100 mg/m^2 per d d 1– 4	30 mg/m^2 IV d 1	30 mg/m^2 IV d 1	–
M-2 (Case et al. 1977[d]) (ECOG modification)	0.03 mg/kg IV d 1	0.25 mg/kg d 1–7	10 mg/kg IV d 1	0.5 mg/kg IV d 1	–	Pred 1 mg/kg d 1–7
MOCCA[d]	0.03 mg/kg IV d 1	0.25 mg/kg d 1–7	10 mg/kg IV d 1	CCNU 40 mg po d 1	–	0.8 mg/kg po d 1–7
VAD[d] (Barlogie et al. 1984)	0.2 mg/m^2 per d d 1–4 CI	–	–	–	9 mg/m^2 per d d 1–4 CI	Dex 40 mg/d d 1–4, 9–12, 17–20
VAMP* (Forgeson et al. 1988)	0.4 mg/d CI d 1–4	–	–	–	9 mg/m^2 per d CI	Methylpred 1 g/m^2 per d d 1–4

ABCM, VBAP/VMCP without vincristine or prednisone; ADR, doxorubicin (Adriamycin); BCNU, carmustine; CI, continuous infusion; CP, cyclophosphamide and prednisone; CTX, cyclophosphamide; d, day; gluco, corticosteroid; IV, intravenous; Mel, melphalan; MOCCA, VBMCP with CCNU replacing BCNU; M-2, VBMCP; MP, melphalan and prednisone; po, by mouth; q, every; qod, every other day; VAD, vincristine, doxorubicin, and dexamethasone; VAMP, vincristine, doxorubicin, and methylprednisolone; VBAP, vincristine, BCNU, doxorubicin, and prednisone; VCR, vincristine; VMCP, vincristine, melphalan, cyclophosphamide, and prednisone; wk, week.

[a] Repeated at 4- or 5-week intervals.

[b] VMCP and VBAP are commonly alternating every 3 weeks.

[c] AB and CM portions of regimen are given alternating every 3 weeks.

[d] Repeated every 5 weeks.

(1975), Eastern Cooperative Oncology Group (ECOG) (Oken et al. 1996a), and IBMTR/ABMTR (Bladé et al. 1998). Although all take into account hemoglobin, calcium, bone changes, and bone marrow plasmacytosis, the main distinction among them is their consideration of the serum and urine M components. With the exception of the old SWOG criteria (McLaughlin and Alexanian 1982), a partial response has been considered to be a 50% reduction in serum M component and a >50% to 90% reduction in urine M component. In the

Table 3.6. Response criteria

| Response | Study | % BMPC | M protein | | Duration, wk |
			Serum	Urine	
Complete response	CLMTF (Chronic Leukemia-Myeloma Task Force 1973)		Not defined		
	SWOG (McLaughlin and Alexanian 1982)	<1[a]	IF −	IF −	8
	IBMTR[b] (Bladé et al. 1998)	<5	IF −	IF −	6
Objective response	SWOG		↓≥75%[c]	↓≥90%	8
Improvement	SWOG		↓≥50%[c]	↓≥75%	8
	CLMTF[d]		↓≥50%	↓≥50%[e]	–
	ECOG		↓≥50%	↓≥90%	6
	IBMTR		↓≥50%	↓≥90%[f]	6
Stable, no change, or no response	SWOG		<±25%[c]	<±25%	–
	ECOG		Not CR, NCR, or PR		
	IBMTR		Neither MR nor progression		–
Plateau	ECOG		<±20%	<±20%	4
	IBMTR		<±25%	<±25%	12
Progression	SWOG		>25%[c]	>25%	–
	ECOG		≥50%[g]	≥50%[h]	–
	IBMTR	>25[i]	>25%[j]	>25%[h]	–

Other special categories include:

ECOG NCR, which includes <5% BMPC or CR by serum and urine but no confirmatory BM performed.

SWOG VGPR, which includes <5% BMPC, ≥90% reduction of serum M protein and ≤100 mg of urinary light chain excretion.

IBMTR/ABMTR MR, which includes 25% to 49% reduction of serum M protein and 50% to 89% reduction of 24-hour urinary light chain excretion, which still exceeds 200 mg per 24 hours.

BMPC, bone marrow plasma cells; CLMTF, Chronic Leukemia-Myeloma Task Force; CR, complete response; ECOG, Eastern Cooperative Oncology Group; IBMTR, International Blood and Bone Marrow Transplant Registry; IF, immunofixation; MR, minimum response; NCR, near complete response; PR, partial response; SWOG, Southwest Oncology Group.

[a] Clonal plasma cells as measured by cytoplasmic immunoglobulin flow cytometry.

[b] Makes allowance for nonsecretory myeloma and plasmacytomas.

[c] Change in synthetic index and not monoclonal protein concentration.

[d] Response also takes into account reduction in size of plasmacytomas, >2 g/dL Hb rise, weight gain, correction of calcium, renal function, albumin.

[e] If pretreatment value greater than 1 g/24 hours, then decrease to 50% or less of pretreatment value; if pretreatment value 0.5 to 1 g/24 hours, then decrease to less than 0.1 g/24 hours; otherwise, if pretreatment value less than 0.5 g/24 hours, variable should not be used to measure response.

[f] Or <200 mg/24 hours.

[g] Absolute increase must be at least 2 g/dL.

[h] Absolute increase must be greater than 200 mg/24 hours.

[i] Absolute increase must be at least 10%.

[j] Absolute increase must be greater than 0.5 g/dL.

earliest literature, response included such factors as increasing hemoglobin concentration or performance status, or decreasing blood urea nitrogen. Some authors have included a minimal response (25% to 49% reduction in serum M protein) as a response. Neither the CLMTF or SWOG originally had a complete response category, because it was unusual for the M protein to disappear completely. It was not until the advent of high-dose melphalan that investigators like Selby et al. (1987) began to define a complete remission category. Their definition, unlike more modern definitions, only included disappearance of M protein by electrophoresis, which is less sensitive than immunoelectrophoresis or immunofixation. Subsequent definitions have required immunofixation negativity to qualify as complete remission (Bladé et al. 1998). Up until about 1990, an SWOG objective response was a 75% reduction in the *tumor mass index* and an improvement was a 50% to 74% reduction in the tumor mass index (McLaughlin and Alexanian 1982).

The early Medical Research Council Myelomatosis trial evaluated the efficacy of treatment, not by the degree of paraprotein reduction but by the proportion of patients achieving plateau (MacLennan et al. 1992). There has been a new iteration of the SWOG response criteria over the last decade, and the M component (rather than the tumor mass index) is used as the primary measurement of the plasma cell burden. Currently, the serum and urine protein response groups include: 1) a partial response is a 50% reduction in the serum and urine M components, 2) a remission is a 75% reduction in the serum and a 90% reduction in the urine M components, and 3) a complete remission is total absence of any monoclonal protein by immunofixation of the serum or urine (personal communication with John Crowley). At Mayo, we have adopted the IBMTR/ABMTR criteria, and we incorporated the IFM's very good partial response category.

The roving denominator also creates challenges in interpreting therapeutic studies. Often an intention to treat analysis is not used to describe response rates or survival, which artificially inflates these end points. Definitions of evaluable patients may often include only those patients who received an adequate trial (3 or 6 months) of therapy, thereby excluding patients with early deaths or progression. In addition, in a steroid-responsive tumor like myeloma, coincident use of prednisone or dexamethasone as an antiemetic or therapy for hypercalcemia may seriously confound the results. Finally, the striking heterogeneity of prognosis in myeloma patients cannot be excluded as a major confounding factor in interpreting both phase 2 and 3 trials. Several prognostic indicators have been identified, including stage, β_2M, labeling index, renal function, and chromosomal abnormalities. Unfortunately, their predictive value is limited, only skimming the surface of myeloma biology and prognosis.

3.8.1.3 Efficacy of Single Chemotherapeutic Agents

3.8.1.3.1 Single Agent Efficacy of Melphalan

Bergsagel et al. demonstrated the benefit of melphalan in 14 of 24 patients with multiple myeloma. Others (Table 3.7) have substantiated that melphalan as a single agent results in response rates of 20% to 34% and median overall survival duration of 15 to 27 months (Bersagel et al. 1967; MacLennan et al. 1992; Rivers and Patno 1969; Sporn and McIntyre 1986).

3.8.1.3.2 Single Agent Efficacy of Cyclophosphamide

Korst et al. (Kyle 2000; Sporn and McIntyre 1986) were the first to report on the activity of oral cyclophosphamide. Twenty-four percent of multiple myeloma patients achieved a partial response (50% M-protein reduction), and 48% had objective improvement, that is, an improvement in the peripheral blood values, bone marrow findings, or serum blood urea nitrogen. Median survival was 24.5 months in all 207 patients and 32 months in the group that received at least 2 months of cyclophosphamide therapy. The single agent activity of cyclophosphamide has been demonstrated in a placebo-controlled trial (Rivers and Patno 1969) and in multiple studies in untreated patients (Medical Research Council's Working Party on Leukaemia in Adults 1980; Sporn and McIntyre 1986) and in those who relapsed or are refractory (Lenhard et al. 1994).

3.8.1.3.3 Single Agent Efficacy of Glucocorticoids

In 1950, Thorn et al. reported the first observations on the beneficial effects of adrenocorticotropic hormone on myeloma. During that decade, it was recognized that adrenocorticotropic hormone, cortisone, and prednisone decreased bone pain, improved hypercalcemia, increased hemoglobin values, and decreased abnormal serum and urine globulin concentrations. Subsequently,

Table 3.7. Early (1969 to 1982) randomized trials – untreated myeloma

Study	Agent	Schedule	N	RR, %	Overall survival, mo
Rivers and Patno, 1969	CTX	2–4 mg/kg per d	54	21	11.5[a]
	Placebo				3.5
Rivers and Patno, 1969	CTX	4 mg/kg per d	49	28	13
	M	0.1 mg/kg per d	54	34	15.5
Alexanian et al., 1969	M qd	0.025 mg/kg per d	35	17	18
	M intermittent	0.25 mg/kg d 1–4	69	32	18
	M alt. P	0.25 mg/kg d 1–4 & 1 mg/kg MWF	28	61	24
	M concurr. P	0.25 mg/kg d 1–4 & 2 mg/kg d 1–4	51	65	17
Medical Research Council's Working Party on Leukaemia in Adults, 1971	CTX	150 mg/d	114	NG	28[b]
	M	4 mg/d	105	NG	24[b]
Costa et al. 1973	M qd	0.15 mg/kg x 7, maintenance 0.05 kg per d	53	20	27 (30, 21)[c]
	M qd & P	M: as above & P: 1.25 mg/kg per d with taper 8 wk	70	39	NG (53, 9)
	M qd, P, & testosterone	M & P: as above & testosterone; 10 g/kg per wk	56	43	NG (36, 4)
Medical Research Council's Working Party on Leukaemia in Adults, 1980	MP	M: 10 mg/d d 1–7; P: 40 mg/d d 1–7 q 3 wk	174	NG	32[b, d]
	CTX IV	600 mg/m² q 3 wk	179	179	24
	MP	See above	71	NG	6[b, e]
	CMLP	C: 250 mg/m² po d 1–3; M: 5 mg/m² d 1–3; L: 50 mg/m² d 4; & P: 40 mg/m² d 1–3 q 4 wk	61	NG	6

Table continues on page 76.

high-dose corticosteroids (Table 3.6) have been shown to produce response rates of 40% to 50% and ~25% in previously untreated and refractory or relapsed patients, respectively (Alexanian et al. 1992; Gertz et al. 1995; Sporn and McIntyre 1986). Despite their contribution to quicker and more abundant responses, the data are conflicting as to whether corticosteroids prolong survival (Sporn and McIntyre 1986). The mechanism of action of this drug class is complex. Corticosteroids suppress the production of cytokines important in myeloma growth, like IL-6 and IL-1β, and reduce nuclear factor κB activity, resulting in enhanced apoptosis.

Table 3.7 (continued)

Study	Agent	Schedule	N	RR, %	Overall survival, mo
Cornwell et al., 1988	MP	M: 0.15 mg/kg d 1–7; P: 0.8 mg/kg with taper	100	44[f]	27
	Carmustine	Carmustine: 150 mg/m^2 IV; P: 0.8 mg/kg with taper	124	34	21
	Lomustine	Lomustine: 100 mg/m^2 qd; P: 0.8 mg/kg with taper	137	30	21

Alt, alternating; concurr., concurrently; CTX, cyclophosphamide; IV, intravenous; L, lomustine; M, melphalan; NG, not given; P, prednisone; po, by mouth; qd, daily.

[a] Overall survival is significant at $P=0.03$. No corticosteroids allowed in trial.

[b] Survival estimated from survival curves.

[c] Patients stratified for good and poor risk; median survival given as all patients (good risk, poor risk). Authors note that much quicker response observed with prednisone but worse survival with prednisone in poor-risk patients.

[d] Patients were required to have BUN ≤10 mM. Difference not significant ($P=0.16$).

[e] All patients had BUN >10 mM.

[f] Response rate between melphalan and lomustine arms significant. Median survival is not different.

3.8.1.3.4 Single Agent Efficacy of Vincristine

Alexanian et al. (1977) suggested that regimens that included vincristine resulted in better patient outcome than protocols not including this agent. The theory behind its posited utility was that after an initial kill by alkylating agents, the observed subsequent increase in mitotic index made myeloma cells more sensitive to vincristine. The report by Case et al. (1977) has been cited as confirmatory evidence for activity of vincristine in myeloma. However, several randomized controlled trials do not support this premise (Sporn and McIntyre 1986; Tribalto et al. 1985). The most compelling of these is the MRC IV Trial in Myelomatosis, which randomized 530 newly diagnosed myeloma patients to monthly melphalan and prednisone, with or without monthly vincristine. Median survival in both arms was 26 months (MacLennan et al. 1992). Although never evaluated as a single agent in newly diagnosed myeloma, vincristine has little activity as a single agent in refractory disease. Twenty-one patients were treated with 0.5 mg bolus followed by 0.25 to 0.5 mg/m^2 per day as a continuous infusion over 5 days on a 3-week schedule. Two patients had transient responses (1.2 and 2.2 months). Finally, the activity credited to vincristine as a maintenance therapy is also ambiguous.

3.8.1.3.5 Single Agent Efficacy of Anthracyclines

Doxorubicin is the most commonly used anthracycline in the treatment of myeloma, but it has not been studied as a single agent in newly diagnosed myeloma patients. Its activity as a single agent in relapsed or refractory disease is modest, with response rates of about 10% (Alberts et al. 1976). A phase 2 trial of mitoxantrone as a single agent yielded a partial response rate of 3% (1 of 35 patients). An additional 4 patients showed clinical improvement lasting 4 to 7 months. Idarubicin is another anthracycline that has been studied in the context of multiple myeloma. Response rates of 0% to 27% have been observed in relapsed and refractory patients with single agent oral regimens.

3.8.1.3.6 Single Agent Efficacy of Etoposide

In relapsed and refractory disease, single agent etoposide has minimal activity; in 85 patients the response rate was <5%. However, Barlogie et al. (1989) treated 14 patients with 200 mg/m^2 by continuous infusion, and 2 responded. In addition, there are 2 anecdotal reports of activity of low-dose oral etoposide.

3.8.1.3.7 Single Agent Efficacy of Nitrosoureas

The nitrosoureas have single agent activity in myeloma. In a randomized trial of 361 previously untreated patients (Table 3.7), objective response frequency with carmustine (BCNU) (40%) and lomustine (CCNU) (42%) was lower than that of melphalan (59%), although the survivals for all groups were not significantly different (Sporn and McIntyre 1986).

3.8.1.3.8 Single Agent Efficacy of Interferon

Since the original report by Mellstedt et al. of activity of human leukocyte interferon in patients with myeloma, multiple studies have confirmed the findings with daily human leukocyte interferon (3–9 MU/day) and with recombinant interferon-α. Although the earliest studies suggested response rates of up to 60%, subsequent studies yielded rates of 15% to 20% (Myeloma Trialists' Collaborative Group 2001). Toxicity was not inconsequential. In vitro activity had good predictive value for in vivo clinical response in 26 patients studied. In vitro, interferon has a stimulatory effect in about one-third of patients' myeloma samples.

3.8.1.3.9 Single Agent Efficacy of Thalidomide

Recognition of the role of increased angiogenesis in the pathogenesis and progression of myeloma and evidence of thalidomide's antiangiogenic properties led to clinical trials in multiple myeloma. The observed responses in patients without high-grade angiogenesis suggest that thalidomide may act via other mechanisms. The actual antitumor mechanism is likely complex. In vitro data suggest that the drug and its metabolites may inhibit angiogenesis, modulate adhesion molecules of myeloma cells and their surrounding stroma, modulate cytokines, and affect natural killer cells. There is recent evidence that thalidomide and its analogs induce apoptosis and G_1 growth arrest in myeloma cells.

Multiple studies have confirmed the initial observation of Singhal et al. that thalidomide as a single agent in relapsed myeloma produces response rates in the range of 25% to 45%. Median response duration is 9 to 12 months, and 2-year progression-free survival is 10% to 20%. Thalidomide is now considered a standard therapy for multiple myeloma, although Food and Drug Administration approval for this indication is pending.

3.8.1.3.10 Single Agent Efficacy of Other Agents

Barlogie et al. (1989) explored the utility of cisplatin therapy for patients with myeloma. Fourteen patients were treated with 10 mg/m² for 7 days by continuous infusion, and 2 responded. The drug has been incorporated into other regimens for relapsed disease (Barlogie et al. 1989) and induction (Barlogie et al. 1999).

Cytosine arabinoside, teniposide, topotecan, deoxycoformycin, and paclitaxel have been reported to produce response rates of 7%, 28%, 16%, 0% to 15%, and 15% to 29%, respectively. Topotecan induces significant toxicity including $\geq$ grade 3 granulocytopenia and thrombocytopenia in 93% and 53% of patients, respectively. Patients treated with paclitaxel were premedicated with 40 mg of dexamethasone every 21 days, bringing into question whether the observed responses were to dexamethasone or paclitaxel.

Agents that do not appear to have any activity in myeloma include drugs that are interesting from a historical perspective and drugs that have known activity in other diseases. Agents in the former category include diamidines like stilbamidine, 1-aminocyclopentanecarboxylic acid, amsacrine, aclarubicin, chlorozotocin, hexamethylmelamine, and azaserine. Other commonly used agents without activity against myeloma include methotrexate, 6-mercaptopurine, 6-thioguanine, 5-fluorouracil, fluorodeoxyuridine, hydroxyurea, mitomycin C, vinblastine, vindesine, carboplatin, bleomycin, ATRA (all trans-retinoic acid), fludarabine, and 2-chlorodeoxyadenosine. Although Durie et al. reported a 57% response rate with clarithromycin, subsequent reports did not verify this response rate, and the activity observed in the original report was attributed to concurrent corticosteroid therapy.

3.8.1.4   Induction Chemotherapy Regimens

3.8.1.4.1   Single Agent With or Without Corticosteroids for Induction

3.8.1.4.1.1 Melphalan as Induction Therapy

Since early reports by Blokhin et al. and Bergsagel et al., various schedules of melphalan have been tried, including continuous daily dose, 6 to 10 mg/day for 2 to 3 weeks, followed by maintenance therapy of 0.01 to 0.03 mg/kg per day; intermittent total doses of 0.25 mg/day given for 4 days every 4 to 8 weeks; or 0.15 mg/kg per day for 7 days every 6 weeks. Several studies suggest that the intermittent schedule is superior to continuous daily dosing (Sporn and McIntyre 1986).

The combination of melphalan and prednisone (Table 3.7) has been studied extensively. Response rates are 40% to 60% and anticipated median survivals are 18 to 42 months (Medical Research Council's Working Party on Leukaemia in Adults 1980; Myeloma Trialists' Collaborative Group 1998). Because of the variable gastrointestinal tract absorption of melphalan, intravenous regimens of 15 to 25 mg/m² every 4 weeks along with oral prednisone or dexamethasone have been tried and resulted in response rates of 50% to 82%.

Not until the report by McElwain and Powles (1983) on the successful use of high-dose melphalan (140 mg/m² intravenously) had dose intensity been studied in myeloma. In previously untreated patients, Selby et al. (1987) confirmed a 78% response rate, including 27% of patients whose M component was no longer visible by protein electrophoresis. This dose intensity without stem cell salvage was associated with prolonged, severe thrombocytopenia and leukopenia (lasting a median of 24 and 28 days, respectively). Treatment-related mortality was 19%. The benefit of melphalan dose intensification was confirmed by others who have used attenuated doses (50 to 70 mg/m²) and reported response rates of 50% to 85% (Barlogie et al. 1988).

3.8.1.4.1.2 Cyclophosphamide as Induction Therapy

Since the original report by Korst et al. (Kyle 2000; Sporn and McIntyre 1986) of the utility of cyclophosphamide in myeloma patients, several single agent induction regimens have been studied. Despite documented equivalency for low-dose oral regimens of cyclophosphamide and melphalan, induction therapies of melphalan and prednisone tend to be preferred over those of cyclophosphamide and prednisone. The focus of study of cyclophosphamide for myeloma has been as an agent in multidrug combinations for induction, in relapse, and in stem cell mobilization. For newly diagnosed myeloma, however, oral daily dosing of cyclophosphamide (150 mg/d) or intravenously at dose levels of 600 mg/m² every 3 weeks with or without prednisone has resulted in a response rate of approximately 25% and median survival of 24 months (Sporn and McIntyre 1986).

3.8.1.4.1.3 Corticosteroids as Induction Therapy

In previously untreated patients, approximately 43% have a 75% decrement in their *tumor mass index* with single agent high-dose dexamethasone therapy (Table 3.8) (Alexanian et al. 1992), which is only 15% lower than for vincristine, doxorubicin, and dexamethasone (VAD). Dexamethasone, in lieu of VAD for induction, in those patients destined for stem cell collection may be potentially advantageous. With single agent dexamethasone, insertion of a long-term central venous catheter can be postponed until conditioning for the stem cell transplantation, thereby reducing the likelihood of catheter-related complications (ie, thrombosis and infection). This strategy has been used successfully in this context, resulting in adequate collection of peripheral blood stem cells without any apparent adverse effect on complete remission rate or progression-free survival in a single-arm study.

3.8.1.4.1.4 Interferon as Induction Therapy

Although the earliest studies of interferon suggested response rates of up to 60%, subsequent studies produced rates of 15% to 20% (Myeloma Trialists' Collaborative Group 2001). Ahre et al. randomized 55 patients to either melphalan and prednisone or interferon (3–6 MU daily); response rates in the melphalan and prednisone arm were significantly higher than in the interferon arm (44% versus 14%, $P < 0.001$).

3.8.1.4.1.5 Thalidomide as Induction Therapy

Thalidomide represents a new and distinct class of agents with significant activity against myeloma. When thalidomide is used as a single agent in previously untreated patients, response rates of about 35% may be achieved (Rajkumar et al. 2001; Weber et al. 2003). The combination of thalidomide and dexamethasone in previously untreated patients results in response rates of 68% to 72% (Rajkumar et al. 2002; Weber et al. 2003). Limited use of thalidomide pre-stem cell mobilization does not appear to impair stem cell collection or engraftment, although we tend to collect stem cells in patients after approximately 4 months of treatment. We typically suggest that patients have at least a 2-week washout period prior to stem cell mobilization efforts.

Table 3.8. Corticosteroids

Study	Agent	Schedule	Disease status	N	RR, %	Overall survival, mo
Adams and Skoog (Kyle 2000)	Cortico-steroids	Various	All	NG	NG	NG
McIntyre et al. (Sporn and McIntyre 1986)	Pred	1.2 mg/kg per day → 70-day taper	Untr	32	44	21
Alexanian et al., 1992	Dex	40 mg/d d 1–4, 9–12, & 17–20; repeat every 42 d	Untr	112	43 [a]	NG
Salmon et al., 1998	Pred	200 mg qod×8 wk → 100 mg qod ×4 → 50 mg qod	Ref, rel	10	80	NG
Alexanian et al. (Alexanian et al. 1992)	Pred	60 mg/m² d 1–5, 9–14, & 17–21; repeat every 42 d	Ref, rel	11	19 [a]	NG
Alexanian et al., 1992	Dex	40 mg d 1–4, 9–12, 17–20 q 5 wk	Ref Rel	30 19	27 [a] 21 [a]	NG
Forgeson et al., 1988	Methylpred	1 g/m² (max 1.5 g) d 1–5 q 21 d	Res Rel All	10 4	10 25	 10
Gertz et al., 1995	Methylpred	2 g tiw×8 wk, → 2 g/wk	Ref, rel	20	25	NG

Dex, dexamethasone; methylpred, methylprednisolone; NG, not given; po, by mouth; q, every; qd, daily; qod; every other day; ref, refractory; rel, relapsed; res, resistant; tiw, 3 times a week; untr, untreated.

[a] According to SWOG response criteria, response according to tumor mass index.

3.8.1.4.2 Combination Chemotherapy (CCT) for Induction

A combination of the multiple active agents in an effort to achieve synergy was a logical corollary. For expediency, these regimens can be separated into 4 categories: alkylator-based without anthracycline, anthracycline-containing regimen, anthracycline-containing with intensified doses of corticosteroids, and induction regimens incorporating interferon. Thirty years of study indicate that multiagent combination chemotherapy as initial therapy results in higher response rates, but not longer overall survival, than standard melphalan and prednisone (Myeloma Trialists' Collaborative Group 1998). Although there has been a suggestion that patients with more advanced disease benefit from combination chemotherapy as compared to melphalan (Cooper et al. 1986; MacLennan et al. 1992), that hypothesis has not been borne out (Myeloma Trialists' Collaborative Group 1998). In time, when we are better able to ascertain biologic differences between myeloma patients and properly classify them in a similar fashion to what is done in the field of lymphoma, a survival benefit with multiagent chemotherapy may be detected in particular subgroups.

3.8.1.4.2.1 Alkylator-based Combination Chemotherapy Without Anthracycline for Induction

The 1970s and 1980s were a testing ground for various combinations of alkylators, corticosteroids, and doxorubicin. Melphalan/cyclophosphamide/prednisone, carmustine/cyclophosphamide/prednisone, melphalan/cyclophosphamide/carmustine/prednisone (MCBP), and vincristine/melphalan/cyclophosphamide/prednisone

(VMCP) resulted in response rates of 47%, 37% to 50%, 49% to 68%, and 62%, respectively (Alexanian et al. 1977). Median survivals with these regimens were 25 to 36 months. Case et al. (1977) introduced the 5-drug regimen of vincristine/carmustine/melphalan/cyclophosphamide/prednisone (VBMCP or the M-2 regimen), which included the same 4 drugs as MCBP plus vincristine; dose intensities, however, were different in these 2 regimens. Response rate for VBMCP was about 85% in previously untreated patients with a median survival of 38 months (Case et al. 1977). The success of the VBMCP regimen supported the value of vincristine. However, the MRC IV trial, which randomized 530 previously untreated patients with myeloma to melphalan and prednisone versus melphalan/vincristine/prednisone, revealed no difference in either response rate or overall survival between the 2 arms (MacLennan et al. 1992). VBMCP has not produced any response or survival advantage over melphalan and prednisone. Finally, the MOCCA regimen, which is essentially VBMCP with CCNU replacing BCNU, results in response rates similar to those for VBMCP (75%), but again a survival no different from melphalan and prednisone (Myeloma Trialists' Collaborative Group 1998).

Although subsequent randomized trials have substantiated the superior response rates of VBMCP over standard melphalan and prednisone (Table 3.9), they have not demonstrated superior survival. In fact, the meta-analysis performed by the Myeloma Trialists' Collaborative Group (1998), which included 6,633 patients and 27 randomized trials, revealed a superior response rate (60.2% versus 53.2%, $P < 0.000001$, 2-tailed) but no survival benefit for combination chemotherapy over standard melphalan and prednisone. A prior meta-analysis of 18 published trials (3,814 patients) also demonstrated no benefit for combination chemotherapy in terms of survival (Fig. 3.9). There might be a survival advantage in the subgroup of patients with more aggressive disease, but this has not been substantiated (Myeloma Trialists' Collaborative Group 1998).

3.8.1.4.2.2 Combination Chemotherapy With Anthracycline for Induction

Alkylator- and doxorubicin-based combination chemotherapy arose from the report that the combination of doxorubicin and BCNU was beneficial in patients who had become resistant to melphalan (Alberts et al. 1976). Regimens like MAP (melphalan, doxorubicin,

and prednisone), CAP (cyclophosphamide, doxorubicin, and prednisone), VCAP (vincristine and CAP), and VBAP (vincristine, BCNU, doxorubicin, and prednisone) were tried; by SWOG response criteria, objective response rates were 41%, 46%, 64%, and 61% (Alexanian et al. 1977). Median survival ranged from 30 to 32 months; subsequent analysis demonstrated a superior median survival for the VBAP arm of 37 months (Crowley et al. 2001).

Enthusiasm for alternating VMCP and VBAP (or VCAP) was generated by the SWOG study of 237 patients randomized to melphalan and prednisone or these other 2 regimens (Table 3.9). Response rates were superior in the alternating combination chemotherapy arms compared to the melphalan arm. Survival was also superior in the combination chemotherapy arms (43 months versus 23 months for melphalan and prednisone, $P = 0.004$). A subsequent analysis with longer follow-up showed less separation of the survival curves (median survival, 25 versus 36 months) (Crowley et al. 2001). The extent of survival benefit of this initial study has not been reproduced (Myeloma Trialists' Collaborative Group 1998).

The V MRC myelomatosis trial randomized patients to ABCM (VBAP/VMCP without the vincristine or prednisone) or melphalan as a single agent on the basis of their findings in the IV MRC trial, which demonstrated an absence of benefit of vincristine. Median survival in the ABCM group was superior to that of the melphalan only arm (32 versus 24 months, $P = 0.0003$) (MacLennan et al. 1992).

3.8.1.4.2.3 Combination Chemotherapy With Doxorubicin and Dose-Intensive Corticosteroids for Induction

The next level of combination chemotherapy includes those programs that include anthracycline and also contain high-dose corticosteroids. VAD-like regimens are commonly used as induction therapy pre–stem cell collection and transplantation. These regimens include VAP, VAD (Barlogie et al. 1984), VAMP (vincristine, doxorubicin, methylprednisolone), and C-VAMP (cyclophosphamide and VAMP) (Forgeson et al. 1988), all of which had been tried with salutary effect in relapsed disease. Subsequently, several of these regimens were applied in previously untreated patients and response rates were 50% to 84% (Alexanian et al. 1990). Median survival for patients treated initially with VAD is about

Table 3.9. MP vs. combination chemotherapy as induction: selected randomized trials

Study	Regimen	N	RR, %[a]	Overall survival, mo	P (RR)	P (OS)
SWOG 727/1972	MP	125	40[b]	28	NS	NS
	MP-Pcb	116	47	31		
SECSG 343/1984	MP	187	29	36	NS	NS
	BCP	186	37	36		
CALGB 7161/1979	MP	126	56	NG	0.047	NS
	MCBP	124	68			
NCI-C-MY1/1979	MP	125	40[b]	28	NS	NS
	MCBP	239	39	31		
ECOG 4472/1982	MP	92	40	19	NS	NS
	BCP	96	50	25		
GATLA3-M-73/1980 & 1988	MP	67	40	38	NS	NS
	CP-MeCCNU	83	40	30		
GATLA3-M-77/1984 & 1988	MP	145	33	42	NS	NS
	MPCV-MeCCNU	115	44	44		
Pavia MM-75/1986	MP	39	41	54	NS	0.039
	Pept-VP	36	58	26		
SWOG 7704/1983 & 1986	MP	77	32[b]	23		
	VMCP/VCAP	80	58	43	0.001	0.004[c]
	VMCP/VBAP	80	49	43	0.028	
MDA7704/1984	MP	30	53[b]	38	NS	NS
	VMCP/VCAP	42	55	27		
	VMCP/VBAP	34	60	28		
CALGB 7761/1986	MP (IV)	146	47	34	NS	[d]
	MCBP	140	56	29		
	Seq-MCBP	148	47	22		
	MCBPA	157	44	26		
IMMSG M-77/1985	MP	47	19[b]	30	NS	NS
	VMCP	53	19	45		
	BC-Pept	33	3	58		
Gentofte, Denmark/1985	MP	31	45	21	NS	NS
	VMP	32	73	30		
	VBMCP	33	58	21		
ECOG 2479/1997	MP	230	51	27	< 0.0001	NS
	VBMCP	235	72	29	1	
MRC MYEL-4/1985	MP	261	NG	26	NS	NS
	VMP	269		26		
Finnish MM80/1987	MP	66	54	41	<0.02	NS
	MOCCA	64	75	45		
Norwegian trial/1986 & 1988	MP	48	48	29	NS	NS
	VBMCP	44	54	33		

Table 3.9 (continued)

Study	Regimen	N	RR, %[a]	Overall survival, mo	P (RR)	P (OS)
MGCS stage III/1989	MP	44	61	28	NS	NS
	VMCP/VBAP	42	52	24		
GMTG MM01/1988 & 1991	MP	170	33[b]	60%	NS	<0.02
	VMCP	150	33	4 y		
MGCS stage II/1990	MP	29	69	46	NS	NS
	VMCP	25	56	33		
MGCS stage III/1990	MP	55	58	26	NS	NS
	VMCP/VBAP	53	57	24		
IMMSG M-83/1991	MP	146	64	37	0.02	NS
	VMCP/VBAP	158	77	32		
PETHEMA 85/1993	MP	247	32	27	0.004	NS
	VMCP/VBAP	241	45	32		
Pavia 1986/1994	MP	87	24	All 24	NS	NS
	Pept-VP	83	24			
NMSG/1993	MP	74	64	31	NS	0.02
	NOP	77	60	14		
GMTG MM02/1995	MP (IV)[e]	99	43	~37	0.01	NS
	VBAMD[e]	105	64			
Meta-analysis (Myeloma Trialists' Collaborative Group 1998)	MP vs. CCT	6633	53	29	<0.00001	NS
			60	29		

A, doxorubicin; B, BCNU or carmustine; C, cyclophosphamide; CCT, combination chemotherapy; D, dexamethasone; IV, intravenous; M, melphalan; MeCCNU, methyl-CCNU; MOCCA, the additional C is for CCNU (lomustine); NG, not given; NOP, mitoxantrone, vincristine, and prednisone; NS, not significant; P, prednisone; Pcb, procarbazine; Pept, peptichemo; V, vincristine.

[a] Except where stated, response is according to Myeloma Task Force criteria or modification.

[b] SWOG response criteria.

[c] Significantly superior survival in combination chemotherapy arms compared to MP in the 174 stage III patients but not in the 74 stage I or II patients.

[d] The sequential arm was significantly worse than either the MP (P=0.01) or the MCBP (P=0.02) and marginally worse than MCBPA (P=0.09).

[e] Part of an interferon trial; stage III patients only.

Data from Myeloma Trialists' Collaborative Group (1998).

36 months. The complete response rate of C-VAMP is higher than for VAMP alone, but survival is no different. Several other variations have been reported in which alternative anthracyclines or corticosteroids were used.

In a randomized trial of 151 patients comparing the NOP regimen (mitoxantrone, vincristine, and high-dose prednisone) to melphalan and prednisone, response rates were equivalent (~60%), but overall survival was inferior in the NOP arm (14 versus 31 months,

P=0.02). Response rates of 80% have also been achieved using the CAD (cyclophosphamide, doxorubicin, dexamethasone) regimen. The addition of etoposide to C-VAD appears to contribute only toxicity.

3.8.1.4.2.4 Combination Chemotherapy With Interferon for Induction

Interferon has been combined with melphalan and prednisone; VMCP; VMCP/VBAP; prednisone, cyclophos-

Fig. 3.10. Interferon (*IFN*) chemotherapy as induction or maintenance therapy influences progression-free and overall survival curves from the meta-analysis by the Myeloma Trialists' Collaborative Group. Results from 24 randomized trials and 4,012 patients. Interferon curves include patients who received interferon as part of induction or of maintenance program. *A,* Progression-free survival after 23 months with interferon and 17 months without. *B,* Overall median survival after 40 months with interferon and 36 months without. (From the Myeloma Trialists' Collaborative Group [2001]. By permission of Blackwell Science.)

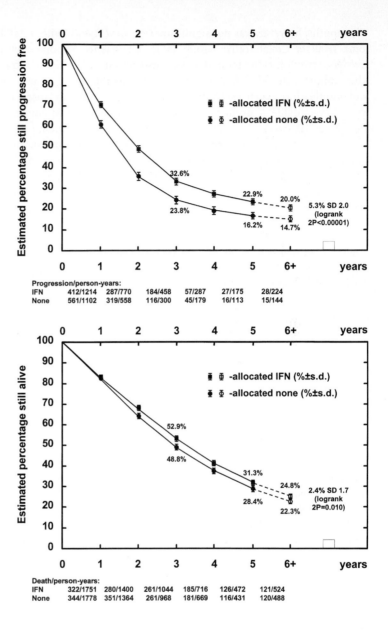

Progression/person-years:
IFN   412/1214   287/770   184/458   57/287   27/175   28/224
None   561/1102   319/558   116/300   45/179   16/113   15/144

Death/person-years:
IFN   322/1751   280/1400   261/1044   185/716   126/472   121/524
None   344/1778   351/1364   261/968   181/669   116/431   120/488

phamide, doxorubicin (Adriamycin), and carmustine (BCNU) (PCAB); VAD; VBMCP; VBAP; and cyclophosphamide as part of an induction regimen. Results have been mixed. Two meta-analyses have been performed in an attempt to reconcile these conflicting results (Ludwig and Fritz 2000; Myeloma Trialists' Collaborative Group 2001). The first, published in 2000 by Ludwig and Fritz, used published data and included 17 induction trials with 2,333 evaluable patients; the second, reported by the Myeloma Trialists' Collaborative Group in 2001, used primary data from 12 induction trials involving 2,469 pa-

tients. Overall, the results were similar. In the former analysis, the benefits of inclusion of interferon in an induction regimen were a 6.6% higher response rate (*P* < 0.002) and a 4.8-month and 3.1-month prolongation of relapse-free (*P* < 0.01) and overall survival (*P* < 0.01) (Ludwig and Fritz 2000). In the second meta-analysis, patients receiving interferon had a slightly better response rate (57.5% versus 53.1%, *P* = 0.01) and progression-free survival (30% versus 25% at 3 years, *P* < 0.0003), with a superior median time to progression of about 6 months (Fig. 3.10). The survival advantage of 2 months, however, was not significant ($P = 0.1$) (Myeloma Trialists' Collaborative Group 2001). A cost-effectiveness estimation for induction was also performed. The authors concluded that interferon administration and monitoring expenses amounted to $US 41,319.28 to save a year of life of myeloma patients, assuming a dosage of 12.1 MU/week (Ludwig and Fritz 2000).

These meta-analyses suggest that incorporation of interferon into induction provides a modest prolongation of response and possibly of survival (Fig. 3.10). The question remains, however, whether these significant differences are clinically relevant.

3.8.2 Hematopoietic Stem Cell Transplantation

3.8.2.1 Autologous Transplant

To overcome resistance of the myeloma cells to conventional-dose chemotherapy, McElwain and Powles (1983) pioneered the use of high-dose melphalan to treat multiple myeloma and plasma cell leukemia. The treatment was complicated by prolonged myelosuppression, and bone marrow (and later peripheral blood stem cell) support was subsequently incorporated. Barlogie et al. (1988) used a regimen combining high-dose melphalan with total body irradiation supported by autologous bone marrow transplantation in multiple myeloma patients refractory to VAD.

Cure rarely if ever occurs, and almost all patients relapse after autologous stem cell transplantation. Although high-dose therapy followed by autologous stem cell transplantation is not curative, it improves response rate and survival (Barlogie et al. 1988; Dalton et al. 2001; Hahn et al. 2003; Harousseau and Attal 2002). Response rates with transplantation are 75% to 90%, and complete response rates are 20% to 40%. The results of single institution and phase 2 trials are difficult to analyze because selection of patients for transplantation is subject to selection bias regarding the stage of disease, performance status, age, and renal function.

The Intergroupe Français du Myelome (Attal et al. 1996) published the first randomized trial comparing high-dose chemotherapy followed by autologous bone marrow transplantation with conventional chemotherapy (Fig. 3.11). Two hundred patients with previously untreated multiple myeloma were randomized to receive high-dose chemotherapy followed by an autologous bone marrow transplantation or a combination of intravenous chemotherapy. The 5-year event-free survival (28% vs. 10%) and overall survival rates (52% vs. 12%) were higher

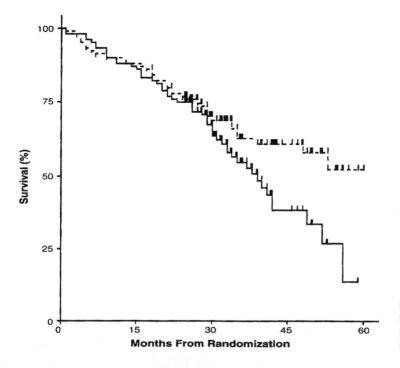

Fig. 3.11. Attal transplant curve. Dashed curve, high dose; solid curve, low dose. (From Attal et al. [1996]. By permission of the Massachusetts Medical Society.)

in the transplantation group. An updated analysis with a median follow-up of 7 years confirmed that high-dose chemotherapy improves event-free survival (median, 28 months vs. 18 months) as well as overall survival (median, 57 months vs. 44 months) (Dalton et al. 2001).

Autologous peripheral blood stem cell transplantation has replaced autologous bone marrow transplantation because engraftment is more rapid and there is less contamination with myeloma cells (Hahn et al. 2003). Hematopoietic stem cells should be collected before the patient is exposed to alkylating agents, because prolonged prior melphalan exposure predicts impaired collection of peripheral blood stem cells when either chemotherapy/growth factor or growth factor alone (Hahn et al. 2003) mobilization strategy is used. Even after 4 to 6 cycles of VMCP/VBAP, which is a regimen containing low doses of melphalan, in approximately 10% of patients, sufficient stem cells could not be collected for stem cell transplantation (Attal et al. 1996). In contrast, successful stem cell collection is achieved in 95% to 100% of multiple myeloma patients treated with VAD before mobilization with high-dose cyclophosphamide. The absolute number of $CD34^+$ cells/kg is the most reliable and practical method for determining the adequacy of a stem cell collection. The mortality rate from autologous stem cell transplantation is currently less than 5%. Age older than 65 years is not a contraindication for transplantation, although there are no randomized data proving or disproving its utility in this age group. Such patients are candidates for transplantation if they have good functional status and limited comorbidity (Hahn et al. 2003) (Fig. 3.8).

3.8.2.1.1 Transplantation for Primary Refractory Myeloma

In contrast to the experience with malignant lymphoma, stem cell transplantation appears to be effective for patients with primary resistant disease (Hahn et al. 2003). Patients with multiple myeloma in whom first-line therapy such as VAD fails can be sensitive to high-dose chemotherapy with stem cell reconstitution. In 1995 Alexanian et al. reported a decrease of 75% in tumor burden in 56% of patients and a marked improvement in survival compared with matched historical controls. Rajkumar et al. also looked at stem cell transplantation in primary refractory disease in 1999 and found no differences in overall and complete response rates between patients with primary refractory and relapsed disease.

The median survival of the entire cohort from diagnosis was 53 months.

3.8.2.1.2 Single Versus Double Transplantation

The role of double or tandem autologous stem cell transplantation is controversial. Barlogie and colleagues at the University of Arkansas advocate this approach of tandem (double) autologous stem cell transplantation to improve complete response rates and survival (Barlogie et al. 1999; Hahn et al. 2003). In tandem transplantation, patients receive a second planned transplant on recovery from the first procedure. In a study of 231 patients with newly diagnosed myeloma, the overall survival with this approach was 68 months (Barlogie et al. 1999). About 50% of patients in this cohort were age 50 years or younger and had less than stage III disease. These results have prompted several studies of stem cell transplantation in myeloma.

Preliminary data from 4 different randomized trials indicated a slight increase in response rates and possibly event-free survival with tandem transplantation (Dalton et al. 2001), but no clear improvement in overall survival (Table 3.10). As presented at the American Society of Hematology in 1997, with 2-year follow-up, there was no difference in event-free or overall survival between double and single autologous stem cell transplant in the IFM 94 trial that included 403 patients from France. In another evaluation of this study (Dalton et al. 2001), a subgroup of patients – those receiving stem cells derived from the peripheral blood rather than the bone marrow – had a modest overall survival benefit with tandem transplantation. There is no obvious explanation for the observed difference in survival between the groups. Most recently, the authors have reported in abstract form that this study is positive. Though the response rate was not significantly different between the 2 groups (complete response and very good partial response 42% in the single-transplant arm versus 50% of patients in the double-transplant group, $P = 0.15$), both event-free survival and overall survival were improved in the double-transplant arm. Median survival in the 2 arms was not different, but the 7-year postdiagnosis probability of event-free survival was 20% (95% CI, 14–26) in the double-transplant arm versus 10% (95% CI, 5–15) in the single-transplant arm ($P < 0.03$). Respective 7-year postdiagnosis overall survival rates were 42% (95% CI, 34–49) and 21% (95% CI, 13–29, $P < 0.01$). In this trial 4 factors were associated with a

Table 3.10. Single versus double hematopoietic stem cell transplantation, randomized trials

Study	N	FU, mo	Event-free survival, % (years FU)			Overall survival, % (years FU)		
			Single	Double	P	Single	Double	P
IFM	403	60	19 (6)	28 (6)	0.03	26 (6)	46 (6)	0.02
Hovon	255	29	35 (3)	36 (3)	NS	47 (4)	43 (4)	NS
Bologna	178	30	21 mo (median)	29 mo (median)	NS	74 (4)	71 (4)	NS
MAG	193	27	41 events	43 events	NS	27 deaths	22 deaths	NS

FU, follow-up; NS, not significant.

Modified from Dalton et al. (2001). By permission of the American Society of Hematology.

longer survival: low β_2-microglobulin at diagnosis ($P<0.01$), young age ($P<0.05$), low LDH at diagnosis ($P<0.01$), and treatment arm ($P<0.05$). The final results of this and the other 3 trials listed in Table 3.10 will provide a definitive answer to the question of tandem transplantation. Because the role of tandem or double transplantation is not settled, it is reasonable to harvest enough stem cells for 2 transplants.

3.8.2.1.3 Timing of Transplantation

The timing of the transplantation, either up front as consolidation therapy or as salvage therapy at the time of relapse, is also a point of controversy. In one study (Fermand et al. 1998), 185 patients were treated with 1 to 2 cycles of intensified CHOP followed by PBSC collection and then randomized to 3 or 4 courses of VAMP followed by high-dose chemotherapy and autologous stem cell transplantation or to conventional chemotherapy (VMCP) until stable plateau, followed by autologous transplantation at disease progression. The median survival was essentially the same in both groups (65 months vs. 64 months). From the time of randomization, the median event-free survival in the early transplant group was 39 months compared with 13 months in the delayed transplant group. The main advantage of early transplantation was the avoidance of the inconvenience and cost of chemotherapy (Fermand et al. 1998). The North American Intergroup Study (S9321) is a larger randomized trial comparing early to late transplantation. It met its accrual goal of approximately 1,000 patients in October 2000. Results of this trial are not yet available.

3.8.2.1.4 Conditioning Therapy and Stem Cell Transplantation

In an effort to improve autologous stem cell transplantation, various preparative regimens have been used. There has been only one prospective randomized controlled trial comparing conditioning regimens in patients with myeloma (Moreau et al. 2002). Moreau et al. (2002) randomized 282 patients to either melphalan (140 mg/m²) plus total body irradiation or melphalan alone (200 mg/m²). There was no difference in response rate or event-free survival. Survival at 45 months favored the melphalan alone arm (65.8% vs. 45.5%, $P = 0.05$). Toxicity with melphalan alone was significantly less. Most investigators have now discontinued the use of total body irradiation and give only melphalan (200 mg/m²) as the preparative regimen. Studies are being conducted with skeletal targeted radiation, ie, beta-emitting phosphonates that localize to bone.

3.8.2.1.5 The Role of Purging

In the setting of autologous stem cell transplant, there was concern regarding the role of potentially contaminated autograft in relapse. Purging marrow with cyclophosphamide derivatives or with monoclonal antibodies (Hahn et al. 2003) has proven feasible although associated with prolonged myelosuppression after transplantation. Schiller et al. demonstrated that CD34⁻ selection of peripheral blood progenitor cells could provide effective hematopoietic support in a group of 55 patients with advanced multiple myeloma after myeloablative chemotherapy. Subsequently, 2 large phase 3 randomized trials have shown no clinical benefit to using CD34⁺ selected autologous peripheral blood stem cells.

3.8.2.2 Allogeneic Transplant

Allogeneic transplantation eliminates the problem of tumor cell contamination of the stem cells that is inevitable with autologous stem cell transplantation. Further, there is evidence of a graft-versus-myeloma effect with allografting (Tricot et al. 1996). Allogeneic transplantation can lead to prolonged disease-free survival in a relatively small percentage of patients (Hahn et al. 2003). The high treatment-related mortality (approximately 30%) and significant toxicity from graft-versus-host disease have limited the role of this procedure in the treatment of myeloma (Bensinger et al. 1996; Gahrton et al. 1991) (Table 3.11). There have been 4 case-control or cohort-control studies comparing autologous to allogeneic stem cell transplant. The largest of these is that of Bjorkstrand et al. In their retrospective analysis of data compiled by the European Blood and Marrow Transplantation Group, there was inferior survival for myeloma patients treated with allogeneic bone marrow transplant compared to case-matched controls treated with autologous transplant (18 months versus 36 months) (Bjorkstrand et al. 1996). The 3 other smaller studies, which had relatively short follow-up, have shown mixed results with regard to progression-free survival and overall survival; transplant-related mortality, however, is consistently higher in the allogeneic groups (19%–25%).

In an effort to reduce transplant-related mortality, Lokhorst et al. (2000) (Table 3.11) compared autologous stem cell transplant to T-cell–depleted allogeneic stem cell transplant (Hahn et al. 2003). Myeloma patients were eligible if they had chemotherapy-sensitive disease. Genetic randomization was used. After 44 months median follow-up, overall survival had not yet been reached in either group. Transplant-related mortality in the allogeneic group was 18% compared with 4% in the autologous group.

In one series, only 5 of 80 patients were alive without evidence of disease at 4 to 7 years after an allogeneic bone marrow transplantation for their multiple myeloma (Bensinger et al. 1996). It must be emphasized that the majority of these patients had chemotherapy-resistant disease before transplantation. Outcomes have improved over time (Hahn et al. 2003). Gahrton et al. reported that of 690 allogeneic, matched, sibling donor transplants for multiple myeloma reported to the European Group for Blood and Marrow Transplantation registry, 334 were performed between 1983 and 1993 (all with bone marrow) and 356 between 1994 and 1998. The 3-year overall survival was 35% for transplant recipients during the earlier period and 55% for recipients of bone marrow transplants during the later period. The improvement in survival since 1994 was the result of a significant reduction in transplant-related mortality, from 46% to 30% at 2 years.

Table 3.11. Nonrandomized comparisons of autologous and allogeneic hematopoietic stem cell transplantation for multiple myeloma

Study	N	TRM, %	MS, mo	P
Bjorkstrand et al., 1996	189 Auto	13	34	0.001
	189 Allo	41	18	
Varterasian et al., 1997 (Hahn et al. 2003)	24 Auto	12	33.5	NS
	24 Allo	25	38.6	
Couban et al., 1997 (Hahn et al. 2003)	40 Auto	5	>48	<0.001
	22 Allo	27	7	
Reynolds et al., 2001 (Hahn et al. 2003)	35 Auto	6	>15	NS
	21 Allo	19	>27	
Lokhorst et al., 1999 (Hahn et al. 2003)	50 Auto [a]	4	>44	NS
	11 Allo [a,b]	18	>44	

MS, median survival; NS, not significant; TRM, treatment-related mortality.

[a] Chemotherapy-sensitive patients only.

[b] T-cell–depleted allogeneic stem cells.

Table 3.12. Nonmyeloablative regimens for multiple myeloma

Study	N	Diagnosis to NMA, mo (range)	Sibling/MUD allograft	Age, y (range)	NMA regimen[a]
Badros et al. (2002)	31	29 (8–164)	25/6	56 (38–69)	Melphalan 100
Giralt et al. (2002)	22	36 (3–135)	13/9	51 (45–64)	FM
Maloney et al. (2002)	54	2 [b, c]	NS	55 (39–71)	Auto → NMA (TBI 200 cGy; MMF)
Kroger et al. (2002)	17	11 [b, e]	9/8	51 (32–64)	Auto → NMA (FM-ATG-MTX)

ATG, antithymocyte globulin; CR, complete response; FM, fludarabine and melphalan; FU, follow-up; MM, multiple myeloma; MMF, mycophenolate; MTX, methotrexate; MUD, matched unrelated donor; NMA, nonmyeloablative transplant; NS, not stated; OS, overall survival; PFS, progression-free survival; PR, partial response; TBI, total body irradiation; TRM, treatment-related mortality.

[a] All studies used cyclosporine as part of the graft-versus-host prophylaxis program.

[b] Patients had NMA after induction (most commonly vincristine, doxorubicin, and dexamethasone) and a standard autologous peripheral blood stem cell transplantation.

Table continues on page 89.

Allogeneic transplantation produces higher rates of molecular complete responses. In a series of 229 myeloma patients, Martinelli et al. demonstrated that allogeneic transplantation resulted in a complete response from 38% compared with 22% after autologous transplantation (*P* <0.01) (Hahn et al. 2003). Among patients achieving a clinical complete response, 50% of the allogeneic transplant group had a molecular complete response compared with only 17% of those who had received an autologous transplant. The median relapse-free survival for those who had a molecular complete remission was 110 months compared with 35 months for those who did not. Moreover, in those with a molecular complete remission, the relapse rate was only 16% in the allogeneic group and 41% in the autologous group. This is strong evidence that molecular complete responses are associated with a longer relapse-free survival.

3.8.2.3 Donor Lymphocyte Infusions

A graft-versus-myeloma effect has been noted after the administration of donor peripheral blood mononuclear cells for relapse after allogeneic transplantation (Tricot et al. 1996). Eight of 13 patients with myeloma relapse after an allogeneic bone marrow transplant responded to donor lymphocyte infusions. Four of the patients had a complete response. In a larger group of patients with a prolonged follow-up period, the factors that were correlated with response to donor lymphocyte infusions were a T-cell dose of more than 1×10^8 cells/kg, response to reinduction therapy, and chemotherapy-sensitive dis-

ease before the allogeneic transplantation (Lokhorst et al. 2000).

3.8.2.4 Nonmyeloablative Allogeneic Transplant

Despite a significant decrease in the relapse rate and graft-versus-myeloma effects, allografts have been associated with inferior survival in nearly all comparisons because of high peritransplantation mortality, late complications of chronic graft-versus-host disease (GVHD), and late infections. The mortality rate for allogeneic transplantation must be reduced before it can assume a major role in the treatment of multiple myeloma. Promising approaches include nonmyeloablative conditioning ("mini") regimens for selected patients with myeloma, either at relapse or immediately after autologous stem cell transplantation.

Investigators from the University of Arkansas reported results of nonmyeloablative allogeneic stem cell transplantation in 31 poor-risk myeloma patients (Badros et al. 2002) (Table 3.12). Twenty-five were human leukocyte antigen-matched compatible siblings and 6 were unrelated and matched. The conditioning consisted of melphalan at 100 mg/m^2 for related and melphalan at 100 mg/m^2 plus total body irradiation (250 cGy) plus fludarabine for unrelated allografts. Donor lymphocyte infusions were initially given on days 21, 42, and 112 to patients with no clinical evidence of GVHD. However, because of a high incidence of GVHD, donor lymphocyte infusion was reserved to attain full donor chimerism or to eradicate residual disease. All

Median FU, mo	Patients in CR/PR, no.	TRM	MM deaths, no.	OS	PFS
6	12/10	9/31	3/31	31% at 24 mo	15 mo (median)
15	7/9	9/22	7/22	10 mo (median)	19% at 24 mo
18[d]	NS	8/32	2/54	79% at 18 mo[d]	NS
17[d]	11/3	2/17	1/17	74% at 24 mo	56% at 24 mo

[c] Time between autologous and NMA transplants.
[d] Time measured from autologous stem cell transplantation.
[e] Time to autologous transplant; time between transplants was 119 days.

but one patient had received 1 or more than 2 prior autologous transplants. Fifty-five percent of the patients had progressive disease at the time of the allograft. Acute GVHD developed in 18 patients. Ten patients progressed to chronic GVHD, limited in 6 and extensive in 4 patients. Two patients failed to engraft even after a second allogeneic peripheral blood stem cell infusion. At a median follow-up of 6 months, 12 patients achieved complete remission and another 7 near complete remission, and 3 achieved partial remission. There were 3 treatment-related deaths during the first 100 days and another 6 after 100 days, for an overall treatment-related mortality of 28%. Three patients died of progressive myeloma. Patients with progressive disease who received transplants or who had received more than 1 autograft had a statistically higher mortality rate. The authors also compared their nonmyeloablative transplant experience to their prior standard allogeneic experience and found that the nonmyeloablative group had a lower mortality during the first year ($P = 0.09$), most notably the subset who had received only 1 prior autograft ($P = 0.05$).

Maloney and colleagues (2002) reported results on 54 newly diagnosed myeloma patients who were treated with a planned tandem autologous/nonmyeloablative allogeneic stem cell transplantation (Table 3.12). After induction with 4 cycles of VAD chemotherapy, followed by autologous stem cell transplantation using melphalan 200 mg/m^2 as conditioning, patients underwent a nonmyeloablative allograft. The conditioning for the second transplant was with total body irradiation (200 cGy).

Matched sibling donor peripheral blood stem cells were infused immediately after the total body irradiation. Postgrafting immunosuppression included mycophenolate and cyclosporine. Fifty-two of the 54 patients received the planned nonmyeloablative transplant, with a median time between autologous and allogeneic transplant of 62 days. The granulocyte and platelet nadirs after the nonmyeloablative transplant were 760 cells/μL and 95,000 cells/μL, respectively. Acute GVHD was seen in 38% of patients and was grade II in all but 4 cases. Forty-six percent of patients developed chronic GVHD that required therapy. All patients achieved donor engraftment. Fifty-seven percent of patients not in complete response at the time of the second transplant achieved a complete response. With a median follow-up of surviving patients of 18 months, 8 patients (15%) have died of transplant-related complications, 2 of progressive myeloma, and 1 of lung cancer.

Kroger et al. (2002) have applied a similar strategy of a planned standard intensity autograft (melphalan 200 mg/m^2) followed by a dose-reduced regimen (fludarabine 180 mg/m^2, melphalan 100 mg/m^2, and antithymocyte globulin 3×10 mg/kg) before allografting (Table 3.12). GVHD prophylaxis included cyclosporine and mini-methotrexate. Nine patients received allografts from related donors and 8 from unrelated donors. Acute GVHD stage II-IV occurred in 6 patients (38%). Chronic GVHD developed in 40% of the patients, but only 1 patient experienced extensive chronic GVHD requiring further immunosuppressive therapy. The 100-day mortality rate was 11%, and with a median follow-up of 17 months after autologous and 13 months after allogeneic transplantation, 13 patients (76%) are alive. The rate of complete remission with negative immunofixation increased from 18% after autografting to 73% after allografting, and 12 remain free of relapse or progression.

Until further refinements are made and additional confirmatory studies are completed, the role of nonmyeloablative allogeneic stem cell transplantation as initial therapy in myeloma must be considered investigational. See Table 3.12 for additional preliminary data.

3.8.2.4.1 Maintenance Therapy

Maintenance therapy strategies can be divided into 2 broad categories: 1) continued induction therapy ad infinitum, and 2) addition of a novel therapy after induction therapy. The former strategy was prevalent until recognition of the risk of alkylator-induced myelodysplastic syndrome and leukemia. The latter strategy has predominantly applied immune modulators, including prednisone, interferon, and cellular therapies.

3.8.2.4.1.1 Maintenance Chemotherapy

Through the 1970s and 1980s, several randomized studies established that alkylator-based maintenance therapy does not produce a survival benefit (Belch et al. 1988; Cohen et al. 1986; MacLennan et al. 1992; Riccardi et al. 2000; Southwest Oncology Group Study 1975). In general, unmaintained patients had similar to slightly shorter remission duration than those receiving maintenance (Alexanian et al. 1978; Belch et al. 1988; Cohen et al. 1986; Riccardi et al. 2000) but had higher rates of second remission (Alexanian et al. 1978; Belch et al. 1988). In some studies there has been a trend toward longer survival in patients not receiving maintenance chemotherapy (MacLennan et al. 1992; Southwest Oncology Group Study 1975). Induction therapy is commonly discontinued after plateau is reached (no change in M protein more than 25% for 4 to 6 months). In the context of standard therapy, the ability to achieve a plateau is as important, if not more important, as depth of response to therapy (Bladé et al. 1994; Corso et al. 1999; Finnish Leukaemia Group 1999; Riccardi et al. 2000). No benefit has been documented for treatment beyond 12 months, although it has been suggested – but not validated – that prolonged primary chemotherapy may be beneficial in patients achieving less than a partial response, ie, a minimal response or stable disease (Oivanen et al. 1999).

Patients who relapse off chemotherapy have response rates of 25% to 80% with resumption of the original regimen (Alexanian et al. 1978; Belch et al. 1988; Riccardi et al. 2000). Second response rates are lower in patients who progress or relapse during maintenance than in those who relapse during no maintenance (Alexanian et al. 1978; Cohen et al. 1986). In a study of 115 newly diagnosed patients treated with the M-2 regimen (VBMCP) for about 1 year, an initial response rate of 82% was achieved, with a median duration of response of 22 months. After a first relapse, 26 of 38 patients (68%) responded again and had a median duration of response of 11 months. After a second relapse, 7 of 16 patients (44%) responded, with a duration of response of 3.5 months (Paccagnella et al. 1991).

3.8.2.4.1.2 Corticosteroids as Maintenance Therapy?

There are 4 studies that refer to the topic of corticosteroids as maintenance therapy. None justify a recommendation of prednisone as a standard maintenance regimen for all patients.

The most recent study (SWOG 9210) compared prednisone 10 mg every other day to prednisone 50 mg every other day in patients who had responded (SWOG PR or better) to 6 to 12 months of a VAD-based program, that is, a corticosteroid-intensive program. From the time of the randomization to the 2 different alternate-day prednisone schedules, the median progression-free survival for the higher-dose prednisone arm was 14 months compared with 5 months ($P = 0.003$). Survival was also marginally better at 37 and 26 months ($P = 0.05$) (Berenson et al. 2002). Although the more dose-intensive corticosteroid maintenance strategy does provide a longer progression-free survival in corticosteroid-responsive patients, these data cannot be generalized and must be placed into context. By comparison, after alkylator-based therapy the median unmaintained progression-free survival is 12 months in responding patients (Cohen et al. 1986).

An earlier randomized study, which compared dexamethasone maintenance to interferon maintenance after induction with melphalan and dexamethasone, demonstrated equivalence to inferiority of dexamethasone compared with interferon. Patients received maintenance treatment with interferon-a (3 MU 3 times a week) or dexamethasone (20 mg/m^2 orally each morning for 4 days, repeated monthly) until relapse. Remission duration was identical (10 months); however, significantly more patients responded on reinstitution of the melphalan and dexamethasone at disease relapse in the interferon group than in the dexamethasone group (82% versus 44%, $P=0.001$) (Alexanian et al. 2000).

The CALGB 7461 study as reported by Cornwell et al. (1988) addressed this issue less directly. Patients were treated initially with alkylator therapy and randomized to observation or vincristine and prednisone as maintenance. Survival and response rates were significantly longer and higher in the vincristine-prednisone maintenance group who had received up-front melphalan (median, 35.3 months versus 27.0 months; $P=0.003$) but not in patients who had received up-front BCNU or CCNU (Sporn and McIntyre 1986).

Finally, SWOG 8624, which evaluated the influence of corticosteroid dose intensity on response and survival, indirectly provides data on corticosteroid maintenance. Higher objective response rate and median survival were observed in patients who received prolonged administration of glucocorticoids (prednisone 50 mg every other day) between chemotherapy courses. Patients given VMCP/VBAP with and without alternate day prednisone had median overall survivals of 40 months versus 31 months, respectively ($P=0.02$). The survival advantage may have been confounded by the complexity of the study; different treatment plans were assigned after 12 months of induction therapy, determined by tumor response. Moreover, one could argue that the corticosteroid was more a part of the induction than of the maintenance program.

3.8.2.4.1.3 Interferon as Maintenance Therapy

3.8.2.4.1.3.1 After Conventional Chemotherapy

The initial findings by Mandelli et al. in 1990 of a superior disease-free and overall survival in chemotherapy-responsive patients randomized to maintenance interferon-a have been challenged by multiple subsequent studies. Ludwig and Fritz (2000) analyzed 1,615 patients from 13 maintenance trials, and the Myeloma Trialists' Collaborative Group (2001) used the individual data of 1,543 patients enrolled in 12 randomized maintenance trials for meta-analysis. Results were similar in that the first group found a 4.4-month and 7.0-month prolongation of relapse-free ($P<0.01$) and overall survival ($P<0.01$), respectively (Ludwig and Fritz 2000). The latter group reported that interferon-a prolonged the med-

ian time to progression by about 6 months ($P<0.00001$) and overall survival by approximately 7 months ($P = 0.04$) (Myeloma Trialists' Collaborative Group 2001) (Fig. 3.8). Survival from progression to death was significantly worse in the interferon group than in the control group (odds ratio 1.21, $P = 0.007$). No factors analyzed predicted for the interferon benefit (ie, pretreatment hemoglobin, calcium, β_2M, creatinine, sex, performance status, or immunoglobulin isotype). The level of response (complete response, partial response, stable disease) or interferon dose intensity (<12 MU/week versus $\geqslant$ 12 MU/week) also did not predict for interferon effect (Myeloma Trialists' Collaborative Group 2001). The cost in 2000 of the 1-year survival benefit in patients treated with interferon as maintenance was \$US 18,968.16, assuming a dose of 11.6 MU/week (Ludwig and Fritz 2000).

3.8.2.4.1.3.2 In Combination With Corticosteroids

Corticosteroids have been added to maintenance interferon in an attempt to intensify the program. Small numbers of patients have been treated with standard maintenance interferon and either dexamethasone or prednisone (Salmon et al. 1998). In one small randomized study, the progression-free survival was longer in the corticosteroid plus interferon arm than in the interferon only arm, although median survival was not different (Salmon et al. 1998). The combination can also induce further partial remissions in more than half of responding patients treated.

3.8.2.4.1.3.3 After High-Dose Chemotherapy With Stem Cell Support

Fewer data are available about the utility of interferon after autologous stem cell transplantation. There is one small randomized trial of 85 patients and a larger retrospective analysis of registry data by the European Group for Blood and Marrow Transplantation (EBMT). The use of interferon in this setting cannot be recommended outside of clinical trials.

After high-dose chemotherapy with stem cell support, Cunningham et al. (1998) randomly assigned 85 patients to interferon at 3 MU/m^2 3 times weekly or to observation. The median progression-free survival in the 43 patients randomized to interferon-a was 46 months compared with 27 months in the control patients ($P<0.025$). Although there was a significant survival advantage at 54 months, at which time 12% of patients in the interferon group and 33% of patients in the no interferon group had died ($P = 0.006$), this survival advantage was no longer evident at a median follow-up of 77 months (Cunningham et al. 1998).

The EBMT registry study data included 473 patients who had received maintenance and 419 who had not. Unfortunately, the 2 groups were poorly matched. The patients who did not receive interferon had significantly more prior therapy, a higher stage at diagnosis, and a longer time to transplantation. They were also significantly older and a higher percentage had received total body irradiation-containing conditioning regimens (Bjorkstrand et al. 2001). Although these factors were "statistically corrected for" in the survival analysis, this imbalance makes interpretation of this retrospective collection of registry patients problematic. Prognostic factors like $\beta_2 M$, C-reactive protein, cytogenetics, and PCLI were not included in the analysis. Overall survival was significantly better in the patients who received interferon (78 versus 47 months, $P = 0.007$). Curiously, there was a more prominent survival benefit in those patients who achieved partial response (97 versus 46 months for interferon versus no interferon, $P = 0.03$) rather than complete response (64 versus 51 months, $P = 0.1$). Paradoxically, the partial response group had a better overall survival than the complete response group.

3.8.2.4.1.4 Immunotherapy as Maintenance Therapy

3.8.2.4.1.4.1 Dendritic Cell-based Vaccination

In an effort to prolong duration of response and hopefully survival, idiotype-treated dendritic cell vaccines are being explored as a therapeutic modality for myeloma patients. B-cell malignancies, including multiple myeloma, are unique in their expression of immunoglobulin. The immunoglobulin on malignant cells can be distinguished from that on normal B cells or plasma cells by virtue of specific idiotypic determinants. Dendritic cells are the only known natural cells that can present antigen to naive T cells. Antigen pulsed dendritic cells can successfully induce both humoral and cytotoxic cellular immune responses.

Idiotypic vaccinations alone have met with limited success in human trials. However, dendritic cell-based vaccination appears to be a more potent way to induce antitumor immunity than vaccines with peptide alone. Trials are ongoing looking at dendritic cell-based vacci-

nations for multiple solid tumors as well as for myeloma, non-Hodgkin lymphoma, chronic myelogenous leukemia, and other hematologic malignancies. Preliminary evidence suggests that idiotype pulsed dendritic cells can stimulate anti-idiotype responses (Titzer et al. 2000). Clinical responses have also been observed by us and other investigators in the setting of relapsed disease and after hematopoietic stem cell transplantation (Titzer et al. 2000).

3.8.2.4.2 Management of Relapsed or Refractory Disease

Relapsed and refractory myeloma likely have distinct biologies but are commonly grouped together in discussions of chemotherapy regimens and trials. Differentiation between relapses occurring on therapy and off therapy should be made, with the former having a poorer prognosis. Similarly, primary refractory – the condition in which the disease has not responded to initial therapy – and secondary refractory (or resistant) disease – should be differentiated. Finally, with the growing list of active agents, clarification should be made as to which class of agents or modality the myeloma is refractory.

Before the advent of high-dose chemotherapy with stem cell support and of thalidomide, treatment guidelines were more straightforward. If the relapse had occurred during an unmaintained remission, resumption of the patient's original therapy was a good rule. Fifty percent to 60% of patients respond again to repeat treatment if relapse occurs after unmaintained remission (Alexanian et al. 1978; Belch et al. 1988; Paccagnella et al. 1991). Median survival is about 10 months (Alexanian et al. 1978). The myeloma cell doubling time and duration of response tend to decrease with each subsequent course of therapy (Paccagnella et al. 1991). In the cases of primary refractory disease or acquired resistance on therapy, the mainstays of treatment had been clinical trials, anthracycline-based, corticosteroid-based, and alkylator-based regimens, which might vary in schedule and dose intensity.

3.8.2.4.2.1 Single Agent Glucocorticoids for Relapsed or Refractory Disease

Salmon et al. described clinical improvement in 7 of 9 relapsed or refractory patients treated with high-dose (200 mg) prednisone every other day. Subsequently, these observations (Table 3.8) were confirmed and extended using prednisone, methylprednisolone, and dexamethasone in pulsed or alternate-day schedules (Alexanian et al. 1990; Gertz et al. 1995). Doses are typically high, with the exception of one small study in which continuous low-dose dexamethasone (4 mg/day) was administered to a small cohort of patients, with a resultant 40% response rate. Overall, approximately 25% of relapsed or refractory patients respond; median survival of responding patients is 16 to 22 months (Alexanian et al. 1990; Gertz et al. 1995). In reviewing their experience with single agent dexamethasone and VAD, Alexanian et al. noted that in patients with refractory disease, response rates with single agent dexamethasone are comparable to those with VAD (27% versus 32%). In contrast, in relapsed disease, response rates achieved with single agent dexamethasone are inferior to those with VAD (Alexanian et al. 1990). These data are not randomized but rather serial observations. On occasion, patients who do not respond to high-dose dexamethasone can be salvaged with intermittent high-dose methylprednisolone (Gertz et al. 1995).

3.8.2.4.2.2 Thalidomide for Relapsed or Refractory Disease

The first published report of the utility of thalidomide in patients with relapsed myeloma was by Singhal et al. Eighty-four patients with relapsed myeloma, 76 of whom had relapsed after high-dose chemotherapy with stem cell support, were treated with escalating doses of thalidomide. Patients were started on 200 mg each evening; the dose was escalated every 2 weeks if tolerated to a final maximal dose of 800 mg daily. Twenty-five percent of patients had at least a 50% reduction in their serum myeloma protein, and an additional 6 patients had a 25% reduction in their serum myeloma protein (minimal response). Preliminary evidence of response was apparent within 2 months in more than three-quarters of the patients who did respond. An update by Barlogie et al. of the original report, including 169 patients with advanced myeloma, verified a 30% response rate (50% reduction in the myeloma protein). Two-year event-free and overall survival rates were 20% and 48%, respectively. These findings have been substantiated by other investigators (Rajkumar et al. 2000).

The role of dose intensity in thalidomide effectiveness is unclear. In the original reports, the highest dose tolerated was administered. In high-risk patients there was a suggestion that response rates were higher and

survival longer in those patients receiving high doses of thalidomide (greater than or equal to 600 mg/day). However, in some patients, responses may be seen with doses as low as 50 to 100 mg/day.

There is synergy with thalidomide and dexamethasone. Response rates of 41% to 55% (Dimopoulos et al. 2001; Palumbo et al. 2001) have been observed in patients with resistant myeloma. Patients who are resistant to dexamethasone-based or thalidomide-based regimens can respond to the combination of these 2 agents (Dimopoulos et al. 2001). Coleman et al. described a 100% response rate for relapsed or refractory disease treated with clarithromycin, low-dose thalidomide, and dexamethasone. These results have yet to be substantiated by other investigators, and clarithromycin alone is not an effective treatment.

Toxicities associated with thalidomide include fetal malformations, constipation, weakness or fatigue, somnolence, skin problems, and sensory neuropathy in more than one-third of patients. There is also an increased risk of thrombosis in patients treated with thalidomide, which appears to be exacerbated by the use of concurrent combination chemotherapy, with rates as high as 28%. Other life-threatening complications have included Stevens-Johnson syndrome and hepatitis.

3.8.2.4.2.3 Chemotherapy for Relapsed or Refractory Disease

The subject of chemotherapy for relapsed or refractory disease will be divided into 4 sections: alkylator-based regimens, anthracycline-based regimens with or without dose-intensified corticosteroids, and other less commonly used regimens.

3.8.2.4.2.3.1 Alkylator-based Regimens for Relapsed or Refractory Disease

There is cross-resistance among the alkylators, but it is not absolute and may be circumvented by increasing dose intensity. Without extreme dose intensification, 5% to 20% of patients with melphalan-resistant disease respond to cyclophosphamide and BCNU as single agents or in combination with prednisone. About one-third of patients will respond if prednisone is administered with the cyclophosphamide (de Weerdt et al. 2001).

Higher doses of cyclophosphamide (eg, 600 mg/m² intravenously for 4 consecutive days) result in response rates of 29% to 43% (Lenhard et al. 1994). Both response duration and overall survival tend to be short, approximately 3 and 9 months, respectively. Consolidating the chemotherapy into a 1-day schedule rather than a 4-day schedule did not improve response rate, but it did increase the toxicity.

Dose intensification of melphalan can also be quite effective and is the basis for high-dose therapy with stem cell support (McElwain and Powles 1983). Selby et al. (1987) reported that 66% of patients with resistant disease treated with 140 mg/m² without stem cell support responded, but median response duration was 6 months, with all patients relapsing within a year. Median times to leukocyte and platelet recovery were 42 and 37 days, respectively, and the regimen-related toxicity was 13%. Doses of 30 to 70 mg/m² have also been explored.

VBMCP (the M-2 regimen) or MOCCA provides responses in 20% to 30% of refractory patients, with a median survival of about 11 months.

3.8.2.4.2.3.2 Anthracycline-based Regimens Without Corticosteroid Dose Intensification for Relapsed or Refractory Disease

Various permutations of doxorubicin-containing chemotherapy regimens – doxorubicin and cyclophosphamide (Alberts et al. 1976); doxorubicin, BCNU, cyclophosphamide, and prednisone; CAP; VCAP; VBAP; and BAP – have been tried in patients with relapsed and refractory disease, resulting in response rates of 7% to 28% (Bonnet et al. 1982; Kyle et al. 1982). Response duration and survival tend to be short – less than 6 and 12 months, respectively. Responding patients tend to live 7 to 10 to even 22 months longer than nonresponders. Patients who have relapsed disease, rather than resistant or refractory disease, have higher response rates (i.e., close to 30%).

3.8.2.4.2.3.3 Anthracycline-based Regimens With Corticosteroid Dose Intensification for Relapsed or Refractory Disease

Another approach to treating relapsed or refractory myeloma is supplementation of the anthracycline and vincristine with high-dose corticosteroids. Alexanian et al. (Barlogie et al. 1984) described VAP (bolus vincristine 1.5 mg day 1, doxorubicin 35 mg/m² day 1, and prednisone 45 mg/m² for 5 days repeated every 8 days for 3 corticosteroid pulses); response rates were 47%. Barlo-

gie et al. (1984) published their experience with VAD, and numerous variants have followed. The overall response rate with VAD in 29 patients who had refractory or resistant disease was 59%, according to SWOG criteria. In the 20 patients who had not received prior doxorubicin, the response rate was 70%. VAD differed from VAP in that the former included continuous infusion vincristine and doxorubicin and a 6-fold corticosteroid dose intensification. The activity of VAD has been substantiated by others. Infection is the most important complication, with 38% of patients having fever and 28%, a documented infectious agent. Early catheter removal may occur in approximately 16% of patients as a result of thrombosis or infection.

Variants of VAD include regimens that alter the type or dose of corticosteroid, schedule of administration, and type of anthracycline and additional drugs. The effectiveness of VAMP (methylprednisolone in place of dexamethasone) appears comparable to VAD, with a response rate and overall survival of 36% and 20 months in patients with resistant disease (Forgeson et al. 1988).

Alternative anthracyclines have been tried, including mitoxantrone (NOP or mitoxantrone, vincristine, and dexamethasone), epirubicin, and liposomal doxorubicin. Several investigators have added additional drugs to the VAD-base without measurable benefit. Concurrent interferon (Gertz et al. 1995) adds nothing to response rate or overall survival. In single-arm studies, there does not appear to be any advantage to the addition of cyclophosphamide to VAD, VAMP, or vincristine, epirubicin, and dexamethasone (VED) (Alexanian et al. 1992; Forgeson et al. 1988).

3.8.2.4.2.3.4 Other Regimens for Relapsed or Refractory Disease

After studying high-dose cytosine arabinoside, cisplatin, and etoposide as single agents, Barlogie et al. (1989) did preliminary studies of DAP (dexamethasone, cytosine arabinoside, and cisplatin) and later EDAP (etoposide and DAP). In patients with refractory disease, response rates with these treatments were 7%, 14%, 17%, 0%, and 40%, respectively. Median survival in patients treated with EDAP was 4.5 months. This regimen is extremely myelosuppressive, with more than half of treated patients requiring platelet transfusions and 80% requiring hospitalization for neutropenic fever. In the first month, treatment-related mortality was 15%. EDAP is part of Barlogie's "Total Therapy II."

As part of Total Therapy II, before 2 cycles of EDAP, 55% and 9% of patients had achieved objective response and complete response, respectively; after EDAP, 65% and 15% had objective response and complete response (Barlogie et al. 1999).

Dimopoulos et al. explored a combination of high-dose cyclophosphamide (3 g/m²) and etoposide (900 mg/m²) followed by granulocyte-macrophage colony-stimulating factor. Of the 52 patients with advanced and refractory multiple myeloma treated, 42% responded. Median time to granulocyte recovery was 19 days, and the median remission duration was 8 months.

Combinations of cisplatin with BCNU, cyclophosphamide, and prednisone have produced response in heavily pretreated patients; however, the addition of cisplatin and bleomycin to VBAP did not appear to produce better outcomes than standard VBAP (Barlogie et al. 1989).

3.8.2.4.3 Clinical Trials and New Agents

Until myeloma is a curable disease in all patients, clinical trials will play a critical role in the treatment of these patients. They will assist in defining a better classification system for the disease, clarify which treatments offer the most value, and bring new effective agents into standard clinical practice.

The 2 most promising new agents for the treatment of multiple myeloma are PS-341 and CC-5013 (Richardson et al. 2002), both of which are still in clinical trials. PS-341 is a small molecule that selectively inhibits cellular proteasomes, offering a novel pathway for targeted anticancer therapy. The proteasome has a key role in protein degradation, cell-cycle regulation, and gene expression. Tumor cells, including multiple myeloma, are heavily dependent on proteasome-regulated proteins for their growth and interaction with stromal cells. PS-341 generally has been well tolerated in phase 1 trials, with apparent clinical activity in patients with multiple myeloma. PS-341 represents a novel anticancer agent with an acceptable safety profile and evidence of anti-tumor activity in multiple myeloma. Partial or complete responses are observed in 27% of patients with relapsed or refractory disease or both (Richardson et al. 2003).

CC-5013, a small molecule derivative of thalidomide and a member of the immunomodulatory drug (IMiD) class, is more potent than thalidomide in mediating direct cytokine-related and immunomodulatory effects

against human multiple myeloma cell lines and patient-derived cells in vitro. During the 2 recently completed phase 1 studies, activity has been documented in patients with refractory or relapsed multiple myeloma. Approximately 25% of relapsed or refractory patients have achieved a partial response. Another 25% to 35% of patients have had a minimal response (25%–49% reduction in serum M component). No significant somnolence, constipation, or neuropathy has been seen (Richardson et al. 2002).

The human anti-CD20 antibody has demonstrated some effect in patients with myeloma. About 20% of patients with myeloma have CD20 expression on their plasma cells. Preliminary data suggest that use of this agent may be beneficial in this subset of patients.

3.8.3 Radiation

As early as the mid-1920s there was recognition that external beam radiation therapy could promote immediate relief of pain, healing of pathologic fractures, and resolution of extramedullary plasmacytomas (Geschickter and Copeland 1928). Until the 1950s, radiation therapy was the only effective treatment available for the management of plasma cell tumors. With the advent of systemic chemotherapy, indications for irradiation were primarily palliation of bone pain and solitary plasmacytomas. Concern for maintaining bone marrow reserve also constrains the use of radiation in patients with multiple myeloma. The majority of patients receiving concentrated local doses of 3,500 cGy or more showed persistent localized marrow aplasia. One must administer enough radiation to provide palliation, without jeopardizing opportunities for further systemic therapy.

3.8.4 Sequential Half-body (Hemibody) Irradiation

The first report of using whole body irradiation to treat myeloma was by Medinger and Craver in 1942. Partial or complete relief of pain was noted in the majority of patients. Once effective systemic chemotherapy came into wide use, this approach became less popular until 1971 when Bergsagel postulated that sequential hemibody radiation could be a means to debulk tumor. He suggested that if a dose of approximately 725 cGy were given to the upper half of the body and 1,000 cGy to the lower half, a theoretical 3-log kill could be achieved and survival prolonged. After a series of retrospective studies and a randomized study (Salmon et al. 1990) evaluating its role in the earlier phases of myeloma, irradiation has once again largely fallen out of favor. In patients who have end-stage disease, with poor pain control, this treatment may still be important.

The majority of series involving hemibody or sequential hemibody radiation are retrospective and include patients who were either resistant to or relapsing from alkylator-based therapy. Significant relief of bone pain occurred in 80% to 90% of patients, and median duration of survival was 5 to 11 months. Objective biochemical response occurred in 25% to 50%. Pain relief typically occurred 1 to 2 days after institution of therapy, with maximal response in 1 to 2 weeks. The most common side effects were moderate myelosuppression, pneumonitis, nausea, vomiting, diarrhea, and stomatitis. If an oral lead shield was not used, mucositis also occurred. Nadirs occurred within 3 weeks, and white cell count and platelet count recovery occurred by about 6 weeks. Decrements in pulmonary function of 20% occurred in about half of treated patients. The most serious complication was radiation-induced pneumonitis, which was seen in 14% of patients. The option of sequential half-body radiation therapy must be balanced against unpredictable and varying degrees of pancytopenia and alternative treatment options.

Bergsagel's postulate and preliminary data from several small studies led 2 cooperative group studies (SWOG 8229 and CALGB 8003) to incorporate systemic radiation therapy as consolidation therapy. Neither study demonstrated meaningful advantage to patients receiving adjuvant hemibody radiation (Salmon et al. 1990), and hemibody radiation is used only for pain palliation in end-stage chemotherapy-refractory myeloma patients.

3.9 Staging and Prognosis

Survival of multiple myeloma patients varies from months to more than a decade. There are no precise methods of identifying the subset of newly diagnosed patients who are best served by standard intensity therapies, by maintenance therapies, by novel therapies, or by more intensive regimens such as hematopoietic stem cell transplantation. Prognostic factors are needed for patient counseling, therapeutic decision making, and clinical trial stratification.

Staging is one form of prognostic modeling. The Durie-Salmon system (Table 3.13), which is the most widely accepted multiple myeloma staging system, separates patients predominantly by tumor burden and renal function (Durie and Salmon 1975). As the biology of myeloma is better understood, novel markers reflecting myeloma cell kinetics, signaling, genetic aberrations, and apoptosis have eclipsed the prognostic significance of tumor burden as a predictor of survival.

Although the Durie-Salmon system has some prognostic value (Durie and Salmon 1975), other biologic variables appear to be more valuable (Bataille et al. 1992; Crowley et al. 2001; Greipp et al. 1993; Konigsberg et al. 2000). At the time of its inception, the Durie-Salmon staging system was an elegant system that incorporated information about immunoglobulin production and half-life, hemoglobin, calcium, creatinine, and extent of bone disease to derive mathematically the total myeloma cell burden. Quantification of bone lesions used in this staging system, however, is not always reliable as a prognostic factor in that patients classified as stage III only because of bone lesion criteria do not have a poorer prognosis.

Other variables, including patient age, performance status, serum albumin, immunoglobulin isotype, and bone marrow plasma cell infiltration, have long been recognized to predict survival, and subsequent models have incorporated these factors (Bartl et al. 1987; Finnish Leukaemia Group 1999; Medical Research Council's Working Party on Leukaemia in Adults 1980) (Table 3.14). Myeloma biology is better addressed by increased concentrations of serum $\beta_2 M$, C-reactive protein, circulating plasma cells by peripheral blood labeling index, other serum markers, bone marrow PCLI, and chromosomal abnormalities (Bataille et al. 1992; Crowley et al. 2001; Greipp et al. 1993; Konigsberg et al. 2000). Each of these systems has value, but the goal is to reach a consensus and to standardize discussions and comparisons among clinical trials and outcomes. An international consensus panel is addressing this. When designing a new staging system, the dilemma exists regarding the use of readily available, inexpensive markers – which frequently describe the host more than the intrinsic properties of the myeloma – or more esoteric, expensive markers – which reflect the individual patient's myeloma biology. Table 3.14 summarizes several investigators' efforts to introduce more meaningful staging systems.

Table 3.13. Durie-Salmon staging system

Criterion	Measured myeloma cell mass, cells $\times$ $10^{12}/m^2$
Stage I	
All of the following	< 0.6 (low)
Hemoglobin >10 g/dL	
Serum calcium <12 mg/dL	
On radiograph, normal bone structure (scale 0)[a] or solitary bone plasmacytoma only	
Low M-component production rates	
IgG <5 g/dL	
IgA <3 g/dL	
Urine light chain M component on electrophoresis <4 g/24 hours	
Stage II	
Fitting neither stage I or III	0.6–1.2 (intermediate)
Stage III	
One or more of the following	>1.2 (high)
Hemoglobin <8.5 g/dL	
Serum calcium >12 mg/dL	
Advanced lytic bone lesions	
High M-component rates	
IgG >7 g/dL	
IgA >5 g/dL	
Urine light chain M component on electrophoresis >12 g/24 hours	
Subclassification	
A: Serum creatinine <2 mg/dL	
B: Serum creatinine ≥2 mg/dL	

[a] Scale of bone lesions: normal bones, 0; osteoporosis, 1; lytic bone lesions, 2; and extensive skeletal destruction and major fractures, 3. Modified from Durie and Salmon (1975). Copyright © 1975 American Cancer Society. By permission of Wiley-Liss.

3.9.1 Individual Prognostic Markers With Standard Intensity Chemotherapy

3.9.1.1 β_2-Microglobulin

β_2M concentration is the strongest and most reliable prognostic factor for multiple myeloma that is available routinely. It depends not only on tumor burden but also on renal function. Increased β_2M values predict early death (Bataille and Harousseau 1997; Bataille et al. 1992; Greipp et al. 1993). Formulas to correct the β_2M concentration for renal insufficiency have not improved its predictive value; the β_2M value is still prognostic in myeloma patients with normal renal function. The British Medical Research Council has shown that after 2 years of survival, the initial β_2M concentration loses its prognostic value. β_2M value also predicts high-dose therapy outcome (ie, event-free and overall survival) (Hahn et al. 2003).

3.9.1.2 C-reactive Protein

French investigators first showed that C-reactive protein was useful as a univariate and multivariate (Bataille et al. 1992) prognostic marker in multiple myeloma. These findings were substantiated in groups of patients from Mayo Clinic and from ECOG clinical trials (Greipp et al. 1993; Rajkumar and Greipp 1999). C-reactive protein concentration does not appear to be useful as a marker of disease status. C-reactive protein value also predicts high-dose therapy outcome.

3.9.1.3 Lactate Dehydrogenase

Increased lactate dehydrogenase values identify a group of patients with poor prognosis and aggressive disease, sometimes a lymphoma-like disease characterized by tumor masses and retroperitoneal adenopathy with a short clinical course. Fewer than 11% of patients with newly diagnosed myeloma have an increased concentration of lactate dehydrogenase (Kyle et al. 2003), thereby limiting its utility.

3.9.1.4 Bone Marrow Plasma Cell Number and Morphology

The quantity, growth patterns, and morphologic features of bone marrow plasma cells have been evaluated as prognosticators for patients with myeloma with vari-

Table 3.14. Prognostic and staging systems in newly diagnosed multiple myeloma patients (prognostic categories defined in patients treated with standard intensity chemotherapy, unless stated otherwise)

Study	Patients no.	Risk or stage	Patients %	Features	Median OS, mo
Durie and Salmon (1975)	150	IA	11	Defined in Table 3.13	61
		IIA & IIB	27		54
		IIIA	50		30
		IIIB	13		15
Medical Research Council's Working Party on Leukaemia in Adults (1980)	485	Low	22	BUN ≤8 mM and Hb >10 g/dL	>48
		Intermediate	56	Not meeting other criteria	~34
		High	22	BUN >10 mM and Hb ≤7.5 g/dL	~24
Bartl et al., 1987	674	Low grade	71	Marschalko and small PC[a]	40
		Intermediate grade	28	Cleaved, polymorphous asynchronous PC	20
		High grade	2	Plasmablastic PC	8
Bataille et al. (1992)	162	Low	50	β_2M and CRP <6 mg/L	54
		Intermediate	35	β_2M or CRP ≥6 mg/L	27
		High	15	β_2M and CRP ≥6 mg/L	6
Greipp et al. (1993)	107	Low	14	PCLI <1% and β_2M <2.7 mg/L	71
		Intermediate	54	PCLI ≥1% or β_2M ≥2.7 mg/L	40
		High	32	PCLI ≥1% and β_2M ≥2.7 mg/L	17
Finnish Leukaemia Group (1999)	324	I	61	Hb ≥10 g/dL and BMPC <70%	57
		II	25	Hb <10 g/dL or BMPC ≥70%	45
		III	14	Hb <10 g/dL and BMPC ≥70%	25
Konigsberg et al. (2000)	88	Low	36	No FISH del 13q and β_2M ≤4 mg/L	102
		Intermediate	40	No FISH del 13q or β_2M >4 mg/L	46
		High	24	No FISH del 13q and β_2M >4 mg/L	11
Crowley et al. (2001)	1,026	SWOG I	13	β_2M <2.5 mg/L	53
		II	43	β_2M ≥2.5 but <5.5 mg/L	41
		III	33	β_2M ≥5.5 mg/L and alb >3 g/dL	24
		IV	11	β_2M ≥5.5 mg/L and alb <3 g/dL	16

Alb, albumin; β_2M, β_2-microglobulin; BMPC, bone marrow plasma cells; BUN, blood urea nitrogen; CRP, C-reactive protein; ECOG, Eastern Cooperative Oncology Group; FISH, fluorescence in situ hybridization; PC, plasma cells; PCLI, plasma cell labeling index; SWOG, Southwest Oncology Group.

[a] See text for details. The Bartl staging system is a plasma cell morphology-based staging system.

able results (Bartl et al. 1987; Rajkumar and Greipp 1999). Bartl et al. (1987) constructed an intricate study of bone marrow characteristics of myeloma patients. The architectural pattern of growth – including interstitial, interstitial/sheets, interstitial/nodular, nodular, and packed – correlates with survival, as does the plasma cell morphology. According to these authors, myeloma cell histologic features can be classified into 6 types: 1) Marschalko type – predominantly normal-appearing plasma cells with a mean size of 21 microns; 2) small cell type – small, round, and lymphoplasmacytoid with mean size of 13 microns; 3) cleaved type – notched, cleaved, or even convoluted nuclei of variable size; 4) polymorphous type – marked cellular polymorphism and multinuclearity, with interspersed giant plasma cells and cytoplasmic inclusions; 5) asynchronous type – marked asynchronous maturation of nucleus and cytoplasm, large eccentric nuclei, frequent nucleoli, and pronounced perinuclear hof; and 6) blastic type – plasmablasts with large nuclei, prominent centrally located nucleoli with a moderate rim of basophilic cytoplasm, and a faint perinuclear hof (Table 3.14). Neither of these morphologic features – architecture or plasma cell histologic features – has been applied widely.

Other investigators have demonstrated the powerful prognostic significance of immature or plasmablastic plasma cells. Plasmablastic morphology is associated with a high PCLI, a higher level of sIL-6R, and *ras* mutations (Rajkumar and Greipp 1999). Electron microscopy confirms that immature nuclear morphology and nuclear cytoplasmic asynchrony correlate with one another and with poor prognosis. Nuclear immaturity and 3 cytoplasmic abnormalities – scattered pattern of mitochondria, single-sac looplike structures, and numerous intramitochondrial granules – have been associated with poor outcome.

3.9.1.5 Plasma Cell Labeling Index

The PCLI of the bone marrow plasma cells is a reproducible and powerful prognostic factor in multiple myeloma (Greipp et al. 1993; Rajkumar and Greipp 1999). The PCLI is determined from an immunofluorescence slide-based assay (Greipp et al. 1993). Cells in DNA S phase of the cell cycle incorporate bromodeoxyuridine, which can be recognized by using a monoclonal antibody. S-phase cells are then marked with a second antibody, and plasma cells are recognized by morphology and reactivity with antihuman immunoglobulin kappa and lambda light chain. An increased PCLI predicts short remission and survival but does not predict response to therapy. All large studies published to date have confirmed the independent prognostic value of the PCLI for survival after treatment with conventional chemotherapy (Boccadoro et al. 1989; Greipp et al. 1993) or high-dose therapy. Other methods for determining proliferation include Ki67 immunohistochemical staining and determination of S phase by flow cytometry.

3.9.1.6 Cytogenetics, Fluorescence In Situ Hybridization, and Other Genetic Abnormalities

Nearly all myeloma patients have abnormal chromosomes by fluorescence in situ hybridization (FISH), including deletions, aneuploidy, and translocations, although abnormal karyotypes are seen in only 18% to 30% of cases. This apparent contradiction is explained by the generally low proliferative rate of myeloma cells and the requirement of obtaining plasma cells in metaphase (and not just the rapidly dividing normal myeloid precursors) to generate conventional cytogenetics (Rajkumar and Greipp 1999). Therefore, any abnormality in conventional cytogenetics identifies a group with a higher proliferative rate and a particularly poor prognosis. There is an excellent correlation between abnormal conventional cytogenetics and high plasma cell proliferative rate (Zojer et al. 2000).

By interphase FISH, aneuploidy is present in the majority of newly diagnosed patients. Aneuploidy is characterized predominantly by a gain of chromosome numbers, but monosomy is not uncommon. With interphase FISH, several chromosomal abnormalities, such as immunoglobulin heavy chain translocations and deletion of chromosome 13, are observed at equal frequencies among the spectrum of plasmaproliferative disorders from MGUS to multiple myeloma to PCL (Avet-Loiseau et al. 2002).

Monoallelic loss of chromosome 13 (del 13) or its long arm (del 13q), when determined by cytogenetics, is a powerful adverse prognostic factor in patients treated with high-dose chemotherapy and hematopoietic stem cell transplantation (Barlogie et al. 1999). Approximately 50% of newly diagnosed multiple myeloma patients have del 13 or del 13q by FISH (Facon et al. 2001; Zojer et al. 2000). Our group has shown that del 13q is associated with specific biologic features, including a higher frequency of λ-type multiple myeloma, slight female predominance, higher PCLI, and higher frequency of serum M component of less than 1 g/dL (Fonseca et al. 2003). Patients with the deletion by FISH have a worse overall survival with standard chemotherapy (Fonseca et al. 2003; Konigsberg et al. 2000; Zojer et al. 2000), high-dose therapy (Facon et al. 2001), and interferon treatment. The absence of abnormalities of chromosome 13 and 11 by conventional cytogenetics is associated with longer complete response duration, event-free survival, and overall survival in patients treated with high-dose therapy (Barlogie et al. 1999). The prognostic significance of del 13q by FISH is less than that for del 13 by conventional cytogenetics, because the latter test incorporates both the chromosomal abnormality and a high rate of plasma cell proliferation, whereas the former captures only the chromosomal abnormality.

Hypodiploid myeloma has a worse prognosis than diploid or hyperdiploid myeloma. This has been demonstrated by flow cytometric methods and metaphase cytogenetics (Smadja et al. 2001). Controversy exists about whether the deletion 13q adds any additional prognostic information to a hypodiploid karyotype (Smadja et al. 2001).

Up to 75% of patients with multiple myeloma have translocations involving the heavy chain gene on chromosome 14. These translocations include illegitimate switch recombinations of the variable regions of the immunoglobulin heavy chain gene at 14q32. Partners of the translocations into the IgH switch region on chromosome 14 include chromosomes 11, 4, 6, and 16 (Avet-Loiseau et al. 2002). Occurring in 16% of myeloma patients, t(11;14)(q13;q32), which increases expression of cyclin D1, is the most common translocation in multiple myeloma (Avet-Loiseau et al. 2002). Previous publications had suggested that this translocation was associated with an adverse outcome in multiple myeloma (Barlogie et al. 1999; Konigsberg et al. 2000), but more recent data refute this hypothesis. The t(4;14)(p16.3;q32) is present in 10% to 20% of multiple myeloma patients (Avet-Loiseau et al. 2002). This translocation results in the upregulation of fibroblast growth factor receptor 3 (FGFR3) and in the hybrid transcript IgH/MMSET (Avet-Loiseau et al. 2002). The t(14;16)(q32;q23) is also seen in a small subset (~5%) of patients with multiple myeloma (Fonseca et al. 2003). In one study there was a tight association of del 13 abnormalities and high β_2M values with the unfavorable t(4;14) and t(16;14) abnormalities. The frequency of high β_2M or del 13 was one-half that in patients with the t(11;14) abnormality. This suggests that the poor prognosis associated with del 13 may be because of other nonrandom, associated chromosomal abnormalities. Three distinct staging groups can be defined based on the presence of t(14;16)(q32;q23), t(4;14)(p16.3;q32), deletion 17p13, and del 13q by FISH (Fonseca et al. 2003).

Mutations of ras have been noted in 30% to 50% of multiple myeloma patients (Hallek et al. 1998), with increasing prevalence in the advanced stages of the disease and shorter survival (K-ras). Mutations of ras were first observed in fulminant disease but have also been observed in 27% to 39% of newly diagnosed cases. Patients with ras mutations had a median survival of 2.1 years versus 4 years for patients with wild-type ras.

Inactivating mutation of p53, locus 17p13, is rare in freshly explanted myeloma cells but is common in human myeloma cell lines and in patients with a terminal phase of myeloma. Such mutations have been observed in ~5% of cases of early multiple myeloma versus 20% to 40% of cases of PCL. Deletions of p53 as detected by FISH are present in 9% to 33% of patients with newly diagnosed myeloma and confer a poorer median survival (15.9 months versus >38 months).

Epigenetic phenomena, such as methylation of the p16 (Met-p16) promoter region, have been associated with progression in the plasma cell dyscrasias. Met-p16 is uncommon in MGUS/smoldering multiple myeloma, increases in frequency with advancing stages of the disease, and is common in extramedullary multiple myeloma, including PCL.

3.9.1.7 Angiogenesis

Several studies have demonstrated prognostic significance of increased microvessel density (ie, angiogenesis) in multiple myeloma. The first description was a comprehensive study of multiple myeloma and MGUS that showed a strong association with diagnosis and with increased S-phase fraction of plasma cells measured by the PCLI.

3.9.1.8 Lymphocyte Subsets

Low numbers of CD4 (helper T) cells at diagnosis are associated with a worse prognosis; the prognostic importance of CD4 T cells is present throughout the course of disease, including after the completion of chemotherapy and at relapse.

In the posttransplantation setting, the number of circulating lymphocytes appears to be an important prognostic factor. Porrata et al. (2001) demonstrated lower relapse rates and prolonged survival for patients with higher absolute lymphocyte counts after autologous stem cell transplantation, suggesting an early graft-versus-tumor effect. The median overall survival and progression-free survival for myeloma patients were significantly longer in patients with an absolute lymphocyte count $\geqslant$ 500 cells/μL on day 15 than for patients with an absolute lymphocyte count < 500 cells/μL (33 vs. 12 months; 16 vs. 8 months). Desikan et al. at the University of Arkansas made a similar observation. In a trial designed to evaluate the role of more intense conditioning, lymphocyte recovery, evaluated as a surrogate for immune recovery, was inferior in more intensively treated patients. Despite identical complete remission rates, event-free survival and overall survival were significantly decreased among patients receiving more intensive conditioning in 2000.

3.9.1.9 Other Prognostic Factors

Other factors that have adverse prognostic value include (Rajkumar and Greipp 1999) decreased staining of bone marrow plasma cells for acid phosphatase; increased circulating plasma cells as measured by the peripheral blood labeling index; apoptotic index; increased sIL-6R; serum neopterin; a_1-antitrypsin; c-terminal telopeptide of Type I collagen; serum bone sialoprotein; B_{12} binding protein; sCD56; soluble Fc receptor (CD16); soluble syndecan or CD138; and serum IL-6 levels. Although IL-6 is known to have a major role in myeloma pathogenesis, C-reactive protein levels correlate well with this more expensive and less readily available prognostic test.

3.9.1.10 Drug Resistance

One form of drug resistance is marked by multidrug resistance-1 expression on plasma cells by immunocytochemistry. The presence of this P-glycoprotein in the cell membrane of plasma cells of patients with multiple myeloma is associated with a poor prognosis. Drug resistance measured by immunocytochemical detection of lung resistance protein is highly correlated with failure of response to melphalan and poor subsequent survival.

3.9.2 Significance of the Extent of Response After Therapy

3.9.2.1 Significance of Response After Standard Intensity Chemotherapy

Response is often used as a measure of efficacy, and it is often assumed that complete remissions are a prerequisite for cure. Indeed, patients treated with standard intensity chemotherapy with responsive disease tend to live a median of 18 months longer than do patients with resistant disease (Bergsagel et al. 1967; Bladé et al. 1994). However, tumor response may speak more to a patient's tumor biology than it does to the therapy in question. Most standard intensity chemotherapy studies suggest that the degree of response does not correlate with survival (Bladé et al. 1994; Oivanen et al. 1999). Rather, the ability to achieve a plateau of at least 6 months' duration is as important, if not more important, as the degree of response to therapy (Corso et al. 1999; Finnish Leukaemia Group 1999). The data from only 3 of 27 randomized induction trials would suggest that a higher response rate translates into longer overall survival (Myeloma Trialists' Collaborative Group 1998).

The importance of response kinetics is also a controversial topic. Some data support the premise that those with the most rapid responses with alkylator-based therapy have a shorter remission duration and survival (Belch et al. 1988), and other data contradict this premise (Bladé et al. 1994).

3.9.2.2 Significance of a Complete Response After High-Dose Therapy

It is controversial whether the achievement of a complete response, as defined by the disappearance of the M protein by immunofixation of the serum and urine after high-dose therapy with hematopoietic stem cell support, is of prognostic value. Multiple studies have produced inconsistent results (Attal et al. 1996; Bjorkstrand et al. 2001; Davies et al. 2001; Gahrton et al. 1991; Lahuerta et al. 2000). Several of these studies (Attal et al. 1996; Gahrton et al. 1991) did not use the more stringent definition of complete response; they relied on the absence of an M protein on electrophoretic pattern rather than immunofixation negativity. These studies should be interpreted with caution because they do not include several of the most powerful determinants of prognosis – PCLI and conventional cytogenetics (Barlogie et al. 1999; Greipp et al. 1993).

One of these is a retrospective study of 344 patients with multiple myeloma treated with high-dose chemotherapy followed by autologous stem cell transplantation. Patients were not treated uniformly. The 5-year overall survival was 48% in those who had no M protein on immunofixation and 21% in those with a persistent M protein (Lahuerta et al. 2000). In 2001 Alexanian et al. (Hahn et al. 2003) reported on a series of 68 patients treated with dexamethasone-based induction therapy followed by early high-dose therapy; results were compared to those of 50 patients who were unable to receive high-dose therapy because of socioeconomic reasons. Those patients who achieved immunofixation-negative complete response by either means (ie, high-dose or standard chemotherapy) had a superior overall survival to that of patients who achieved a partial response or less. The implication of these data is that complete response may be an important surrogate marker of long survival and less aggressive myeloma biology. This study was also lacking important baseline prognostic information (ie, PCLI and cytogenetics). In yet another study, Davies and colleagues (2001) reported a series of 96 patients who received high-dose therapy and were assessed for the effect of response on survival. Although there was a trend toward an improved progression-free survival among patients with an immunofixation-negative complete response compared with patients with a partial response (49.4 months vs. 41.1 months, $P = 0.26$), there was no improvement in overall survival. Finally, Rajkumar et al. reported a complete response in 33% of 126 multiple myeloma patients who underwent stem cell transplantation. There was no difference in the overall survival or progression-free survival between patients who achieved a complete response and those who did not; rather, overall survival was significantly influenced by the level of the PCLI.

3.9.3 New Staging Systems

Durie-Salmon stage has been the standard of prognosis in multiple myeloma (Durie and Salmon 1975). Deficiencies in this system include the subjectivity of interpretation of the severity of bone lesions and their questionable prognostic value, as well as the limited value of hypercalcemia as a prognostic indicator. Other investigators have designed staging systems (Table 3.14) including other variables: β_2M, C-reactive protein, PCLI, serum albumin, hemoglobin, renal function, del 13q, bone marrow plasma cell involvement, and bone marrow morphology (including plasmablastic morphology) (Bartl et al. 1987; Bataille et al. 1992; Crowley et al. 2001; Facon et al. 2001; Finnish Leukaemia Group 1999; Greipp et al. 1993; Konigsberg et al. 2000; Medical Research Council's Working Party on Leukaemia in Adults 1980). Each of these systems has value, but the goal is to reach a consensus and to standardize discussions and comparisons among clinical trials and outcomes. An international consensus panel is addressing this.

At Mayo Clinic and ECOG (Greipp et al. 1993), the PCLI is heavily relied on. It has been incorporated into 3 different staging systems. There has been no analysis in which the PCLI was included that it was not one of the most – if not the most – important predictor of survival (Boccadoro et al. 1989, Greipp et al. 1993).

Barlogie et al. (1999) proposed a prognostic system for high-dose chemotherapy patients that incorporates "unfavorable cytogenetics" (abnormalities of chromosomes 13 and 11 by conventional cytogenetics) and β_2M values greater than 4 mg/L. The small subset of patients with both unfavorable cytogenetics and increased β_2M values has median event-free and overall survival of only 1.7 and 2.1 years, respectively, compared with 4.2 and 7.0 plus years for patients without unfavorable cytogenetics and any β_2M value. The combination of del 13 by FISH and β_2M was recently proposed as a new staging system in patients receiving high-dose chemotherapy (Facon et al. 2001).

3.10 Treatment of Complications and Supportive Care

3.10.1 Treatment of Myeloma Bone Disease

Myeloma bone disease is a significant contributor to morbidity. The standard method of following patients is with periodic (every 6 to 12 months) skeletal radiographs; the use of more sophisticated imaging modalities is being explored. Cross-linked N-telopeptides of Type I collagen, which can be measured in the serum or urine, appear to be a sensitive indicator of bone turnover, and urinary levels show a strong positive correlation with the dynamic histomorphometric indices of bone resorption. Despite careful monitoring, patients are at risk for skeletal events.

Monthly intravenous administration of pamidronate has been shown to reduce the likelihood of a skeletal event by almost 50% in patients with multiple myeloma (Berenson et al. 1998). In this study, 392 patients with stage III myeloma and at least 1 lytic lesion received either placebo or pamidronate, 90 mg intravenously administered as a 4-hour infusion monthly for 21 cycles. Skeletal events (pathologic fracture, radiation or surgery, and spinal cord compression) and hypercalcemia were assessed monthly. The mean number of skeletal events per year was less in the pamidronate group (1.3) than in placebo-treated patients (2.2; $P=0.008$), and the proportion of patients who developed any skeletal event was lower in the pamidronate group ($P=0.015$). A recent study demonstrated equivalency of pamidronate and zoledronic acid (Rosen et al. 2001). Median time to the first skeletal-related event was approximately 1 year in each treatment group, and the proportion of patients with at least 1 skeletal-related event was similar in all treatment groups.

When a lytic bone lesion is present, significant risk factors for fracture of a long bone include increased pain with use and involvement by more than two-thirds the diameter of the bone. These lesions should be treated prophylactically with surgery if they are situated in weight-bearing bones. Endosteal resorption of one-half the cortical width of the femur weakens the bone by 70%. Surgical treatment should be considered for these lesions as well. Once a bone has fractured, healing can occur, especially if proper internal fixation is performed and if patients have an anticipated survival of >6 months. Much of these data regarding malignant bone disease are derived from patients with carcinoma rather than multiple myeloma. In patients with carcinoma metastatic to bone, modest postoperative radiation doses ($\leqslant 3,000$ cGy) as adjuvant therapy are associated with better healing, but the role of adjuvant radiation therapy in this setting in multiple myeloma patients is less clear. Multiple myeloma is often chemotherapy sensitive; adjuvant systemic chemotherapy in multiple myeloma patients may be more appropriate than adjuvant radiation therapy. In general, radiation therapy should be used for pain relief in chemotherapy-refractory disease, because it relieves pain in 80% to 90% of patients with bony metastases, long-term in 55% to 70%.

Percutaneous vertebroplasty is occasionally an option for patients with vertebral body compression fracture. Pain relief is generally apparent within 1 to 2 days after injection and persists for at least several months up to several years. Complications are relatively rare, although some studies reported a high incidence of clinically insignificant leakage of bone cement into the paravertebral tissues. Compression of spinal nerve roots or neuralgia due to the leakage of polymer and pulmonary embolism have also been reported.

3.10.2 Spinal Cord Compression

Spinal cord compression, however, remains an important and emergent subject. The usual standard treatment is high-dose corticosteroids and radiation therapy. On rare occasions, surgical decompression may be considered. Because most myelomatous lesions arise from the vertebral body, an anterior surgical approach is generally used, which may contribute to additional morbidity. The 1 small randomized trial addressing the question of radiation versus laminectomy and radiation showed no benefit from laminectomy; similarly, a larger retrospective series found no benefit. If the deficit is due to compression by the plasma cell tumor (rather than a bone fragment retropulsed by a pathologic compression fracture), outcomes with radiation therapy are probably equal to (or superior to) surgical intervention in a radiosensitive tumorlike myeloma.

High-dose corticosteroids may provide immediate pain palliation and improvement in neurologic function. The optimal corticosteroid dose has not been established, but common dose schedules for metastatic disease include dexamethasone in an initial bolus of 10 mg intravenously or 100 mg intravenously followed by 4 mg orally 4 times daily or 100-mg intravenous bolus followed by 96 mg in 4 divided doses for 3 days followed by a dose taper.

3.10.3 Hypercalcemia

Patients with multiple myeloma are at risk for severe hypercalcemia that can precipitate acute renal failure, hypertension, nausea, vomiting, pancreatitis, cardiac arrhythmia, coma, and death. The extracellular volume depletion associated with hypercalcemia should be corrected by vigorous hydration followed by an antiresorptive agent such as intravenous bisphosphonate. Serum calcium value usually declines rapidly, reaching the normal range within 2 to 3 days in more than 80% of cases. It occasionally goes below normal at the nadir. Corticosteroids can also reduce serum calcium concentration in about 60% of patients with hypercalcemia.

Gallium nitrate, mithramycin, and calcitonin are interesting from a historical perspective. Since the advent of bisphosphonates, they are generally not used.

3.10.4 Hematologic Complications Including Anemia, Secondary Leukemia, Hyperviscosity, and Cryoglobulinemia

3.10.4.1 Anemia

The anemia of multiple myeloma can result from many factors. For patients with anemia due solely to myelomatous bone marrow infiltration, chemotherapy remedies the problem. Other patients have a relative erythropoietin deficiency related to renal injury due to the myeloma or to age-related changes. In these patients, as in any patient with renal insufficiency, modest doses of recombinant erythropoietin are effective. For patients with chemotherapy-induced anemia, recombinant erythropoietin may be effective at higher doses (150 to 300 IU/kg thrice weekly or 40,000 units weekly) (Garton et al. 1995). An inappropriately low endogenous erythropoietin concentration is the most important factor predicting response.

3.10.4.2 Secondary Myelodysplasia and Acute Leukemia

The most ominous cause of anemia in the setting of previously treated multiple myeloma is secondary myelodysplastic syndrome or acute leukemia. In the late 1960s and early 1970s investigators noted that cytotoxic agents can induce myelodysplasia and acute myeloid leukemia. The risk of secondary myelodysplastic syndrome or acute leukemia is approximately 3% at 5 years and 10% at 8 to 9 years (Cuzick et al. 1987). The extremes of estimates range from an actuarial risk of 25% at 5 years to 0.7% over 10 years, with multiple other estimates somewhere in between. A reasonable guideline is that the 10-year risk of myelodysplastic syndrome or acute myeloid leukemia is about 3% for every year of melphalan treatment (Cuzick et al. 1987). Some authors have suggested that higher cumulative doses of melphalan are implicated as a risk for acute leukemia; others have shown no difference in incidence based on the number of courses of chemotherapy or the cumulative melphalan dose between the patients who did and did not develop acute leukemia. Investigators from the Finnish Leukaemia Study showed that mean number of chemotherapy cycles was 19.7 and 18.5 in patients with and without secondary leukemia; mean cumulative melphalan doses were 1,440 and 1,400 mg, respectively. Although cyclophosphamide has been shown to be leukemogenic, data suggest that it is less so than melphalan (Cuzick et al. 1987). After secondary leukemia is diagnosed, median survival tends to be short – about 2 months.

The occurrence of multiple cases of acute leukemia in multiple cases of myeloma suggests that there may be a proclivity for acute leukemia to develop in patients with myeloma. After stem cell transplantation for myeloma, the risk of myelodysplastic syndrome appears to be related to prior chemotherapy rather than to the transplant itself, at least in one retrospective series.

3.10.4.3 Cryoglobulinemia

Approximately 5% of myeloma gamma globulins exhibit reversible precipitation in the cold, so-called cryoglobulins, forming either a flocculent precipitate or a gel-like coagulum when the serum is cooled.

3.10.4.4 Hyperviscosity

Plasmapheresis relieves the symptoms of hyperviscosity, but the benefit of this treatment in the absence of concurrent chemotherapy is short-lived.

3.10.5 Renal Failure

A normal creatinine value is present in approximately half of multiple myeloma patients at diagnosis (Kapadia 1980; Kyle et al. 2003). Only 15% to 25% have a creatinine value above 2 mg/dL. If the renal insufficiency reverses, as it does in more than half of cases, survival is 4-fold to 7-fold higher than in those in whom it does not. Factors predicting for renal function recovery include serum creatinine < 4 mg/dL, serum calcium value 11.5 mg/dL, proteinuria <1 g/24 h, and adequate rehydration. For patients with multiple myeloma and severe renal failure who survive the first 2 months on dialysis, 40% have an objective response to chemotherapy and a median survival of almost 2 years. Factors that increase renal tubular cast formation include dehydration, infection, and hypercalcemia. Maintaining a 24-hour fluid intake of at least 3 liters can improve renal function.

Because light chains with the lowest isoelectric points tend to be more nephrotoxic in animal models, avoidance of a low or acidic urinary pH is recommended. Give either oral or intravenous bicarbonate in the setting of acute renal failure. The MRC III myelomatosis trial randomized multiple myeloma patients with significant renal failure to oral sodium bicarbonate to neutralize urine pH (or not), and there was a trend toward better survival in the bicarbonate recipients.

The use of plasmapheresis in the setting of renal failure remains controversial. One small randomized study of patients with active myeloma and progressive renal failure suggested benefit of plasmapheresis in a subset of patients (Johnson et al. 1990). Twenty-one patients were randomized to either forced diuresis and chemotherapy (10 patients) or forced diuresis, chemotherapy, and plasmapheresis (11 patients). There was a trend toward better outcome in the plasmapheresis group, but the difference was not statistically significant. It is unclear whether the lack of significance is due to the small sample size (underpowered) or to an equivalence of the 2 therapeutic strategies. The study did demonstrate that the severity of myeloma cast formation directly correlated with lack of improvement regardless of treatment strategy.

3.10.6 Infection Management

Infections are a major cause of morbidity in myeloma patients. Pneumonias and urinary tract infections caused by *Streptococcus pneumoniae*, *Haemophilus influenzae*, and *Escherichia coli* are most frequent. The susceptibility to infection varies with the phase of illness. In one prospective study, the overall serious infection rate was 0.92 infections per patient-year and was 4 times higher during periods of active disease (1.90) than in plateau phase myeloma (0.49). In a retrospective study evaluating the sequential incidence of infection, the first 2 months of initial chemotherapy emerged as a particularly high-risk period, with nearly half of the patients experiencing at least 1 clinically significant infection. Infections late in the course of multiple myeloma may be an inevitable result of long-standing immunosuppression and overwhelming tumor burden. Prevention of infection is a critical goal for improving survival.

Prevention of infections by use of vaccines is an attractive strategy. Unfortunately, responses to vaccines are poor among myeloma patients. Patients with myeloma were investigated to assess whether immunologic risk factors predisposing to serious infection could be identified. Specific antibody titers to pneumococcal capsular polysaccharides and tetanus and diphtheria toxoids were significantly reduced compared with the control population. Low antipneumococcal and anti–*Escherichia coli* titers correlated with risk of serious infection. In addition, among 41 immunized patients, responses to pneumococcus vaccine and tetanus and diphtheria toxoids were poor. IgG subclass levels were significantly reduced, and a poor IgG response to pneumococcus vaccine immunization was associated with an increased risk of septicemia. The predominant site of infection was the respiratory tract. Decreased concentrations of the uninvolved immunoglobulins were significantly associated with at least 1 serious infection.

The most common prevention strategy consists of prophylaxis with antibiotics (Oken et al. 1996b). A randomized, placebo-controlled trial of trimethoprim-sulfamethoxazole (TMP-SMX) demonstrated a significant decrease in severe infections among newly diagnosed myeloma patients randomized to TMP-SMX compared with controls (Oken et al. 1996b). Fifty-seven patients about to begin chemotherapy for multiple myeloma were randomly assigned to prophylaxis for 2 months or to no prophylaxis (control). Antibiotic prophylaxis consisted of TMP-SMX (160/800 mg orally every 12 hours) administered for the first 2 months of initial chemotherapy. Bacterial infection occurred in 11 control patients but in only 2 patients assigned to receive TMP-SMX ($P = 0.004$). Eight severe infections occurred in controls compared with 1 in a TMP-SMX patient ($P = 0.010$). Severe infections included 5 cases of pneumonia (3 with sepsis), 2 urinary tract infections with complicating pneumonia or sepsis, 1 diverticulitis with perforation, and 1 staphylococcal scalded skin syndrome. The rate of bacterial infection was 2.43 per patient-year for controls and 0.29 per patient-year for the TMP-SMX group ($P = 0.001$). Toxicity (skin rash in 6 patients, nausea in 1 patient) was not life-threatening but required discontinuation of TMP-SMX in 25% of patients.

References

Alberts DS, Durie BG, Salmon SE (1976) Doxorubicin/B.C.N.U. chemotherapy for multiple myeloma in relapse. Lancet 1:926–928

Alexanian R (1980) Localized and indolent myeloma. Blood 56:521–525

Alexanian R, Salmon S, Bonnet J, Gehan E, Haut A, Weick J (1977) Combination therapy for multiple myeloma. Cancer 40:2765–2771

Alexanian R, Gehan E, Haut A, Saiki J, Weick J (1978) Unmaintained remissions in multiple myeloma. Blood 51:1005–1011

Alexanian R, Barlogie B, Tucker S (1990) VAD-based regimens as primary treatment for multiple myeloma. Am J Hematol 33:86–89

Alexanian R, Dimopoulos MA, Delasalle K, Barlogie B (1992) Primary dexamethasone treatment of multiple myeloma. Blood 80:887–890

Alexanian R, Weber D, Dimopoulos M, Delasalle K, Smith TL (2000) Randomized trial of alpha-interferon or dexamethasone as maintenance treatment for multiple myeloma. Am J Hematol 65:204–209

Attal M, Harousseau JL, Stoppa AM, Sotto JJ, Fuzibet JG, Rossi JF, Casassus P, Maisonneuve H, Facon T, Ifrah N, Payen C, Bataille R (1996) A prospective, randomized trial of autologous bone marrow transplantation and chemotherapy in multiple myeloma. Intergroupe Français du Myélome. N Engl J Med 335:91–97

Avet-Loiseau H, Facon T, Grosbois B, Magrangeas F, Rapp MJ, Harousseau JL, Minvielle S, Bataille R, for the Intergroupe Francophone du Myélome (2002) Oncogenesis of multiple myeloma: 14q32 and 13q chromosomal abnormalities are not randomly distributed, but correlate with natural history, immunological features, and clinical presentation. Blood 99:2185–2191

Badros A, Barlogie B, Siegel E, Cotter-Fox M, Zangari M, Fassas A, Morris C, Anaissie E, Van Rhee F, Tricot G (2002) Improved outcome of allogeneic transplantation in high-risk multiple myeloma patients after nonmyeloablative conditioning. J Clin Oncol 20:1295–1303

Barlogie B, Smith L, Alexanian R (1984) Effective treatment of advanced multiple myeloma refractory to alkylating agents. N Engl J Med 310:1353–1356

Barlogie B, Dicke KA, Alexanian R (1988) High dose melphalan for refractory myeloma: the M.D. Anderson experience. Hematol Oncol 6:167–172

Barlogie B, Velasquez WS, Alexanian R, Cabanillas F (1989) Etoposide, dexamethasone, cytarabine, and cisplatin in vincristine, doxorubicin, and dexamethasone-refractory myeloma. J Clin Oncol 7:1514–1517

Barlogie B, Jagannath S, Desikan KR, Mattox S, Vesole D, Siegel D, Tricot G, Munshi N, Fassas A, Singhal S, Mehta J, Anaissie E, Dhodapkar D, Naucke S, Cromer J, Sawyer J, Epstein J, Spoon D, Ayers D, Cheson B, Crowley J (1999) Total therapy with tandem transplants for newly diagnosed multiple myeloma. Blood 93:55–65

Bartl R, Frisch B, Fateh-Moghadam A, Kettner G, Jaeger K, Sommerfeld W (1987) Histologic classification and staging of multiple myeloma. A retrospective and prospective study of 674 cases. Am J Clin Pathol 87:342–355

Bataille R, Harousseau JL (1997) Multiple myeloma. N Engl J Med 336:1657–1664

Bataille R, Boccadoro M, Klein B, Durie B, Pileri A (1992) C-reactive protein and beta-2 microglobulin produce a simple and powerful myeloma staging system. Blood 80:733–737

Belch A, Shelley W, Bergsagel D, Wilson K, Klimo P, White D, Willan A (1988) A randomized trial of maintenance versus no maintenance melphalan and prednisone in responding multiple myeloma patients. Br J Cancer 57:94–99

Bensinger WI, Buckner CD, Anasetti C, Clift R, Storb R, Barnett T, Chauncey T, Shulman H, Appelbaum FR (1996) Allogeneic marrow transplantation for multiple myeloma: an analysis of risk factors on outcome. Blood 88:2787–2793

Berenson JR, Lichtenstein A, Porter L, Dimopoulos MA, Bordoni R, George S, Lipton A, Keller A, Ballester O, Kovacs M, Blacklock H, Bell R, Simeone JF, Reitsma DJ, Heffernan M, Seaman J, Knight RD (1998) Long-term pamidronate treatment of advanced multiple myeloma patients reduces skeletal events. Myeloma Aredia Study Group. J Clin Oncol 16:593–602

Berenson JR, Crowley JJ, Grogan TM, Zangmeister J, Briggs AD, Mills GM, Barlogie B, Salmon SE (2002) Maintenance therapy with alternate-day prednisone improves survival in multiple myeloma patients. Blood 99:3163–3168

Bergsagel DE, Griffith KM, Haut A, Stuckey WJ Jr (1967) The treatment of plasma cell myeloma. Adv Cancer Res 10:311–359

Bjorkstrand B, Svensson H, Goldschmidt H, Ljungman P, Apperley J, Mandelli F, Marcus R, Boogaerts M, Alegre A, Remes K, Cornelissen JJ, Bladé J, Lenhoff S, Iriondo A, Carlson K, Volin L, Littlewood T, Goldstone AH, San Miguel J, Schattenberg A, Gahrton G (2001) Alpha-interferon maintenance treatment is associated with improved survival after high-dose treatment and autologous stem cell transplantation in patients with multiple myeloma: a retrospective registry study from the European Group for Blood and Marrow Transplantation (EBMT). Bone Marrow Transplant 27:511–515

Bjorkstrand BB, Ljungman P, Svensson H, Hermans J, Alegre A, Apperley J, Bladé J, Carlson K, Cavo M, Ferrant A, Goldstone AH, de Laurenzi A, Majolino I, Marcus R, Prentice HG, Remes K, Samson D, Sureda A, Verdonck LF, Volin L, Gahrton G (1996) Allogeneic bone marrow transplantation versus autologous stem cell transplantation in multiple myeloma: a retrospective case-matched study from the European Group for Blood and Marrow Transplantation. Blood 88:4711–4718

Bladé J, Kyle RA (1999) Nonsecretory myeloma, immunoglobulin D myeloma, and plasma cell leukemia. Hematol Oncol Clin North Am 13:1259–1272

Bladé J, Lopez-Guillermo A, Bosch F, Cervantes F, Reverter JC, Montserrat E, Rozman C (1994) Impact of response to treatment on survival in multiple myeloma: results in a series of 243 patients. Br J Haematol 88:117–121

Bladé J, Samson D, Reece D, Apperley J, Bjorkstrand B, Gahrton G, Gertz M, Giralt S, Jagannath S, Vesole D (1998) Criteria for evaluating disease response and progression in patients with multiple myeloma treated by high-dose therapy and haemopoietic stem cell transplantation. Myeloma Subcommittee of the EBMT. European Group for Blood and Marrow Transplant. Br J Haematol 102:1115–1123

Boccadoro M, Marmont F, Tribalto M, Fossati G, Redoglia V, Battaglio S, Massaia M, Gallamini A, Comotti B, Barbui T, Campobasso N, Dammacco F, Cantonetti M, Petrucci MT, Mandelli F, Resegotti L, Pileri A (1989) Early responder myeloma: kinetic studies identify a patient subgroup characterized by very poor prognosis. J Clin Oncol 7:119–125

Bonnet J, Alexanian R, Salmon S, Bottomley R, Amare M, Haut A, Dixon D (1982) Vincristine, BCNU, doxorubicin, and prednisone (VBAP) combination in the treatment of relapsing or resistant multiple myeloma: a Southwest Oncology Group study. Cancer Treat Rep 66:1267–1271

Case DC Jr, Lee DJ III, Clarkson BD (1977) Improved survival times in multiple myeloma treated with melphalan, prednisone, cyclophosphamide, vincristine and BCNU: M-2 protocol. Am J Med 63:897–903

Cohen HJ, Bartolucci AA, Forman WB, Silberman HR (1986) Consolidation and maintenance therapy in multiple myeloma: randomized comparison of a new approach to therapy after initial response to treatment. J Clin Oncol 4:888–899

Committee of the Chronic Leukemia-Myeloma Task Force NCI (1973) Proposed guidelines for protocol studies. I. Introduction. II. Plasma cell myeloma. III. Chronic lymphocytic leukemia. IV. Chronic granulocytic leukemia. Cancer Chemother Rep 3 vol 4:141–173

Cooper MR, McIntyre OR, Propert KJ, Kochwa S, Anderson K, Coleman M, Kyle RA, Prager D, Rafla S, Zimmer B (1986) Single, sequential, and multiple alkylating agent therapy for multiple myeloma: a CALGB Study. J Clin Oncol 4:1331–1339

Cornwell GG III, Pajak TF, Kochwa S, McIntyre OR, Glowienka LP, Brunner K, Rafla S, Coleman M, Cooper MR, Henderson E, Kyle RA, Haurani FI, Cuttner J, Prager D, Holland JF (1988) Vincristine and prednisone prolong the survival of patients receiving intravenous or oral melphalan for multiple myeloma: Cancer and Leukemia Group B experience. J Clin Oncol 6:1481–1490

Corso A, Nozza A, Lazzarino M, Klersy C, Zappasodi P, Arcaini L, Bernasconi C (1999) Plateau phase in multiple myeloma: an end-point of conventional-dose chemotherapy. Haematologica 84:336–341

Crowley J, Jacobson J, Alexanian R (2001) Standard-dose therapy for multiple myeloma: the Southwest Oncology Group experience. Semin Hematol 38:203–208

Cunningham D, Powles R, Malpas J, Raje N, Milan S, Viner C, Montes A, Hickish T, Nicolson M, Johnson P, Treleaven J, Raymond J, Gore M (1998) A randomized trial of maintenance interferon following high-dose chemotherapy in multiple myeloma: long-term follow-up results. Br J Haematol 102:495–502

Cuzick J, Erskine S, Edelman D, Galton DA (1987) A comparison of the incidence of the myelodysplastic syndrome and acute myeloid leukaemia following melphalan and cyclophosphamide treatment for myelomatosis. A report to the Medical Research Council's Working Party on Leukaemia in Adults. Br J Cancer 55:523–529

Dalton WS, Bergsagel PL, Kuehl WM, Anderson KC, Harousseau JL (2001) Multiple myeloma. Hematology (Am Soc Hematol Educ Program), pp 157–177

Davies FE, Forsyth PD, Rawstron AC, Owen RG, Pratt G, Evans PA, Richards SJ, Drayson M, Smith GM, Selby PJ, Child JA, Morgan GJ (2001) The impact of attaining a minimal disease state after high-dose melphalan and autologous transplantation for multiple myeloma. Br J Haematol 112:814–819

de Weerdt O, van de Donk NW, Veth G, Bloem AC, Hagenbeek A, Lokhorst HM (2001) Continuous low-dose cyclophosphamide-prednisone is effective and well tolerated in patients with advanced multiple myeloma. Neth J Med 59:50–56

Dimopoulos MA, Zervas K, Kouvatseas G, Galani E, Grigoraki V, Kiamouris C, Vervessou E, Samantas E, Papadimitriou C, Economou O, Gika D, Panayiotidis P, Christakis I, Anagnostopoulos N (2001) Thalidomide and dexamethasone combination for refractory multiple myeloma. Ann Oncol 12:991–995

Dispenzieri A, Kyle RA, Lacy MQ, Rajkumar SV, Therneau TM, Larson DR, Greipp PR, Witzig TE, Basu R, Suarez GA, Fonseca R, Lust JA, Gertz MA (2003) POEMS syndrome: definitions and long-term outcome. Blood 101:2496–2506

Drayson M, Tang LX, Drew R, Mead GP, Carr-Smith H, Bradwell AR (2001) Serum free light-chain measurements for identifying and monitoring patients with nonsecretory multiple myeloma. Blood 97:2900–2902

Durie BG, Salmon SE (1975) A clinical staging system for multiple myeloma. Correlation of measured myeloma cell mass with presenting clinical features, response to treatment, and survival. Cancer 36:842–854

Facon T, Menard JF, Michaux JL, Euller-Ziegler L, Bernard JF, Grosbois B, Daragon A, Azais I, Courouble Y, Kaplan G, LaPorte JP, De Gramont A, Duclos B, Leonard A, Mineur P, Delannoy A, Jouet JP, Bauters F, Monconduit M (1995) Prognostic factors in low tumour mass asymptomatic multiple myeloma: a report on 91 patients. The Groupe d'Etudes et de Recherche sur le Myelome (GERM). Am J Hematol 48:71–75

Facon T, Avet-Loiseau H, Guillerm G, Moreau P, Genevieve F, Zandecki M, Lai JL, Leleu X, Jouet JP, Bauters F, Harousseau JL, Bataille R, Mary JY (2001) Chromosome 13 abnormalities identified by FISH analysis and serum beta$_2$-microglobulin produce a powerful myeloma staging system for patients receiving high-dose therapy. Blood 97:1566–1571

Fermand JP, Ravaud P, Chevret S, Divine M, Leblond V, Belanger C, Macro M, Pertuiset E, Dreyfus F, Mariette X, Boccacio C, Brouet JC (1998) High-dose therapy and autologous peripheral blood stem cell transplantation in multiple myeloma: up-front or rescue treatment? Results of a multicenter sequential randomized clinical trial. Blood 92:3131–3136

Finnish Leukaemia Group (1999) Long-term survival in multiple myeloma: a Finnish Leukaemia Group study. Br J Haematol 105:942–947

Fonseca R, Blood E, Rue M, Harrington D, Oken MM, Kyle RA, Dewald GW, Van Ness B, Van Wier SA, Henderson KJ, Bailey RJ, Greipp PR (2003) Clinical and biologic implications of recurrent genomic aberrations in myeloma. Blood 101:4569–4575

Forgeson GV, Selby P, Lakhani S, Zulian G, Viner C, Maitland J, McElwain TJ (1988) Infused vincristine and Adriamycin with high dose methylprednisolone (VAMP) in advanced previously treated multiple myeloma patients. Br J Cancer 58:469–473

Gahrton G, Tura S, Ljungman P, Belanger C, Brandt L, Cavo M, Facon T, Granena A, Gore M, Gratwohl A, Löwenberg B, Nikoskelainen J, Reiffers JJ, Samson D, Verdonck L, Volin L (1991) Allogeneic bone marrow transplantation in multiple myeloma. European Group for Bone Marrow Transplantation. N Engl J Med 325:1267–1273

Garton JP, Gertz MA, Witzig TE, Greipp PR, Lust JA, Schroeder G, Kyle RA (1995) Epoetin alfa for the treatment of the anemia of multiple myeloma. A prospective, randomized, placebo-controlled, double-blind trial. Arch Intern Med 155:2069–2074

Gertz MA, Garton JP, Greipp PR, Witzig TE, Kyle RA (1995) A phase II study of high-dose methylprednisolone in refractory or relapsed multiple myeloma. Leukemia 9:2115–2118

Geschickter CF, Copeland MM (1928) Multiple myeloma. Arch Surg 16:807–863

Giralt S, Aleman A, Anagnostopoulos A, Weber D, Khouri I, Anderlini P, Molldrem J, Ueno NT, Donato M, Korbling M, Gajewski J, Alexanian R, Champlin R (2002) Fludarabine/melphalan conditioning for allogeneic transplantation in patients with multiple myeloma. Bone Marrow Transplant 30:367–373

Greipp PR, Lust JA, O'Fallon WM, Katzmann JA, Witzig TE, Kyle RA (1993) Plasma cell labeling index and beta 2-microglobulin predict survival independent of thymidine kinase and C-reactive protein in multiple myeloma. Blood 81:3382–3387

Hahn T, Wingard JR, Anderson KC, Bensinger WI, Berenson JR, Brozeit G, Carver JR, Kyle RA, McCarthy PL Jr (2003) The role of cytotoxic therapy with hematopoietic stem cell transplantation in the therapy of multiple myeloma: an evidence-based review. Biol Blood Marrow Transplant 9:4–37

Hallek M, Bergsagel PL, Anderson KC (1998) Multiple myeloma: increasing evidence for a multistep transformation process. Blood 91:3–21

Harousseau JL, Attal M (2002) The role of stem cell transplantation in multiple myeloma. Blood Rev 16:245–253

Hjorth M, Hellquist L, Holmberg E, Magnusson B, Rodjer S, Westin J (1993) Initial versus deferred melphalan-prednisone therapy for asymptomatic multiple myeloma stage I: a randomized study. Myeloma Group of Western Sweden. Eur J Haematol 50:95–102

The International Myeloma Working Group (2003) Criteria for the classification of monoclonal gammopathies, multiple myeloma and related disorders: a report of the International Myeloma Working Group. Br J Haematol 121:749–757

Johnson WJ, Kyle RA, Pineda AA, O'Brien PC, Holley KE (1990) Treatment of renal failure associated with multiple myeloma. Plasmapheresis, hemodialysis, and chemotherapy. Arch Intern Med 150:863–869

Kapadia SB (1980) Multiple myeloma: a clinicopathologic study of 62 consecutively autopsied cases. Medicine (Baltimore) 59:380–392

Konigsberg R, Zojer N, Ackermann J, Kromer E, Kittler H, Fritz E, Kaufmann H, Nosslinger T, Riedl L, Gisslinger H, Jager U, Simonitsch I, Heinz R, Ludwig H, Huber H, Drach J (2000) Predictive role of interphase cytogenetics for survival of patients with multiple myeloma. J Clin Oncol 18:804–812

Kroger N, Schwerdtfeger R, Kiehl M, Sayer HG, Renges H, Zabelina T, Fehse B, Togel F, Wittkowsky G, Kuse R, Zander AR (2002) Autologous stem cell transplantation followed by a dose-reduced allograft induces high complete remission rate in multiple myeloma. Blood 100:755–760

Kyle RA (2000) Multiple myeloma: an odyssey of discovery. Br J Haematol 111:1035–1044

Kyle RA, Greipp PR (1980) Smoldering multiple myeloma. N Engl J Med 302:1347–1349

Kyle RA, Pajak TF, Henderson ES, Nawabi IU, Brunner K, Henry PH, McIntyre OR, Holland JF (1982) Multiple myeloma resistant to melphalan: treatment with doxorubicin, cyclophosphamide, carmustine (BCNU), and prednisone. Cancer Treat Rep 66:451–456

Kyle RA, Therneau TM, Rajkumar SV, Offord JR, Larson DR, Plevak MF, Melton LJ III (2002) A long-term study of prognosis in monoclonal gammopathy of undetermined significance. N Engl J Med 346:564–569

Kyle RA, Gertz MA, Witzig TE, Lust JA, Lacy MQ, Dispenzieri A, Fonseca R, Rajkumar SV, Offord JR, Larson DR, Plevak ME, Therneau TM, Greipp PR (2003) Review of 1,027 patients with newly diagnosed multiple myeloma. Mayo Clin Proc 78:21–33

Lacy MQ, Donovan KA, Heimbach JK, Ahmann GJ, Lust JA (1999) Comparison of interleukin-1 beta expression by in situ hybridization in monoclonal gammopathy of undetermined significance and multiple myeloma. Blood 93:300–305

Lahuerta JJ, Martinez-Lopez J, Serna JD, Bladé J, Grande C, Alegre A, Vazquez L, Garcia-Larana J, Sureda A, Rubia JD, Conde E, Martinez R, Perez-Equiza K, Moraleda JM, Leon A, Besalduch J, Cabrera R, Miguel JD, Morales A, Garcia-Ruiz JC, Diaz-Mediavilla J, San-Miguel

J (2000) Remission status defined by immunofixation vs. electrophoresis after autologous transplantation has a major impact on the outcome of multiple myeloma patients. Br J Haematol 109:438–446

Lenhard RE, Daniels MJ, Oken MM, Glick JH, Ettinger DS, Kalish L, O'Connell MJ (1994) An aggressive high dose cyclophosphamide and prednisone regimen for advanced multiple myeloma. Leuk Lymphoma 13:485–489

Lokhorst HM, Schattenberg A, Cornelissen JJ, van Oers MH, Fibbe W, Russell I, Donk NW, Verdonck LF (2000) Donor lymphocyte infusions for relapsed multiple myeloma after allogeneic stem-cell transplantation: predictive factors for response and long-term outcome. J Clin Oncol 18:3031–3037

Ludwig H, Fritz E (2000) Interferon in multiple myeloma: summary of treatment results and clinical implications. Acta Oncol 39:815–821

MacLennan IC, Chapman C, Dunn J, Kelly K (1992) Combined chemotherapy with ABCM versus melphalan for treatment of myelomatosis. The Medical Research Council Working Party for Leukaemia in Adults. Lancet 339:200–205

Maloney DG, Sandmaier BM, Mackinnon S, Shizuru JA (2002) Non-myeloablative transplantation. Hematology (Am Soc Hematol Educ Program), pp 392–421

McElwain TJ, Powles RL (1983) High-dose intravenous melphalan for plasma-cell leukaemia and myeloma. Lancet 2:822–824

McLaughlin P, Alexanian R (1982) Myeloma protein kinetics following chemotherapy. Blood 60:851–855

Medical Research Council's Working Party on Leukaemia in Adults (1980) Treatment comparisons in the third MRC myelomatosis trial. Br J Cancer 42:823–830

Moreau P, Facon T, Attal M, Hulin C, Michallet M, Maloisel F, Sotto JJ, Guilhot F, Marit G, Doyen C, Jaubert J, Fuzibet JG, François S, Benboubker L, Monconduit M, Voillat L, Macro M, Berthou C, Dorvaux V, Pignon B, Rio B, Matthes T, Casassus P, Caillot D, Najman N, Grosbois B, Bataille R, Harousseau JL (2002) Comparison of 200 mg/m^2 melphalan and 8 Gy total body irradiation plus 140 mg/m^2 melphalan as conditioning regimens for peripheral blood stem cell transplantation in patients with newly diagnosed multiple myeloma: final analysis of the Intergroupe Francophone du Myélome 9502 randomized trial. Blood 99:731–735

MRC Working Party on Leukaemia in Adults (1984) Analysis and management of renal failure in fourth MRC myelomatosis trial. Br Med J (Clin Res Ed) 288:1411–1416

Myeloma Trialists' Collaborative Group (1998) Combination chemotherapy versus melphalan plus prednisone as treatment for multiple myeloma: an overview of 6,633 patients from 27 randomized trials. Myeloma Trialists' Collaborative Group. J Clin Oncol 16:3832–3842

Myeloma Trialists' Collaborative Group (2001) Interferon as therapy for multiple myeloma: an individual patient data overview of 24 randomized trials and 4012 patients. Br J Haematol 113:1020–1034

Oivanen TM, Kellokumpu-Lehtinen P, Koivisto AM, Koivunen E, Palva I (1999) Response level and survival after conventional chemotherapy for multiple myeloma: a Finnish Leukaemia Group study. Eur J Haematol 62:109–116

Oken MM, Kyle RA, Greipp PR, Kay NE, Tsiatis A, Gregory SA, Spiegel RJ, O'Connell MJ (1996a) Complete remission induction with combined VBMCP chemotherapy and interferon (rIFN alpha 2b) in patients with multiple myeloma. Leuk Lymphoma 20:447–452

Oken MM, Pomeroy C, Weisdorf D, Bennett JM (1996 b) Prophylactic antibiotics for the prevention of early infection in multiple myeloma. Am J Med 100:624–628

Paccagnella A, Chiarion-Sileni V, Soesan M, Baggio G, Bolzonella S, De Besi P, Casara D, Frizzarin M, Salvagno L, Favaretto A, Fiorentino MV (1991) Second and third responses to the same induction regimen in relapsing patients with multiple myeloma. Cancer 68:975–980

Palumbo A, Giaccone L, Bertola A, Pregno P, Bringhen S, Rus C, Triolo S, Gallo E, Pileri A, Boccadoro M (2001) Low-dose thalidomide plus dexamethasone is an effective salvage therapy for advanced myeloma. Haematologica 86:399–403

Peest D, Deicher H, Coldewey R, Leo R, Bartl R, Bartels H, Braun HJ, Fett W, Fischer JT, Göbel B, Harms P, Henke R, Hoffmann L, Kreuser ED, Maier WD, Meier CR, Oertel J, Petit M, Planker M, Platzeck C, Respondek M, Schäfer E, Schumacher K, Stennes M, Stenzinger W, Tirier C, Wagner H, Weh HJ, von Wussow P, Wysk J (1995) A comparison of polychemotherapy and melphalan/prednisone for primary remission induction, and interferon-alpha for maintenance treatment, in multiple myeloma. A prospective trial of the German Myeloma Treatment Group. Eur J Cancer 2:146–151

Porrata LF, Gertz MA, Inwards DJ, Litzow MR, Lacy MQ, Tefferi A, Gastineau DA, Dispenzieri A, Ansell SM, Micallef IN, Geyer SM, Markovic SN (2001) Early lymphocyte recovery predicts superior survival after autologous hematopoietic stem cell transplantation in multiple myeloma or non-Hodgkin lymphoma. Blood 98:579–585

Rajkumar SV, Greipp PR (1999) Prognostic factors in multiple myeloma. Hematol Oncol Clin North Am 13:1295–1314

Rajkumar SV, Fonseca R, Dispenzieri A, Lacy MQ, Lust JA, Witzig TE, Kyle RA, Gertz MA, Greipp PR (2000) Thalidomide in the treatment of relapsed multiple myeloma. Mayo Clin Proc 75:897–901

Rajkumar SV, Dispenzieri A, Fonseca R, Lacy MQ, Geyer S, Lust JA, Kyle RA, Greipp PR, Gertz MA, Witzig TE (2001) Thalidomide for previously untreated indolent or smoldering multiple myeloma. Leukemia 15:1274–1276

Rajkumar SV, Hayman S, Gertz MA, Dispenzieri A, Lacy MQ, Greipp PR, Geyer S, Iturria N, Fonseca R, Lust JA, Kyle RA, Witzig TE (2002) Combination therapy with thalidomide plus dexamethasone for newly diagnosed myeloma. J Clin Oncol 20:4319– 4323

Rettig MB, Ma HJ, Vescio RA, Pold M, Schiller G, Belson D, Savage A, Nishikubo C, Wu C, Fraser J, Said JW, Berenson JR (1997) Kaposi's sarcoma-associated herpesvirus infection of bone marrow dendritic cells from multiple myeloma patients. Science 276:1851–1854

Riccardi A, Mora O, Tinelli C, Valentini D, Brugnatelli S, Spanedda R, De Paoli A, Barbarano L, Di Stasi M, Giordano M, Delfini C, Nicoletti G, Bergonzi C, Rinaldi E, Piccinini L, Ascari E (2000) Long-term survival of stage I multiple myeloma given chemotherapy just after diagnosis or at progression of the disease: a multicentre randomized study. Cooperative Group of Study and Treatment of Multiple Myeloma. Br J Cancer 82:1254–1260

Richardson PG, Schlossman RL, Weller E, Hideshima T, Mitsiades C, Davies F, LeBlanc R, Catley LP, Doss D, Kelly K, McKenney M, Mechlowicz J, Freeman A, Deocampo R, Rich R, Ryoo JJ, Chauhan D, Balinski K, Zeldis J, Anderson KC (2002) Immunomodulatory drug CC-5013 overcomes drug resistance and is well tolerated in patients with relapsed multiple myeloma. Blood 100:3063–3067

Richardson PG, Barlogie B, Berenson J, Singhal, S, Jagannath S, Irwin D, Rajkumar SV, Srkalovic G, Alsina M, Alexanian R, Siegel D, Orlowski

RZ, Kuter D, Limentani SA, Lee S, Hideshima T, Esseltine DL, Kauffman M, Adams J, Schenkein DP, Anderson KC (2003) A phase 2 study of bortezomib in relapsed, refractory myeloma. N Engl J Med 348:2609–2617

Rivers SL, Patno ME (1969) Cyclophosphamide vs melphalan in treatment of plasma cell myeloma. JAMA 207:1328–1334

Rosen LS, Gordon D, Kaminski M, Howell A, Belch A, Mackey J, Apffelstaedt J, Hussein M, Coleman RE, Reitsma DJ, Seaman JJ, Chen B-L, Ambros Y (2001) Zoledronic acid versus pamidronate in the treatment of skeletal metastases in patients with breast cancer or osteolytic lesions of multiple myeloma: a phase III, double-blind, comparative trial. Cancer J 7:377–387

Salmon SE, Tesh D, Crowley J, Saeed S, Finley P, Milder MS, Hutchins LF, Coltman CA Jr, Bonnet JD, Cheson B, Knost JA, Samhouri A, Beckford J, Stock-Novack D (1990) Chemotherapy is superior to sequential hemibody irradiation for remission consolidation in multiple myeloma: a Southwest Oncology Group study. J Clin Oncol 8:1575–1584

Salmon SE, Crowley JJ, Balcerzak SP, Roach RW, Taylor SA, Rivkin SE, Samlowski W (1998) Interferon versus interferon plus prednisone remission maintenance therapy for multiple myeloma: a Southwest Oncology Group study. J Clin Oncol 16:890–896

Selby PJ, McElwain TJ, Nandi AC, Perren TJ, Powles RL, Tillyer CR, Osborne RJ, Slevin ML, Malpas JS (1987) Multiple myeloma treated with high dose intravenous melphalan. Br J Haematol 66:55–62

Smadja NV, Bastard C, Brigaudeau C, Leroux D, Fruchart C, on behalf of the Groupe Français de Cytogenetique Hematologique (2001) Hypodiploidy is a major prognostic factor in multiple myeloma. Blood 98:2229–2238

Southwest Oncology Group study (1975) Remission maintenance therapy for multiple myeloma. Arch Intern Med 135:147–152

Sporn JR, McIntyre OR (1986) Chemotherapy of previously untreated multiple myeloma patients: an analysis of recent treatment results. Semin Oncol 13:318–325

Titzer S, Christensen O, Manzke O, Tesch H, Wolf J, Emmerich B, Carsten C, Diehl V, Bohlen H (2000) Vaccination of multiple myeloma patients with idiotype-pulsed dendritic cells: immunological and clinical aspects. Br J Haematol 108:805–816

Tribalto M, Amadori S, Cantonetti M, Franchi A, Papa G, Pileri A, Boccadoro M, Dammacco F, Vacca A, Centurioni R, Leoni P, Martelli M, Aversa F, Tonato M, Deriv L, Guarino S, Neri A, Pericolo Ridolfini F, Mandelli F (1985) Treatment of multiple myeloma: a randomized study of three different regimens. Leuk Res 9:1043–1049

Tricot G, Vesole DH, Jagannath S, Hilton J, Munshi N, Barlogie B (1996) Graft-versus-myeloma effect: proof of principle. Blood 87:1196–1198

Weber D, Rankin K, Gavino M, Delasalle K, Alexanian R (2003) Thalidomide alone or with dexamethasone for previously untreated multiple myeloma. J Clin Oncol 21:16–19

Weber DM, Dimopoulos MA, Moulopoulos LA, Delasalle KB, Smith T, Alexanian R (1997) Prognostic features of asymptomatic multiple myeloma. Br J Haematol 97:810–814

Zojer N, Konigsberg R, Ackermann J, Fritz E, Dallinger S, Kromer E, Kaufmann H, Riedl L, Gisslinger H, Schreiber S, Heinz R, Ludwig H, Huber H, Drach J (2000) Deletion of 13q14 remains an independent adverse prognostic variable in multiple myeloma despite its frequent detection by interphase fluorescence in situ hybridization. Blood 95:1925–1930

Solitary Plasmacytoma of Bone and Extramedullary Plasmacytoma

John A. Lust, M.D., Ph.D.

Contents

4.1 Diagnosis 111

4.2 Clinical and Laboratory Characteristics 112

4.3 Treatment 112

4.4 Disease Progression and Survival 115

4.5 Prognostic Factors 115

4.6 Adjuvant Chemotherapy 115

4.7 Pathogenesis 115

References 117

Plasmacytomas are localized tumors consisting of monoclonal plasma cells that may develop in either the bones or soft tissue. Plasmacytomas may arise during the course of multiple myeloma (MM) when the histologic appearance of the lesion consists of plasma cells identical to those seen in the bone marrow. Plasmacytomas can also occur with no detectable abnormalities in the bone marrow and may be single or multiple. Those patients with a solitary plasmacytoma arising within a bone (solitary plasmacytoma of bone [SPB]) or arising in extraosseous locations (extramedullary plasmacytoma [EMP]) with no evidence of disease elsewhere have a clinical entity distinct from MM and a more favorable prognosis. However, the risk of eventual progression to MM is higher with SPB than with EMP (Alexanian 1980; Bataille and Sany 1981; Bolek et al. 1996; Dimopoulos et al. 1992; Frassica et al. 1989; Galieni et al. 1995, 2000; Holland et al. 1992; Knowling et al. 1983; Kyle 1997; Liebross et al. 1998, 1999; Mehta and Jagannath 2002).

4.1 Diagnosis

Solitary plasmacytoma is diagnosed from a solitary lytic bone lesion or a solitary EMP, histologic confirmation of the lesion consisting of plasma cells identical to those seen in MM, normal bone marrow without evidence of clonal disease, normal results on a skeletal survey with proximal humeri and femora, and a normal magnetic resonance image (MRI) of the spine and pelvis or a normal regional computed tomographic (CT) scan (except for the solitary plasmacytoma). Immunoelectrophoresis and immunofixation of the serum or concentrated urine should show no or a small amount of monoclonal (M) protein. There should be no anemia, hypercalcemia, or renal insufficiency due to myeloma. Recommended criteria for diagnosis of solitary plasmacytoma are detailed in Table 4.1 (Dimopoulos et al. 2000; Mehta and Jagannath 2002).

The studies in the literature differ with respect to the extent of plasmacytosis allowed in the marrow and the radiographic techniques used to eliminate the possibility of disease elsewhere. Several studies included patients with up to 10% plasma cells in the bone marrow (Frassica et al. 1989; Holland et al. 1992; Mayr et al. 1990). Other authors included only patients with normal bone marrow (Bataille and Sany 1981; Bolek et al. 1996; Dimopoulos et al. 1992; Galieni et al. 1995; Knowling et al. 1983; Liebross et al. 1998). Typically, distant plasmacytomas are excluded by a conventional metastatic bone survey with single views of the humeri

Table 4.1. Diagnostic criteria for solitary plasmacytoma of bone and extramedullary plasmacytoma

Solitary osseous lesion or extramedullary lesion due to clonal plasma cells

Normal marrow with no evidence of clonal plasma cells or aneuploidy by flow cytometry

Normal skeletal survey with proximal humeri and femora and a normal magnetic resonance image of the axial skeleton (for solitary plasmacytoma of bone) or a normal regional computed tomographic scan (for extramedullary plasmacytoma)

Absent or low serum or urinary concentration of monoclonal protein

No anemia, hypercalcemia, or renal insufficiency attributable to myeloma

and femora. However, MRI can detect bone lesions not seen on plain radiographs. The group at M.D. Anderson Cancer Center reported on the usefulness of MRI scans in 57 patients with SPB. Among 23 patients with thoracolumbar spine disease, in 7 of 8 patients staged with plain radiographs alone MM developed compared with 1 of 7 patients who also had MRI (Liebross et al. 1998).

It is critical to use all existing methodologies to obtain an accurate diagnosis. Flow cytometry and polymerase chain reaction detection of heavy- and light-chain gene rearrangements are more sensitive than standard morphology and may reveal clonal plasma cells in the bone marrow of some patients who have no evidence of disease on light microscopy. MRI of the axial skeleton and other imaging modalities should be used to exclude other sites of occult disease (Dimopoulos et al. 2000; Mehta and Jagannath 2002).

4.2 Clinical and Laboratory Characteristics

SPB is seen in approximately 5% of patients with plasma cell disorders (Alexanian 1980). The typical patient with SPB is male, presents with bone pain, and is about one decade younger than the average patient with MM (Table 4.2) (Alexanian 1980; Bataille and Sany 1981; Bolek et al. 1996; Dimopoulos et al. 1992; Frassica et al. 1989; Galieni et al. 1995; Holland et al. 1995; Knowling et al. 1983; Liebross et al. 1998). Among the 9 studies summarized in Table 4.2, the median age for patients in each study ranged between 50 and 60 years and the percentage of males

ranged from 65 to 81%. Rarely, SPB may be observed in adolescents (Bertoni-Salateo et al. 1998). Although SPB may involve any bone, it arises in a vertebral body 33 to 60% of the time (Table 4.2). Immunoelectrophoresis and immunofixation of the serum and urine reveal that an M protein may be detected in the serum or urine or both in approximately one-fourth to one-half of patients. Typically, there is no evidence of anemia, hypercalcemia, or renal involvement that could be attributed to occult MM. MRI of the lumbosacral spine has become useful in some patients for clarifying whether they have SPB or early systemic MM. For SPB, MRI shows a focal area of bone marrow replacement. The signal intensity is similar to muscle on T_1-weighted images and hyperintense relative to muscle on T_2-weighted images. An associated soft tissue mass may be present that can impinge on the spinal cord or nerve roots.

EMP typically occurs in the upper respiratory tract, including the nasal cavity and sinuses, nasopharynx, and larynx (Bolek et al. 1996; Galieni et al. 2000; Knowling et al. 1983; Liebross et al. 1999). This was the case 80% to 90% of the time in the 4 series summarized in Table 4.3. Similar to patients with SPB, patients with EMP are usually between 50 and 60 years and male and may show an M protein in the serum or urine. Epistaxis, rhinorrhea, and nasal obstruction are the most frequent presenting symptoms. Occasionally, EMP may be observed in the testis, retroperitoneum, parotid gland, meninges, lymph nodes, eyelid, vocal cord, epiglottis, atria, or skin (Chen et al. 1998; Fischer et al. 1996; Hari and Roblin 2000; Leigh et al. 1997; Lin and Weiss 1997; Olivieri et al. 2000; Rakover et al. 2000; Vujovic et al. 1998; Wan et al. 2001; Welsh et al. 1998). However, EMP can occur in virtually any organ and spread locally or develop into MM.

4.3 Treatment

Treatment of SPB consists of local irradiation in the range of 4,000 to 5,000 cGy over 4 to 5 weeks if allowed by normal tissue tolerances. Treatment fields should be designed to encompass all disease shown by MRI or CT scanning and should include a margin of normal tissue. For spinal lesions, the margin should include at least 1 uninvolved vertebra. The radiologic response may include sclerosis and bone remineralization in up to 50% of patients followed by plain film (Dimopoulos et al. 2000). On MRI, abnormalities of the bone marrow

Table 4.2. Clinical outcome of patients with solitary plasmacytoma of bone

Variable	Alexanian (1980)	Bataille and Sany (1981)	Knowling et al. (1983)	Frassica et al. (1989)	Dimopou- los et al. (1992)	Holland et al. (1992)	Bolek et al. (1996)	Galieni et al. (1995)	Liebross et al. (1998)
Patients, no.	29	18	25	46	45	32	27	32	57
Males, %	72	72	68	65	69	70	70	81	69
Median age, y	52	51	50	56	53	60	55	52	53
Myeloma protein, %	55	33	24	54	67	NA	52	47	72
Spine disease, %	40	60	40	54	33	34	33	40	40
Local recurrence, %	5	11	8	11	5	6	4	9	4
Progression to MM, %	NA	44	48	54	51	53	54	44	51
Disease-free at 10 y, %	30	15	16	25	42	45	46	35	42
Median survival, y	12	NA	7	8	13	11	10	10	11

MM, multiple myeloma; NA, not available.

Table 4.3. Clinical outcome of patients with extramedullary plasmacytoma

Variable	Knowling et al. (1983)	Bolek et al. (1996)	Galieni et al. (2000)	Liebross et al. (1999)
Patients, no.	25	10	46	22
Males, %	84	80	63	86
Median age, y	59	60	55	55
Myeloma protein, %	32	60	21	23
Head and neck disease, %	80	90	80	86
Local recurrence, %	0	4	7	5
Progression to MM, %	8	11	15	32
Disease free at 10 y, %	71	89	78	56
Median survival, y	8	15+	20+	9.5

MM, multiple myeloma.

and an accompanying soft tissue mass may persist even after successful treatment (Dimopoulos et al. 2000; Liebross et al. 1998). Given adequate radiation therapy, virtually all patients achieve pain relief, and the local tumor recurrence rate is typically less than 10%.

For SPB, Mendenhall et al. (1980) reported a 31% incidence of local failure with radiation doses less than 4,000 cGy and 6% with doses of at least 4,000 cGy. Frassica et al. (1989) had no local failures when the radiation therapy dose was 4,500 cGy or greater. In the study by Liebross et al. (1998), the mean radiation therapy dose was 5,000 cGy (range, 3,000-7,000 cGy). Local control was achieved in 96% of patients. One patient had radiographic progression of a rib lesion 1 year after receiving 50 Gy in 25 fractions; the other patient showed recurrence of a thoracic spine tumor 4 years after receiving 41 Gy in 23 fractions and subsequently had a resection. MM did not develop in either patient. There may be a slightly higher proportion of local failures in patients with spinal SPB (Bataille and Sany 1981; Frassica et al. 1989).

The myeloma protein may disappear in up to 50% of patients who receive local radiation therapy (Frassica et al. 1989; Liebross et al. 1998). This disappearance is helpful in following the course of a patient with SPB. Frequent serial measurements of the M protein for at least 6 months after treatment are required to confirm plasmacytoma radiosensitivity. The rate of reduction of the M protein may be slow and continue for several years. The likelihood of disappearance of the M protein is higher in patients in whom the pretreatment value is low. In the series by Liebross et al. (1998), disappearance of the pretreatment serum myeloma protein of 1.0 g/dL or less was achieved in 9 of 22 patients compared with none of 11 patients with a higher concentration; there was no dose-response relationship between radiation dose and disappearance of the M protein (Dimopoulos et al. 2000). Knowling et al. (1983) reported that in 1 SPB patient, an IgGκ M protein of 2.2 g/dL disappeared from the serum within 8 weeks after surgical resection of a 500-g mass on the right fourth rib, with no evidence of recurrence for 16 years.

EMPs are usually sensitive to radiation therapy, and 4,000 to 5,000 cGy is tumoricidal in the majority of patients. Most patients have had surgical intervention; however, complete excision is not required. Knowling and colleagues (1983) reported 5 failures of radiation therapy in their 25 patients with EMP: 1 developed a single bony lesion, 2 progressed to MM, and 2 developed multiple EMP. In this series, the most common dose fractionation was 3,500 cGy in 15 fractions up to 4,500 cGy in 15 to 24 fractions. Table 4.3 summarizes 4 series of patients with EMP who were treated mostly by radiation therapy and surgical resection (Bolek et al. 1996; Galieni et al. 2000; Knowling et al. 1983; Liebross et al. 1999). Local disease recurrence after radiation therapy ranged from 0 to 7% (Table 4.3). Knowling et al. (1983) suggested that consideration be given to include regional lymph nodes in the radiation fields. However, Liebross et al. (1999) found that local control was achieved in 21 of 22 patients (95%), and disease never recurred in regional lymph nodes.

4.4 Disease Progression and Survival

Solitary plasmacytoma may relapse in 3 different forms: 1) local recurrence, 2) development of additional plasmacytomas, and 3) development of MM (Frassica et al. 1989). Progression from solitary plasmacytoma to MM typically consists of new bone lesions, diffuse marrow plasmacytosis, and an increasing M protein concentration in the blood or urine or both. Progression to MM is more frequent with SPB than EMP (Tables 4.2 and 4.3). Knowling et al. (1983) found that 48% of SPB patients progressed to MM compared with 8% of EMP patients. The median time to progression for SPB patients was 6.5 years, and death resulted from progression to MM in most of these patients. However, the median survival of the 2 groups was relatively similar: 86.4 months for SPB and 100.8 months for EMP. Among the 9 series including patients with SPB, 44 to 54% of the patients eventually progressed to MM. In contrast, in the series by Bolek et al. (1996), Galieni et al. (2000), and Liebross et al. (1999), 11, 15, and 32% of the patients with EMP, respectively, progressed to MM. Despite progression to myeloma, the median survival of patients with SPB is still far more favorable than that for patients with MM, often exceeding 10 years in most series. Patients with EMP who are treated with tumoricidal radiation have an even more favorable prognosis. In 2 of the studies, the median survival still had not been reached at 15 years (Bolek et al. 1996; Galieni et al. 2000). Therefore, many patients with EMP are likely to be cured.

4.5 Prognostic Factors

In patients with SPB, factors at presentation that have been associated with systemic recurrence include decreased levels of uninvolved immunoglobulins (Galieni et al. 1995), age (Bataille and Sany 1981), axial lesions (Bataille and Sany 1981), higher M protein values (Dimopoulos et al. 2000), and larger lesions (Holland et al. 1992). In several series, disappearance of the M protein after local radiation therapy was associated with a high probability of long-term stability (Dimopoulos et al. 1999, 2000; Galieni et al. 1995). In the M.D. Anderson series, among 11 patients in whom the M protein disappeared, MM developed in only 2, after 4 and 12 years, whereas MM developed in 57% of patients with a persistent M protein and 63% of those with nonsecretory disease (Dimopoulos et al. 2000; Liebross et al. 1998).

4.6 Adjuvant Chemotherapy

In several series, chemotherapy was administered after completion of local radiation treatment. Mayr et al. (1990) found that none of 5 patients who received adjuvant chemotherapy in their SPB group progressed to MM compared with 9 of 12 patients who did not receive chemotherapy. Holland et al. (1992) reported that adjuvant chemotherapy did not affect the incidence of conversion but did appear to delay conversion to myeloma from 29 to 59 months. In other series, adjuvant chemotherapy had no effect (Bolek et al. 1996; Galieni et al. 1995; Holland et al. 1992). Delauche-Cavallier et al. (1988) administered adjuvant chemotherapy to 7 of 19 patients. In 3 of the 7, acute leukemia eventually developed. Given the favorable long-term survival of most patients with solitary plasmacytoma, the addition of systemic chemotherapy is not recommended. However, this is an area for future clinical investigation, especially in patients with features predictive of a high risk of progression to MM.

4.7 Pathogenesis

The pathogenesis of solitary plasmacytomas in humans is largely unknown. However, Potter (1992) and Potter and colleagues (1973) have detailed the pathogenesis of plasmacytomas in genetically susceptible BALB/c mice. These observations in the mouse system together with results on human samples from individuals with SPB or EMP provide a framework to generate hypotheses that can be tested to better understand the pathogenesis of human SPB and EMP. This framework is detailed in Fig. 4.1.

Early work by Potter (Potter 1992; Potter et al. 1973) demonstrated that paraffin oil or pristane injected into BALB/c mice induced plasmacytomas. The generation of the plasmacytomas depended on development of a c-*myc* translocation in genetically susceptible mice (BALB/c) and factors produced by the inflammatory cells. These cells were subsequently shown to produce interleukin (IL)-6, a potent growth factor for plasmacytomas (Potter 1992). It was shown that avian v-*myc* could replace chromosomal translocation in murine

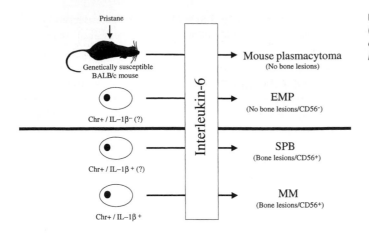

Fig. 4.1. Pathogenesis of solitary plasmacytoma of bone (*SPB*) and extramedullary plasmacytoma (*EMP*). Chr+, chromosome abnormality. (?), hypothesized IL-1β results. *IL*, interleukin; *MM*, multiple myeloma

plasmacytomagenesis (Potter et al. 1987). Transgenic mice (BALB/c) carrying a widely expressed IL-6 transgene developed readily transplantable plasmacytomas with c-*myc* translocations (Kovalchuk et al. 2002). Most importantly, animal studies using IL-6 knockout mice have shown that IL-6 is an essential requirement for the development of B-lineage neoplasms (Hilbert et al. 1995). A uniting feature of human and mouse plasma cell neoplasms is the critical role of IL-6.

Analysis of samples from patients with EMP appears to parallel the pristane mouse model of plasmacytomagenesis. Aalto et al. (1999) found that among 27 specimens from 24 patients with plasmacytoma, all specimens exhibited DNA copy number changes. The most frequent change involved losses at 13q. With immunohistochemical techniques, Vasef et al. (1997) detected cyclin D1 protein in 2 of 12 plasmacytomas. Nishimoto et al. (1994) found that human plasmacytoma cells proliferated in response to IL-6, similar to MM cells. In another study by Sakai et al. (1996), plasma cells from a solitary plasmacytoma in the liver were immunoglobulin light-chain positive for kappa and demonstrated the presence of an IgH gene by Southern blotting. However, the phenotype of the plasma cells was CD38$^+$, CD19$^+$, and CD56$^-$, which represents the pattern observed with normal plasma cells. This contrasts with the typical phenotype of MM cells (CD38$^+$, CD19$^-$, and CD56$^+$). The above observations suggest that a clonal event (chromosomal abnormality) and IL-6 are both required for EMP, similar to the mouse system diagrammed in Figure 4.1.

In contrast, individuals with SPB appear to have a localized, indolent form of myeloma that has a higher rate of progression to active disease compared with EMP. These observations parallel some of the features in the progression from monoclonal gammopathy of undetermined significance to smoldering or indolent MM to active MM. In this regard, we have shown that IL-1β is important in this transition. Normal plasma cells are IL-1β negative; however, the plasma cells from virtually all patients with MM are IL-1β positive at the RNA (Donovan et al. 1998; Lacy et al. 1999; Lust and Donovan 1999) and protein (Carter et al. 1990) levels. It is possible that a major feature that distinguishes the plasma cells in EMP from those in SPB is the amount of IL-1β production. Torcia et al. (1996) have shown that IL-1β is the dominant osteoclast-activating factor in supernatants from patients with active MM. Therefore, patients with SPB may be IL-1β positive as well. The fact that bone lesions are not observed in patients with EMP and in the pristane mouse model suggests that IL-1β is not produced in substantial amounts by these plasma cells.

IL-1β is also a potent inducer of paracrine IL-6 (Carter et al. 1990). In the BALB/c mouse model, pristane is the inducer of IL-6. In humans, other factors important in generating an inflammatory response are likely important in the genesis of EMP. The fact that bone lesions are not observed in either of these 2 processes may be because IL-1β is not produced by the clonal plasma cells. However, in active MM, we and others have shown that IL-1β is produced by the monoclonal plasma cells, and this is likely to be the case with SPB (Carter et al. 1990; Cozzolino et al. 1989; Donovan et al. 1998; Lacy et al. 1999; Yamamoto et al. 1989) (Fig. 4.1). Similar to our recent observations with monoclonal gammopathy of undetermined significance, the amount of IL-1β biologic activity appears to be critical in the progression to active MM, and this may explain why patients with SPB are more likely to progress to active MM (Lust and Donovan 1999).

Plasmacytomas have been observed in patients with human immunodeficiency virus disease and in cardiac transplant patients, suggesting that Epstein-Barr virus may have an etiologic role in selected patients (Herranz et al. 2000; Leigh et al. 1997; Theodossiou et al. 1998; Vallisa et al. 1998). One fascinating case of primary plasmacytoma occurring 12 years after electrical injury was reported by Mongkonsritragoon et al. (1998). Radiographs showed multiple well-circumscribed lytic lesions involving both the right and left tibial diaphyseal regions. A bone biopsy specimen from the left tibial region showed sheets of monoclonal myeloma cells. No evidence of MM was found. The patient was treated with local radiation to both tibias and had no evidence of recurrence 6 years later. These phenomena all stimulate the induction of IL-1β (Dinarello 1991, 1996). Production of IL-1β by the plasma cells in SPB but not by those in EMP offers a potential explanation and a testable hypothesis for the observed differences between SPB and EMP or the mouse plasmacytoma model.

References

Aalto Y, Nordling S, Kivioja AH, Karaharju E, Elomaa I, Knuutila S (1999) Among numerous DNA copy number changes, losses of chromosome 13 are highly recurrent in plasmacytoma. Genes Chromosomes Cancer 25:104–107

Alexanian R (1980) Localized and indolent myeloma. Blood 56:521–525

Bataille R, Sany J (1981) Solitary myeloma: clinical and prognostic features of a review of 114 cases. Cancer 48:845–851

Bertoni-Salateo R, de Camargo B, Soares F, Chojniak R, Penna V (1998) Solitary plasmocytoma of bone in an adolescent. J Pediatr Hematol Oncol 20:574–576

Bolek TW, Marcus RB, Mendenhall NP (1996) Solitary plasmacytoma of bone and soft tissue. Int J Radiat Oncol Biol Phys 36:329–333

Carter A, Merchav S, Silvian-Draxler I, Tatarsky I (1990) The role of interleukin-1 and tumour necrosis factor-alpha in human multiple myeloma. Br J Haematol 74:424–431

Chen TC, Wu JH, Ng KF, Lien JM, Hung CF (1998) Solitary extramedullary plasmacytoma in the retroperitoneum. Am J Hematol 58:235–238

Cozzolino F, Torcia M, Aldinucci D, Rubartelli A, Miliani A, Shaw AR, Lansdorp PM, Di Guglielmo R (1989) Production of interleukin-1 by bone marrow myeloma cells. Blood 74:380–387

Delauche-Cavallier MC, Laredo JD, Wybier M, Bard M, Mazabraud A, Le Bail Darne JL, Kuntz D, Ryckewaert A (1988) Solitary plasmacytoma of the spine: long-term clinical course. Cancer 61:1707–1714

Dimopoulos MA, Goldstein J, Fuller L, Delasalle K, Alexanian R (1992) Curability of solitary bone plasmacytoma. J Clin Oncol 10:587–590

Dimopoulos MA, Kiamouris C, Moulopoulos LA (1999) Solitary plasmacytoma of bone and extramedullary plasmacytoma. Hematol Oncol Clin North Am 13:1249–1257

Dimopoulos MA, Moulopoulos LA, Maniatis A, Alexanian R (2000) Solitary plasmacytoma of bone and asymptomatic multiple myeloma. Blood 96:2037–2044

Dinarello CA (1991) Interleukin-1 and interleukin-1 antagonism. Blood 77:1627–1652

Dinarello CA (1996) Biologic basis for interleukin-1 in disease. Blood 87:2095–2147

Donovan KA, Lacy MQ, Kline MP, Ahmann GJ, Heimbach JK, Kyle RA, Lust JA (1998) Contrast in cytokine expression between patients with monoclonal gammopathy of undetermined significance or multiple myeloma. Leukemia 12:593–600

Fischer C, Terpe HJ, Weidner W, Schulz A (1996) Primary plasmacytoma of the testis: case report and review of the literature. Urol Int 56:263–265

Frassica DA, Frassica FJ, Schray MF, Sim FH, Kyle RA (1989) Solitary plasmacytoma of bone: Mayo Clinic experience. Int J Radiat Oncol Biol Phys 16:43–48

Galieni P, Cavo M, Avvisati G, Pulsoni A, Falbo R, Bonelli MA, Russo D, Petrucci MT, Bucalossi A, Tura S (1995) Solitary plasmacytoma of bone and extramedullary plasmacytoma: two different entities? Ann Oncol 6:687–691

Galieni P, Cavo M, Pulsoni A, Avvisati G, Bigazzi C, Neri S, Caliceti U, Benni M, Ronconi S, Lauria F (2000) Clinical outcome of extramedullary plasmacytoma. Haematologica 85:47–51

Hari CK, Roblin DG (2000) Solitary plasmacytoma of the parotid gland. Int J Clin Pract 54:197–198

Herranz S, Sala M, Cervantes M, Sasal M, Soler A, Segura F (2000) Neoplasia of plasma cells with atypical presentation and infection by the human immunodeficiency virus: a presentation of two cases. Am J Hematol 65:239–242

Hilbert DM, Kopf M, Mock BA, Kohler G, Rudikoff S (1995) Interleukin 6 is essential for in vivo development of B lineage neoplasms. J Exp Med 182:243–248

Holland J, Trenkner DA, Wasserman TH, Fineberg B (1992) Plasmacytoma: treatment results and conversion to myeloma. Cancer 69:1513–1517

Knowling MA, Harwood AR, Bergsagel DE (1983) Comparison of extramedullary plasmacytomas with solitary and multiple plasma cell tumors of bone. J Clin Oncol 1:255–262

Kovalchuk AL, Kim JS, Park SS, Coleman AE, Ward JM, Morse HC III, Kishimoto T, Potter M, Janz S (2002) IL-6 transgenic mouse model for extraosseous plasmacytoma. Proc Natl Acad Sci U S A 99:1509–1514

Kyle RA (1997) Monoclonal gammopathy of undetermined significance and solitary plasmacytoma: implications for progression to overt multiple myeloma. Hematol Oncol Clin North Am 11:71–87

Lacy MQ, Donovan KA, Heimbach JK, Ahmann GJ, Lust JA (1999) Comparison of interleukin-1 beta expression by in situ hybridization in monoclonal gammopathy of undetermined significance and multiple myeloma. Blood 93:300–305

Leigh BR, Larkin EC, Doggett RL (1997) Solitary extramedullary plasmacytoma five years after successful cardiac transplantation: case report and review of the literature. Am J Clin Oncol 20:467–470

Liebross RH, Ha CS, Cox JD, Weber D, Delasalle K, Alexanian R (1998) Solitary bone plasmacytoma: outcome and prognostic factors following radiotherapy. Int J Radiat Oncol Biol Phys 41:1063–1067

Liebross RH, Ha CS, Cox JD, Weber D, Delasalle K, Alexanian R (1999) Clinical course of solitary extramedullary plasmacytoma. Radiother Oncol 52:245–249

Lin BT, Weiss LM (1997) Primary plasmacytoma of lymph nodes. Hum Pathol 28:1083–1090

Lust JA, Donovan KA (1999) The role of interleukin-1 beta in the pathogenesis of multiple myeloma. Hematol Oncol Clin North Am 13:1117–1125

Mayr NA, Wen BC, Hussey DH, Burns CP, Staples JJ, Doornbos JF, Vigliotti AP (1990) The role of radiation therapy in the treatment of solitary plasmacytomas. Radiother Oncol 17:293–303

Mehta J, Jagannath S (2002) Solitary plasmacytoma. In: Mehta J, Singhal S (eds) Myeloma. Martin Dunitz, London, pp 433–444

Mendenhall CM, Thar TL, Million RR (1980) Solitary plasmacytoma of bone and soft tissue. Int J Radiat Oncol Biol Phys 6:1497–1501

Mongkonsritragoon W, Kyle RA, Shreck RR, Greipp PR (1998) Primary plasmacytoma at the site of exit wounds after electrical injury. Am J Hematol 58:77–79

Nishimoto N, Ogata A, Shima Y, Tani Y, Ogawa H, Nakagawa M, Sugiyama H, Yoshizaki K, Kishimoto T (1994) Oncostatin M, leukemia inhibitory factor, and interleukin 6 induce the proliferation of human plasmacytoma cells via the common signal transducer, gp130. J Exp Med 179:1343–1347

Olivieri L, Ianni MD, Giansanti M, Falini B, Tabilio A (2000) Primary eyelid plasmacytoma. Med Oncol 17:74–75

Potter M (1992) Perspectives on the origins of multiple myeloma and plasmacytomas in mice. Hematol Oncol Clin North Am 6:211–223

Potter M, Sklar MD, Rowe WP (1973) Rapid viral induction of plasmacytomas in pristane-primed BALB-c mice. Science 182:592–594

Potter M, Mushinski JF, Mushinski EB, Brust S, Wax JS, Wiener F, Babonits M, Rapp UR, Morse HC III (1987) Avian v-myc replaces chromosomal translocation in murine plasmacytomagenesis. Science 235:787–789

Rakover Y, Bennett M, David R, Rosen G (2000) Isolated extramedullary plasmacytoma of the true vocal fold. J Laryngol Otol 114:540–542

Sakai A, Fujii T, Noda M, Hyodo H, Oda K, Kimura A (1996) Plasma cells composing plasmacytoma have phenotypes different from those of myeloma cells. Am J Hematol 53:251–253

Theodossiou C, Burroughs R, Wynn R, Schwarzenberger P (1998) Plasmacytoma in HIV disease: two case reports and review of the literature. Am J Med Sci 316:351–353

Torcia M, Lucibello M, Vannier E, Fabiani S, Miliani A, Guidi G, Spada O, Dower SK, Sims JE, Shaw AR, Dinarello CA, Garaci E, Cozzolino F (1996) Modulation of osteoclast-activating factor activity of multiple myeloma bone marrow cells by different interleukin-1 inhibitors. Exp Hematol 24:868–874

Vallisa D, Pagani L, Berte R, Civardi G, Viale P, Paties C, Cavanna L (1998) Extramedullary plasmacytoma in a patient with AIDS: report of a case and review of the literature. Tumori 84:511–514

Vasef MA, Medeiros LJ, Yospur LS, Sun NC, McCourty A, Brynes RK (1997) Cyclin D1 protein in multiple myeloma and plasmacytoma: an immunohistochemical study using fixed, paraffin-embedded tissue sections. Mod Pathol 10:927–932

Vujovic O, Fisher BJ, Munoz DG (1998) Solitary intracranial plasmacytoma: case report and review of management. J Neurooncol 39:47–50

Wan X, Tarantolo S, Orton DF, Greiner TC (2001) Primary extramedullary plasmacytoma in the atria of the heart. Cardiovasc Pathol 10:137–139

Welsh J, Westra WH, Eisele D, Hogan R, Lee DJ (1998) Solitary plasmacytoma of the epiglottis: a case report and review of the literature. J Laryngol Otol 112:174–176

Yamamoto I, Kawano M, Sone T, Iwato K, Tanaka H, Ishikawa H, Kitamura N, Lee K, Shigeno C, Konishi J, Asaoku H, Tanabe O, Nobuyoshi M, Ohmoto Y, Hirai Y, Higuchi M, Ohsawa T, Kuramoto A (1989) Production of interleukin 1β, a potent bone resorbing cytokine, by cultured human myeloma cells. Cancer Res 49:4242–4246

Plasma Cell Leukemia

Suzanne R. Hayman, M.D.

Contents

5.1	Epidemiology	120
5.2	Etiology	120
5.3	Screening and Prevention	120
5.4	Molecular Biology and Genetics	120
	5.4.1 Ploidy	120
	5.4.2 Cytogenetics	121
	5.4.2.1 c-myc	121
	5.4.2.2 1q	121
	5.4.2.3 ras	121
	5.4.2.4 Chromosome 13	122
	5.4.2.5 p53	122
	5.4.2.6 Hypermethylation	122
	5.4.3 Immunophenotype	122
5.5	Clinical Presentation of PCL	123
5.6	Classification and Staging	123
5.7	Diagnosis	123
	5.7.1 Laboratory Tests	123
	5.7.1.1 Peripheral Blood	123
	5.7.1.2 Urine	124
	5.7.1.3 Bone Marrow	124
	5.7.2 Imaging	124
	5.7.3 Other	124
5.8	Differential Diagnosis	124
5.9	Second Malignancies	124
5.10	Therapy	124
	5.10.1 Chemotherapy	124
	5.10.1.1 Induction and Combination Chemotherapy	124
	5.10.2 Stem Cell Transplantation	125
	5.10.2.1 Autologous	125
	5.10.2.2 Tandem Transplant	125
	5.10.2.3 PBSCT in Renal Failure	125
	5.10.2.4 Mobilization Chemotherapy	126
	5.10.2.5 Conditioning Regimen	126
	5.10.2.6 Allogeneic Transplantation	126
	5.10.3 Radiation Therapy	126
	5.10.3.1 Conditioning	126
	5.10.3.2 Palliation	126
	5.10.3.3 Radioisotopes	126
	5.10.4 Biologic Therapy	126
	5.10.5 Surgery	127
	5.10.6 Supportive Care	127
	5.10.6.1 Pain Control	127
	5.10.6.2 Constipation	127
	5.10.6.3 Avoidance of Nephrotoxicity	127
	5.10.6.4 Gastrointestinal Tract Side Effects	127
	5.10.7 Other Therapeutic Measures	127
	5.10.7.1 Bisphosphonates	127
5.11	Relapse Therapy	128
	5.11.1 Chemotherapy	128
	5.11.1.1 EDAP	128
	5.11.1.2 VDD	128
	5.11.1.3 CP	128
	5.11.1.4 High-Dose Methylprednisolone	128
	5.11.1.5 High-Dose Dexamethasone	128
	5.11.1.6 Thalidomide	128

5.11.2 Clinical Trials   128
5.11.3 Second Transplant   129

5.12 Prognosis   129

5.13 Quality of Life and Rehabilitation . . .   129

5.14 Emergencies   129

5.14.1 Spinal Cord Compression   129
5.14.2 Infection   129
5.14.3 Acute Renal Failure   129
5.14.4 Hypercalcemia   129

References   130

5.1 Epidemiology

Plasma cell leukemia (PCL) is a variant of multiple myeloma characterized by a fulminant disease course and a poor prognosis. There are no published epidemiologic data because of the rarity of the disease. Its epidemiology is presumed to be similar to that of myeloma. Myeloma represents approximately 10% of all hematologic malignancies in whites, with the incidence being at least 2-fold greater in African Americans (Cohen et al. 1998; Riedel et al. 1991). Males are affected more frequently than females (Cohen et al. 1998). The age at PCL onset is similar to that in myeloma. Primary (de novo) PCL comprises only 2% to 4% of newly diagnosed myelomas (Dimopoulos et al. 1994; Noel and Kyle 1987) and represents approximately 60% of all PCL (Bladé and Kyle 1999). Secondary PCL, the leukemic transformation of a known underlying relapsed or refractory myeloma, comprises the remaining 40%.

5.2 Etiology

No etiologic factors have been established definitively.

5.3 Screening and Prevention

There are no known screening tests or preventive measures.

5.4 Molecular Biology and Genetics

There is considerable overlap in the biology and genetics of myeloma and PCL. Significant differences may still be found in terms of tumor DNA content, frequency and extent of cytogenetic abnormalities, and differential expression of tumor cell adhesion molecules and surface antigens that partially account for differences in clinicopathology, treatment responses, and prognosis between the 2 disease entities.

5.4.1 Ploidy

Ploidy of a cell is its DNA content or chromosome number. Aneuploidy, an imbalance of chromosomes, is thought to arise by carcinogenic exposure or gene mutation or both. Karyotypic instability ensues and an autocatalytic evolution may result in a neoplastic karyotype (Li et al. 2000). Aneuploidy is an established feature of myeloma and PCL (Drach et al. 1995b). Hyperdiploidy (DNA index by flow cytometry >1) is more common in myeloma, 57% vs. 1% for PCL (Garcia-Sanz et al. 1999), and is associated with a significantly better prognosis than for patients with diploid, pseudodiploid, or hypodiploid (DNA index <1) karyotypes, 46 months vs. 21 months overall survival (Avet-Loiseau et al. 2001a; Garcia-Sanz et al. 1995, 1999; Perez-Simon et al. 1998; Seong et al. 1998; Smadja et al. 2001). Diploidy and hypodiploidy are found in virtually all PCL cases (Garcia-Sanz et al. 1999) and correlate with adverse clinical features such as proteinuria, elevated β_2-microglobulin, elevated serum Ca^{2+}, elevated lactate dehydrogenase, decreased renal function, and increased proportion of plasma cells in S phase (Garcia-Sanz et al. 1999).

5.4.2 Cytogenetics

The extent of cytogenetic abnormalities present in myeloma and PCL has been underestimated by traditional conventional karyotyping. More sensitive techniques such as interphase fluorescent in situ hybridization, spectral karyotyping, and comparative genomic hybridization estimate that some form of cytogenetic abnormality exists in 100% of myeloma and PCL cases.

The current schema or paradigm used to represent the projected cytogenetic evolution of myeloma and PCL from a plasma cell clone is as follows.

Monoclonal gammopathy of undetermined significance (MGUS) → Smoldering myeloma → Myeloma → PCL

The initial immortalizing events resulting in a plasma cell clone are thought to be primary, simple, reciprocal chromosomal translocations, involving the Ig heavy chain (IgH) locus at band 14q32 in at least 50% to 60% of cases (Bergsagel et al. 1996; Drach et al. 1995a; Nishida et al. 1997; Sawyer et al. 1995, 1998a; Taniwaki et al. 1994). This translocation is believed to result primarily from errors in isotype class switching and, less frequently, errors in somatic hypermutation in the germinal centers of secondary lymphoid organs during the course of normal B = cell development and antigen selection (Bergsagel and Kuehl 2001). The IgH translocation, which may have multiple partner chromosomes, is believed to culminate in oncogene dysregulation as a result of the juxtaposition of an oncogene with an IgH enhancer. The incidence of IgH translocations increases with disease stage, increasing to 70% to 80% in extramedullary myeloma, suggesting that they may also be present as secondary translocations (Bergsagel and Kuehl 2001). Despite multiple IgH partner chromosomes reported, 3 sets of genes are involved most often in primary translocations.

1) *Cyclin D₁* at 11q13 (Chesi et al. 1996): a higher incidence of t(11;14)(q13;q32), 33% vs. 16%, has been found in patients with PCL than in patients with high cell mass myeloma (Avet-Loiseau et al. 2001a). The effect of this translocation on prognosis remains unsettled (Avet-Loiseau et al. 2001a; Fonseca et al. 1999; Hoechtlen-Vollmar et al. 2000; Lai et al. 1998; Rasmussen et al. 2001).

    Cyclin D₃ at 6p21 (Shaughnessy et al. 2001): t(6;14)(p21;q32) is found in ∼5% of myeloma patients (Bergsagel and Kuehl 2001).

2) *Fibroblast growth factor receptor 3* and *multiple myeloma set domain* at 4p16: simultaneous dysregulation of 2 oncogenes (Chesi et al. 1998b). This translocation is estimated to be present in 15% to 20% of myeloma tumors (Avet-Loiseau et al. 1998; Chesi et al. 1998b; Malgeri et al. 2000). The incidence of t(4;14)(p16;q32) was not significantly differ-

ent in high mass myeloma and PCL (Avet-Loiseau et al. 2001a).

3) *c-Maf* at 16q23 in ∼5% to 10% of myeloma tumors (Chesi et al. 1998a; Sawyer et al. 1998a): t(14;16)(q32;q23) had a significantly higher incidence in PCL than in high cell mass myeloma, 13% vs. 1% (Avet-Loiseau et al. 2001a).

Secondary translocations, those that are thought to be involved with tumor progression rather than initiation, do not involve B-cell DNA modification mechanisms such as somatic hypermutation, VDJ recombination, or isotype class switching (Bergsagel and Kuehl 2001).

5.4.2.1 *c-myc*

Secondary, complex translocations are thought to dysregulate *c-myc* as a late progressive event in myeloma and PCL (Bergsagel and Kuehl 2001; Shou et al. 2000). Rearrangements at the *c-myc* locus were present in ∼15% of patients with myeloma or primary PCL, independent of the disease stage (Avet-Loiseau et al. 2001b). Translocations t(8;14) and t(8;22) represented only 25% of the total *c-myc* rearrangements (Avet-Loiseau et al. 2001b).

5.4.2.2 1*q*

Abnormalities of chromosome 1 are the most common structural derangements in myeloma (Sawyer et al. 1998b). These are believed to be the most common secondary, complex karyotypic findings of myeloma: present in up to 40% of those patients with abnormal cytogenetics (Dewald et al. 1985; Sawyer et al. 1995, 1998b). Unbalanced, nonrandom whole-arm 1q translocations have been reported for patients with aggressive myeloma and may provide a proliferative advantage (Sawyer et al. 1998b). Analysis of differences in genetic changes between myeloma and PCL by comparative genomic hybridization revealed DNA copy number gains of 1q in 36% of myeloma patients and 100% of PCL patients (Gutierrez et al. 2001).

5.4.2.3 *ras*

The frequencies of N- and K-*ras* mutations are relatively independent of stage of myeloma and value of the plasma cell labeling index (PCLI) (Kuehl and Bergsagel 2002). They are believed to be activating mutations and distinguish myeloma from MGUS. A high incidence of these mutations was found at diagnosis in 54.5% of patients with myeloma and 50% of patients with primary PCL (Bezieau et al. 2001).

5.4.2.4 Chromosome 13

Loss of 13q regions usually manifesting as monosomy and, less commonly, interstitial deletion of 13q14 (Avet-Loiseau et al. 2000; Fonseca et al. 2001b) are some of the most frequently found chromosomal aberrations in myeloma and PCL (Avet-Loiseau et al. 2001a; Garcia-Sanz et al. 1999; Seong et al. 1998). Monosomy 13 or interstitial deletion of 13q14 is an independent, adverse prognostic factor in both myeloma and PCL (Avet-Loiseau et al. 2001a; Garcia-Sanz et al. 1999; Seong et al. 1998; Tricot et al. 1995; Zojer et al. 2000). It is associated with significantly shorter survival (24.2 months vs. > 60 months), higher levels of β_2-microglobulin, Durie-Salmon stage III disease, and a higher percentage of bone marrow plasma cells than in myeloma patients without the abnormality (Zojer et al. 2000). Monosomy 13 has been found in 20% to 45% of patients with MGUS (Avet-Loiseau et al. 1999), but it increases in prevalence with disease progression and has been found in 68% to 84% of PCL cases (Avet-Loiseau et al. 2001a; Garcia-Sanz et al. 1999). The presence of chromosome 13 abnormalities is also associated with a significant decrease in survival of patients who have undergone high-dose chemotherapy (Desikan et al. 2000; Facon et al. 2001) and those treated with conventional chemotherapy (Perez-Simon et al. 1998). In a study of 1,000 patients, the presence of chromosome 13 abnormalities reduced 5-year event-free survival from 20% to 0%, and overall survival from 44% to 16% compared to patients without the abnormality (Desikan et al. 2000). The exact role of chromosome 13 abnormalities in the pathogenesis and progression of disease remains unclear. The t(4;14)(p16;q32) has been strongly associated with chromosome 13 abnormalities (Fonseca et al. 2001a).

5.4.2.5 *p53*

Mutations or deletions (or both) of *TP53*, which encodes the *p53* suppressor gene, are associated with advanced myeloma and PCL and are thought to represent late events in disease progression (Corradini et al. 1994; Portier et al. 1992; Preudhomme et al. 1992). Mutations or deletions are present in up to 40% of patients who have advanced myelomas (Corradini et al. 1994). The presence of *TP53* abnormalities is associated with significantly reduced survival from diagnosis compared to patients without the aberration, 13.9 months vs. 38.7 months (Kuehl and Bergsagel 2002).

5.4.2.6 Hypermethylation

Lack of tumor suppressor function may result from gene deletion, mutation, or hypermethylation of 5′CpG islands in tumor suppressor gene promoters, which leads to inactivation of transcription. Derangement of tumor suppressor gene function can result in cell cycle dysregulation. The *p16* gene competes with cyclin D_1 for binding to cyclin-dependent kinase (CDK4/CDK6). It therefore inhibits CDK4/CDK6 activity, leading to dephosphorylation of the retinoblastoma gene (*RB*) and resulting in G_1 growth arrest. In one study evaluating p16^{INK4A} expression in myeloma and PCL, *p16* was expressed in all myeloma patient samples but was undetectable in PCL samples and myeloma cell lines (Urashima et al. 1997). In a larger study, involving 101 untreated myeloma patients and 5 primary PCL patients, 40.5% of the myeloma patients and 80% of the primary PCL patients had evidence for hypermethylation in exon E1*a* of *p16* (Gonzalez et al. 2000).

5.4.3 Immunophenotype

There is considerable immunophenotypic overlap between myeloma and PCL plasma cells, although there are several notable differences that reflect their pathobiologic differences. Myeloma cells in the marrow bind to stromal cells and the extracellular matrix via adhesion molecules, leading to the up-regulation of interleukin-6, which is secreted in a paracrine manner and enhances the proliferation and survival of malignant cells. Loss of the markers, shown in Table 5.1, is associated with interleukin-6 independent, extramedullary spread of plasma cells (Pellat-Deceunynck et al. 1998; Tatsumi et al. 1996; Teoh and Anderson 1997).

Expression of CD11b, which facilitates cell binding to high endothelial venules and migration, is associated with PCL, as is the expression of CD28 and lymphocyte function-associated antigen (Teoh and Anderson 1997).

Up-regulation of CD20 on PCL cells is a significant difference between PCL and myeloma and has been as-

Table 5.1. Surface markers on myeloma cells

Marker	Function
Neural cell adhesion molecule; CD56	Binds heparan sulfate
Very late antigen-5	Binds fibronectin
Surface markers on plasma cells	Adhesion to marrow stroma
Syndecan-1	Mediates adhesion to Type I collagen, fibronectin, and fibroblast growth factor

sociated with a poorer prognosis (Garcia-Sanz et al. 1999; San Miguel et al. 1991). Markers that are expressed significantly more frequently on myeloma cells than PCL cells include CD9, CD56, CD117, and DR (Garcia-Sanz et al. 1999).

5.5 Clinical Presentation of PCL

The clinical presentation of patients who have primary PCL is similar to that seen with advanced-stage multiple myeloma. Constitutional symptoms such as fatigue, anorexia, weight loss, and night sweats are common. Dehydration, hypercalcemia and other electrolyte derangements, cytopenias, a high percentage of Bence Jones proteinuria, renal dysfunction or failure, hypogammaglobulinemia, and extramedullary disease involvement also are frequently noted. Fever and chills are not usually manifestations of the underlying disease and likely suggest concurrent infection. Lytic bone lesions are often present but are less frequently found than with myeloma (Bladé and Kyle 1999). Focal weakness, paresthesias, or pain, and change in bowel or bladder habits may be manifestations of bone lesions or impending fracture or spinal cord compression. Mental status changes may be observed with hypercalcemia, uremia, dehydration, electrolyte abnormalities, or infection.

Adverse prognostic indicators, such as the surrogates for high tumor burden (lactate dehydrogenase and β_2-microglobulin) and plasma cell proliferative rate, fraction of plasma cells in S phase, and PCLI, are often increased on initial presentation.

5.6 Classification and Staging

Classification and staging are the same as for myeloma. Serum protein electrophoresis (SPEP) and urine protein electrophoresis (UPEP) with immunofixation, in addition to bone marrow aspiration and biopsy, establish the isotype class and light chain restriction of the paraprotein. Rarely, the disease may be nonsecretory or not produce immunoglobulin, resulting in negative findings of serum and urine immunofixation. A bone marrow biopsy is then required to establish clonality. Staging is clinical, with the Durie-Salmon system used most often (Durie and Salmon 1975). PCL is most consistent with stage III disease, defined as having 1 or more of the following (Durie and Salmon 1975).

1) Large M-component
   A. IgG >70 g/L
   B. IgA >50 g/L
   C. Urine light chain >12 g/24 h
2) Hemoglobin <85 g/L
3) Extensive, advanced lytic bony disease
4) Serum calcium >12 mg/dL
   Subclassification of stage
   A. Creatinine <2 mg/dL
   B. Creatinine ≥2 mg/dL

5.7 Diagnosis

5.7.1 Laboratory Tests

5.7.1.1 Peripheral Blood

Complete blood cell count with manual differential: required to document the presence of $\geq 2.0 \times 10^9$/L absolute number of plasma cells in the peripheral blood, erythrocyte sedimentation rate, C-reactive protein

Coagulation parameters: prothrombin time and International Normalized Ratio.

Serum chemistry: Na^+, K^+, Cl^-, HCO_3^-, BUN, creatinine, albumin, glucose, total and ionized Ca^{2+}, phosphorus, Mg^{2+}, uric acid, SPEP with immunofixation, β_2-microglobulin, lactate dehydrogenase

Liver function tests

Microbiology: blood cultures as needed

5.7.1.2 Urine

Twenty-four-hour UPEP with immunofixation, urinalysis with microscopy, urine culture, creatinine clearance, and urine electrolytes in the setting of renal failure

5.7.1.3 Bone Marrow

A unilateral bone marrow aspiration and biopsy are needed for assessment of percentage and type of clonal plasma cells and to obtain a PCLI and tissue for conventional cytogenetics or cytogenetic analysis using fluorescent in situ hybridization (or both).

5.7.2 Imaging

Initial imaging studies required on diagnosis include a metastatic bone survey with plain films of long bones to evaluate for the presence of lytic bone lesions. Nuclear bone scans are not useful if looking for lytic lesions. Posteroanterior and lateral chest radiographs are required. Additional imaging depends on an individual patient's presentation. Magnetic resonance imaging is the study of choice to eliminate the possibility of spinal cord compression.

5.7.3 Other

12-lead electrocardiogram

5.8 Differential Diagnosis

The differential diagnosis for primary PCL includes myeloma vs. secondary PCL. The distinction is usually not problematic because either primary or secondary PCL can be distinguished from myeloma by the presence of $\geq 2.0 \times 10^9$/L peripheral blood plasma cells. Patients with the secondary form of the disease have a history of previously diagnosed multiple myeloma.

5.9 Second Malignancies

Second malignancies are not common in PCL. The usual short overall survival precludes systematic assessment of long-term risks of previous therapies, although the small number of patients with longer survival carry increased risks of myelodysplastic syndrome and secondary leukemias as a result of prior treatment with alkylating agents.

5.10 Therapy

The goals of treatment for de novo PCL are to prolong survival and to improve quality of life, given the poor prognosis and disease incurability. There have been no large prospective clinical trials to systematically evaluate different treatments because of the relatively low incidence of PCL. Treatment is therefore empiric or extrapolated and implemented from the myeloma literature. Secondary PCL remains a terminal event for refractory or relapsed myeloma and is usually unresponsive to any treatment modality.

5.10.1 Chemotherapy

5.10.1.1 Induction and Combination Chemotherapy

The current treatment recommendation for eligible patients consists of induction chemotherapy followed by high-dose chemotherapy and stem cell rescue, as for myeloma. There are several combination chemotherapy regimens that have been used as primary therapy for PCL or as induction chemotherapy before bone marrow or peripheral blood stem cell transplantation (PBSCT). No regimen has demonstrated superiority in terms of response or overall survival. Regimens that use an alkylating agent, such as melphalan, are generally avoided in potential transplant candidates before bone marrow or stem cell collection to maximize cell yield. Combination chemotherapy increased overall survival in primary PCL patients compared to therapy with melphalan and prednisone (Bladé and Kyle 1999; Dimopoulos et al. 1994; Garcia-Sanz et al. 1999; Noel and Kyle 1987). In contrast, combination chemotherapy was not significantly different than treatment with melphalan and prednisone for myeloma patients (Myeloma Trialists' Collaborative Group 1998). Response rates for PCL were significantly lower than for myeloma, 38% vs. 68% (Garcia-Sanz et al. 1999).

Combination chemotherapy is the treatment of choice in primary PCL patients unwilling or unable to undergo transplantation.

5.10.1.1.1 VAD

A widely used regimen in the United States, especially for transplant-eligible patients, consists of vincristine, doxorubicin (Adriamycin), and dexamethasone, usually given every 28 days for 2 to 4 cycles to reduce tumor burden. Vincristine (0.4 mg/day) and doxorubicin (9 mg/m² per day) are mixed together in an ambulatory pump and given as an intravenous continuous infusion on days 1–4 of each cycle. Dexamethasone (40 mg/day) is given orally on days 1–4, 9–12, and 17–20 for odd-numbered cycles and days 1–4 only during even-numbered cycles.

5.10.1.1.2 CE

Cyclophosphamide (600 mg/m² per day in 250 mL 0.9% NaCl) given intravenously over 30 minutes and etoposide (180 mg/m² per day), each drug given intravenously on days 1–5 every 28 days.

5.10.1.1.3 VCMP/VBAP

Vincristine (1.2 mg/m²) given as an intravenous push on day 1, cyclophosphamide (400 mg/m² in 250 mL 0.9% NaCl) given intravenously over 20 to 30 minutes on day 1, melphalan (8 mg/m²) given orally on days 1–4, and prednisone (40 mg/m²) given orally on days 1–7 of all cycles and on days 8–14 for the first cycle only, every 35–42 days. VCMP may be given as single therapy or alternated with vincristine (1.4 mg/m²) given as an intravenous push on day 1, carmustine (BCNU) (30 mg/m² in 250 mL dextrose 5% in water [D5W]) given intravenously over 30 minutes on day 1, and doxorubicin (30 mg/m²) given as an intravenous push on day 1 of each cycle, until cardiac side effects are noted or a cumulative dose of 450 mg/m² has been reached. Doxorubicin is discontinued once the lifetime maximum is reached and cyclophosphamide (600 mg/m² in 250 mL 0.9% NaCl) is given intravenously over 30 minutes on day 1, and prednisone (60 mg/m²) is given orally on days 1–5. VBAP is administered every 21 days.

5.10.1.1.4 MP

Standard-dose melphalan (0.15 mg/m²) on days 1–7 and prednisone (15 mg) given orally 4 times a day on days 1–7 every 6 weeks may be used for patients unable to tolerate the side effects of combination chemotherapy.

The use of thalidomide with or without dexamethasone is being investigated in clinical trials as a possibly less toxic and more convenient induction regimen.

5.10.2 Stem Cell Transplantation

5.10.2.1 Autologous

The recommended treatment of myeloma patients younger than age 65 years, and applied to PCL, is high-dose chemotherapy followed by PBSCT, ideally within the context of a clinical trial. This recommendation is largely the result of prospective randomized trial data collected by the Intergroupe Française du Myélome that demonstrated that high-dose chemotherapy with autologous PBSCT is superior to conventional chemotherapy as the initial treatment for myeloma (Attal et al. 1996). Five-year overall survival (52% vs. 12%), 5-year event-free survival (28% vs. 10%), and response rate (81% vs. 57%) were all significantly better in the PBSCT group than in the conventional chemotherapy group, respectively, with similar treatment-related mortality (Attal et al. 1996, 1997). The optimal timing of high-dose chemotherapy remains controversial (Fermand et al. 1998). Poor response to induction chemotherapy should not disqualify an otherwise appropriate candidate from consideration for high-dose chemotherapy. There is an increased risk of graft contamination with malignant plasma cells (Gertz et al. 2000), but even patients with refractory disease can achieve durable responses after high-dose chemotherapy with stem cell rescue (Gertz et al. 1995; Rajkumar et al. 1999; Vesole et al. 1999).

5.10.2.2 Tandem Transplant

Sequential transplantation is being performed currently in some centers (Barlogie et al. 1997, 1999). Final data from a randomized trial comparing single autologous PBSCT with tandem transplantation are pending.

5.10.2.3 PBSCT in Renal Failure

PBSCT is not absolutely contraindicated for patients with renal failure, including those in whom dialysis is required. Prognostic factors and outcomes in this group of patients remain controversial, because study results vary significantly depending on the definitions of renal failure and recovery of function and on the indications for dialysis. Renal failure has generally been considered a poor prognostic factor, although it is unclear whether it is an independent factor or a reflection of aggressive disease. A prospective, nonrandomized study evaluated the pharmacokinetics and toxicity associated with high-dose melphalan for patients with and without renal failure (Tricot et al. 1996). Transplant-associated morbidity was significantly higher in the renal failure group; however, adequacy of stem cell collection, pharmacokinetics, engraftment, and overall survival between the groups was not significantly different (Tricot et al. 1996). A reduction of the conditioning dose of melphalan from 200 mg/m^2 to 140 mg/m^2 may decrease morbidity in these patients.

5.10.2.4 Mobilization Chemotherapy

There is no standard chemotherapy used in the mobilization of stem cells. Most commonly, high-dose cyclophosphamide, which spares stem cells, is used in conjunction with granulocyte or granulocyte-macrophage colony-stimulating factor. A minimum of 2.0×10^6 CD34$^+$ cells/kg body weight is required to maximize the chances of engraftment.

5.10.2.5 Conditioning Regimen

The conditioning regimen used most often for autologous stem cell transplantation is single agent, high-dose melphalan (200 mg/m^2) given intravenously as a single dose the day before reinfusion of stem cells (day –1). An alternative regimen has been melphalan (140 mg/m^2) in addition to total body irradiation (8 Gy). Data from a 2-arm randomized trial, however, suggested that melphalan (200 mg/m^2) alone is less toxic and at least as efficacious as the treatment additionally utilizing total body irradiation (Moreau et al. 2002).

5.10.2.6 Allogeneic Transplantation

Allogeneic transplantation is not routinely recommended treatment for myeloma or PCL. It is also not an option for the majority of patients because of their advanced age at diagnosis. Additionally, it carries a high mortality with no definitive evidence for increased overall survival. In an early series, it was associated with a 40% to 50% treatment-related mortality, a relapse rate of 50% at 5 years, and a 5-year survival of only 30%. It should remain a consideration for PCL patients younger than age 55 years with an appropriate donor, however, given the dismal disease prognosis. Attempts are being made to decrease the treatment-related mortality by altering the preparative regimens and using T-cell-de-

pleted stem cells and by using donor lymphocyte infusions to reduce the risk of graft-versus-host disease (Badros et al. 2001). Allogeneic mini-transplantation after a nonmyeloablative conditioning regimen is being investigated as a less toxic form of transplantation.

5.10.3 Radiation Therapy

5.10.3.1 Conditioning

Total body irradiation has been used in the past as part of transplant conditioning regimens for myeloma. A total dose of 8 Gy plus melphalan (140 mg/m^2) has commonly been used. Its use before autologous stem cell transplantation for patients younger than age 65 years has been questioned seriously by data published by the Intergroupe Francophone du Myélome 9502 randomized trial (Moreau et al. 2002) that compared its toxicity and effectiveness to melphalan at 200 mg/m^2 without total body irradiation. Conditioning with melphalan alone was less toxic and at least as effective.

5.10.3.2 Palliation

Radiation, in the form of limited-field therapy, is indicated for the palliation of pain associated with lytic bony lesions and treatment of impending pathologic fractures. External beam radiation is used in the treatment of extramedullary plasmacytomas and for spinal cord compression.

5.10.3.3 Radioisotopes

The uses of skeletal-targeted radioisotopes, such as samarium (^{153}Sm-EDMTP), to treat painful bony metastases or as part of conditioning before transplantation are being investigated in clinical trials (Dispenzieri et al. 2000).

5.10.4 Biologic Therapy

A wide variety of biologic and immunomodulatory agents are in clinical trials or drug development for possible use in myeloma and PCL. These include thalidomide and its more potent analogs such as 3-aminothalidomide, drugs that influence signal transduction, other antiangiogenic agents, antibodies, dendritic cell vaccines, proteosome inhibitors, and cytokine therapies, alone or in combination with traditional chemotherapeutic or transplantation regimens. Thalidomide is the best studied agent whose mechanism of action is presumed to be antiangiogenic but also likely has an immunomodulatory component to its antimyeloma effect by modulating natural killer cell number and function (Davies et al. 2001).

5.10.5 Surgery

Orthopedic surgery or neurosurgical consultation (or both) should be considered for any impending or actual pathologic bone fracture and in cases of erosive vertebral plasmacytomas that threaten spinal stability, with or without associated spinal cord compression.

5.10.6 Supportive Care

5.10.6.1 Pain Control

Narcotic agents are usually necessary for pain control at some point in the disease process.

5.10.6.2 Constipation

Frequently, constipation is a subsequent problem, and patients should begin a bowel regimen (laxatives, stool softeners, and fiber) on initiation of narcotic therapy.

5.10.6.3 Avoidance of Nephrotoxicity

Nonsteroidal anti-inflammatory drugs, except for acetaminophen, should be avoided and good hydration should be maintained to reduce the risk of nephrotoxicity.

5.10.6.4 Gastrointestinal Tract Side Effects

The use of an H_2 blocker or proton pump inhibitor may alleviate gastrointestinal tract side effects, which are common in patients taking oral steroid preparations.

5.10.7 Other Therapeutic Measures

5.10.7.1 Bisphosphonates

Osteolytic bone lesions as a result of increased osteoclastic bone resorption relative to bone formation are major sources of morbidity and mortality in myeloma and PCL patients. Monthly intravenous administration of bisphosphonates should definitely be used for patients with any lytic bone lesions or osteoporosis or both and can be considered even for patients with stages I and II disease. Oral use of these agents is not recommended, given their poor absorption and bioavailability and frequent gastrointestinal tract intolerability. Pamidronate (second generation) and zoledronic acid (third generation) are nitrogen-containing bisphosphonates used in the treatment of myeloma and PCL bone disease. These medications have antiosteoclastic activity and possible proapoptotic and antiangiogenic effects, in addition to their known calcium-lowering effects. Zoledronic acid is the most potent drug of this class that is commercially available.

An analysis of 2 randomized, double-blind, placebo-controlled trials demonstrated that zoledronic acid (at doses of 4 and 8 mg) produced a higher response rate, faster onset of action, and longer duration of action than pamidronate (90 mg) for treatment of hypercalcemia of malignancy (Major et al. 2001). A randomized, double-blind study of pamidronate vs. placebo in stage III patients by the Myeloma Aredia Study Group showed a significant decrease in the number of skeletal events, an improvement in quality of life measurements, and increased performance status in patients in the pamidronate arm (Berenson et al. 1996). Overall survival, however, was not significantly different. A phase 3 double-blind trial (Rosen et al. 2001) comparing pamidronate with zoledronic acid in the treatment of skeletal metastases associated with myeloma or breast carcinoma showed that zoledronic acid is at least as effective and well tolerated as pamidronate. Current recommendations for administration for the treatment of myeloma or PCL bone lesions or osteoporosis are: pamidronate at 90 mg in 500 mL 0.9% NaCl intravenously over 2 to 4 hours every 28 days indefinitely or zoledronic acid at 4 mg in 100 mL 0.9% NaCl or D5W intravenously over 15 minutes every 28 days indefinitely.

Infusion rates faster than recommended can result in albuminuria or azotemia. Side effects of either drug include fever, bone pain, headache, changes in bowel habits, fatigue, malaise, and nausea.

5.11   Relapse Therapy

5.11.1

Chemotherapy

Conventional regimens are described below.

5.11.1.1 EDAP

Etoposide (100-200 mg/m^2) and cisplatin (20 mg/m^2) are mixed in the same bag. Administer 1/3 of the total daily dose in 1 L D5/0.45% NaCl intravenously over 8 hours as a continuous infusion for a total of 3 bags/day on days 1–4. Cytarabine (1,000 mg/m^2) in 250 mL D5W given intravenously over 3 hours on day 5. Dexamethasone (20 mg/m^2) in 50 mL D5W given intravenously over 10 minutes on days 1–5. The cycle is repeated weekly.

5.11.1.2 VDD

Vincristine (2 mg) given as an intravenous push on day 1; doxorubicin (40 mg/m^2) in 250 mL D5W given intravenously over 1 hour on day 1; and dexamethasone (40 mg/day) given orally on days 1–4, 9–12, and 17–20. Repeat cycle every 28 days.

5.11.1.3 CP

High-dose cyclophosphamide (600 mg/m^2) in 250 mL D5W given intravenously over 30 minutes on days 1–4, and prednisone (100 mg/m^2) given orally daily on days 1–4. Repeat cycle every 5 weeks.

5.11.1.4 High-Dose Methylprednisolone

1 to 2 g given intravenously once or twice each week.

5.11.1.5 High-Dose Dexamethasone

40 mg given orally each day on days 1–4, 9–12, and 17–20 every 28 days alternating with 40 mg given orally every day and on days 1–4 only every 28 days.

5.11.1.6 Thalidomide
(Bladé et al. 2001a; Singhal et al. 1999; Yakoub-Agha et al. 2000)

This may be used as monotherapy or with dexamethasone given orally. Response rates range from 32% to 53% (Bladé et al. 2001b; Singhal et al. 1999) and have been reported to be significantly higher in patients without extramedullary disease than in those with soft tissue masses (Bladé et al. 2001b). Thalidomide is given orally at 200 to 400 mg every day. Dosing starts at 200 mg daily and is titrated to response or side effects to a total of 400 mg given orally every day.

Side effects of thalidomide include somnolence, rash, peripheral neuropathy (can be permanent), orthostatic hypotension and dizziness, and occasional central nervous system effects such as ataxia. Birth defects are a well-established adverse effect of thalidomide. The drug is contraindicated in pregnancy and should not be prescribed to individuals unwilling to use contraception. Hypothyroidism has been associated with thalidomide treatment. There are several reports documenting increased risk of deep vein thrombosis (27%–28%) in patients receiving thalidomide in combination with chemotherapy compared with 4% to 7% in patients not receiving this therapy (Osman et al. 2001; Zangari et al. 2001).

Toxic epidermal necrolysis is a potentially life-threatening condition associated with thalidomide therapy, particularly when it is combined with dexamethasone (Rajkumar et al. 2000). It is clinically manifested by a scalded skin appearance and blistering with full-thickness epidermal necrosis. It is characterized by death of keratinocytes and the separation of the epidermis from the dermis. Thalidomide should be discontinued immediately in the event of this reaction and should not be resumed.

5.11.2   Clinical Trials

Clinical trials may be available that test novel therapeutic modalities such as immunomodulatory agents, signal transduction agents, and monoclonal antibodies, often in some combination with conventional forms of chemotherapy. These trials should be a strong consideration for this group of patients.

5.11.3 Second Transplant

Patients who are eligible for stem cell transplantation may be considered for a second PBSCT if adequate numbers of stored CD34$^+$ cells are available.

5.12 Prognosis

The prognosis for either the primary or secondary form of PCL remains quite poor regardless of treatment. Median survival for de novo PCL after treatment with conventional chemotherapy is 2 to 6 months (Dimopoulos et al. 1994; Garcia-Sanz et al. 1999; Noel and Kyle 1987). Median survival for secondary PCL is approximately 1.3 months (Noel and Kyle 1987).

5.13 Quality of Life and Rehabilitation

The poor prognosis of the disease usually precludes long-term rehabilitation in these patients. Physical therapy may be of benefit in the short term.

5.14 Emergencies

5.14.1 Spinal Cord Compression

Cord compression is one of the most frequently encountered emergencies in PCL or myeloma patients. Suspicion should be raised for symptoms of focal weakness or pain, paresthesias, or change in bowel or bladder habits. Signs may include asymmetric deep tendon reflexes, decreased motor strength, decreased rectal tone on digital examination, or detection of a level of sensory anesthesia. Concern for this possibility necessitates immobilization and administration of high-dose dexamethasone. An initial intravenous bolus of dexamethasone (50 to 100 mg) is given, followed by an oral or intravenous dose of 6 to 8 mg every 6 hours. Steroid therapy should aid in reducing edema and risk of cord ischemia. Magnetic resonance imaging of the pertinent region should be done emergently, followed by a radiation oncology consultation if findings are consistent with compression. If there is concern for the possibility of spine instability in addition to compression, orthopedic surgery or neurosurgery evaluation (or both) may be required.

5.14.2 Infection

Infection is the major cause of death in myeloma and PCL patients and may be the initial presentation of disease. Increased susceptibility to infection is thought to result largely from the polyclonal hypogammaglobulinemia seen in the majority of patients. *Streptococcus pneumoniae*, *Haemophilus influenzae*, and *Staphylococcus aureus* are common pathogenic organisms. The possibility of encountering vancomycin-resistant enterococcus and vancomycin intermediate resistance *Staphylococcus aureus* should be entertained, especially for patients with histories of multiple hospitalizations or transplantation. Patients profoundly immunosuppressed posttransplantation or receiving long-term steroid therapy should be placed on *Pneumocystis carinii* prophylaxis with trimethoprim 160 mg/sulfamethoxazole 800 mg, 1 tablet orally twice daily, twice a week. Aerosolized pentamidine, 300 mg every month, may be used in patients with sulfa drug allergy or intolerance.

5.14.3 Acute Renal Failure

Patients presenting in acute renal failure may require emergent dialysis for signs of uremia, pericarditis, congestive heart failure, or fluid overload not responsive to diuresis, hyperkalemia, or metabolic acidosis. Possible reversible causes of renal failure should be sought and treated, including prerenal azotemia due to dehydration, hypercalcemia, nephrotoxic agents such as nonsteroidal anti-inflammatory agents, angiotensin-converting enzyme inhibitors, hyperuricemia, and interstitial nephritis due to medications.

5.14.4 Hypercalcemia

Nausea, anorexia, vomiting, polyuria, polydipsia, and mental status changes suggest the possibility of hypercalcemia. Prompt initial treatment consists of aggressive hydration with 0.9% NaCl and a forced diuresis. Intensive monitoring and other modifications may need to be made in the event of frank renal failure, given the risk of fluid overload. Administration of a bisphosphonate, pamidronate (60–90 mg in 500 mL 0.9% NaCl intravenously over 2 to 4 hours), or zoledronic acid (4 mg in 100 mL 0.9% NaCl or D5W intravenously over 15 minutes) may also be considered, depending on the calcium value and severity of symptoms.

References

Attal M, Harousseau JL, Stoppa AM, Sotto JJ, Fuzibet JG, Rossi JF, Casassus P, Maisonneuve H, Facon T, Ifrah N, Payen C, Bataille R (1996) A prospective, randomized trial of autologous bone marrow transplantation and chemotherapy in multiple myeloma. Intergroupe Français du Myélome. N Engl J Med 335:91–97

Attal M, Harousseau JL, Stoppa AM, Sotto JJ, Fuzibet G, Rossi JF, Casassus P, Thyss A, Maisonneuve H, Facon T, Ifrah N, Payen C, Bataille R (1997) High dose therapy in multiple myeloma: an updated analysis of the IFM 90 protocol (abstract). Blood 90 Suppl 1:418a

Avet-Loiseau H, Li JY, Facon T, Brigaudeau C, Morineau N, Maloisel F, Rapp MJ, Talmant P, Trimoreau F, Jaccard A, Harousseau JL, Bataille R (1998) High incidence of translocations t(11;14)(q13;q32) and t(4;14)(p16;q32) in patients with plasma cell malignancies. Cancer Res 58:5640–5645

Avet-Loiseau H, Li JY, Morineau N, Facon T, Brigaudeau C, Harousseau JL, Grosbois B, Bataille R (1999) Monosomy 13 is associated with the transition of monoclonal gammopathy of undetermined significance to multiple myeloma. Intergroupe Francophone du Myélome. Blood 94:2583–2589

Avet-Loiseau H, Daviet A, Sauner S, Bataille R (2000) Chromosome 13 abnormalities in multiple myeloma are mostly monosomy 13. Br J Haematol 111:1116–1117

Avet-Loiseau H, Daviet A, Brigaudeau C, Callet-Bauchu E, Terre C, Lafage-Pochitaloff M, Desangles F, Ramond S, Talmant P, Bataille R (2001a) Cytogenetic, interphase, and multicolor fluorescence in situ hybridization analyses in primary plasma cell leukemia: a study of 40 patients at diagnosis, on behalf of the Intergroupe Francophone du Myélome and the Groupe Français de Cytogénétique Hématologique. Blood 97:822–825

Avet-Loiseau H, Gerson F, Magrangeas F, Minvielle S, Harousseau JL, Bataille R (2001b) Rearrangements of the c-myc oncogene are present in 15% of primary human multiple myeloma tumors. Blood 98:3082–3086

Badros A, Barlogie B, Morris C, Desikan R, Martin SR, Munshi N, Zangari M, Mehta J, Toor A, Cottler-Fox M, Fassas A, Anaissie E, Schichman S, Tricot G, Aniassie E (2001) High response rate in refractory and poor-risk multiple myeloma after allotransplantation using a nonmyeloablative conditioning regimen and donor lymphocyte infusions. Blood 97:2574–2579

Barlogie B, Jagannath S, Vesole DH, Naucke S, Cheson B, Mattox S, Bracy D, Salmon S, Jacobson J, Crowley J, Tricot G (1997) Superiority of tandem autologous transplantation over standard therapy for previously untreated multiple myeloma. Blood 89:789–793

Barlogie B, Jagannath S, Desikan KR, Mattox S, Vesole D, Siegel D, Tricot G, Munshi N, Fassas A, Singhal S, Mehta J, Anaissie E, Dhodapkar D, Naucke S, Cromer J, Sawyer J, Epstein J, Spoon D, Ayers D, Cheson B, Crowley J (1999) Total therapy with tandem transplants for newly diagnosed multiple myeloma. Blood 93:55–65

Berenson JR, Lichtenstein A, Porter L, Dimopoulos MA, Bordoni R, George S, Lipton A, Keller A, Ballester O, Kovacs MJ, Blacklock HA, Bell R, Simeone J, Reitsma DJ, Heffernan M, Seaman J, Knight RD (1996) Efficacy of pamidronate in reducing skeletal events in patients with advanced multiple myeloma. Myeloma Aredia Study Group. N Engl J Med 334:488–493

Bergsagel PL, Kuehl WM (2001) Chromosome translocations in multiple myeloma. Oncogene 20:5611–5622

Bergsagel PL, Chesi M, Nardini E, Brents LA, Kirby SL, Kuehl WM (1996) Promiscuous translocations into immunoglobulin heavy chain switch regions in multiple myeloma. Proc Natl Acad Sci USA 93:13931–13936

Bezieau S, Devilder MC, Avet-Loiseau H, Mellerin MP, Puthier D, Pennarun E, Rapp MJ, Harousseau JL, Moisan JP, Bataille R (2001) High incidence of N and K-Ras activating mutations in multiple myeloma and primary plasma cell leukemia at diagnosis. Hum Mutat 18:212–224

Bladé J, Kyle RA (1999) Nonsecretory myeloma, immunoglobulin D myeloma, and plasma cell leukemia. Hematol Oncol Clin North Am 13:1259–1272

Bladé J, Esteve J, Rosinol L, Perales M, Montoto S, Tuset M, Montserrat E (2001a) Thalidomide in refractory and relapsing multiple myeloma. Semin Oncol 28:588–592

Bladé J, Perales M, Rosinol L, Tuset M, Montoto S, Esteve J, Cobo F, Villela L, Rafel M, Nomdedeu B, Montserrat E (2001b) Thalidomide in multiple myeloma: lack of response of soft-tissue plasmacytomas. Br J Haematol 113:422–424

Chesi M, Bergsagel PL, Brents LA, Smith CM, Gerhard DS, Kuehl WM (1996) Dysregulation of cyclin D1 by translocation into an IgH gamma switch region in two multiple myeloma cell lines. Blood 88:674–681

Chesi M, Bergsagel PL, Shonukan OO, Martelli ML, Brents LA, Chen T, Schrock E, Ried T, Kuehl WM (1998a) Frequent dysregulation of the c-maf proto-oncogene at 16q23 by translocation to an Ig locus in multiple myeloma. Blood 91:4457–4463

Chesi M, Nardini E, Lim RS, Smith KD, Kuehl WM, Bergsagel PL (1998b) The t(4;14) translocation in myeloma dysregulates both FGFR3 and a novel gene, MMSET, resulting in IgH/MMSET hybrid transcripts. Blood 92:3025–3034

Cohen HJ, Crawford J, Rao MK, Pieper CF, Currie MS (1998) Racial differences in the prevalence of monoclonal gammopathy in a community-based sample of the elderly. Am J Med 104:439–444

Corradini P, Inghirami G, Astolfi M, Ladetto M, Voena C, Ballerini P, Gu W, Nilsson K, Knowles DM, Boccadoro M (1994) Inactivation of tumor suppressor genes, p53 and Rb1, in plasma cell dyscrasias. Leukemia 8:758–767

Davies FE, Raje N, Hideshima T, Lentzsch S, Young G, Tai YT, Lin B, Podar K, Gupta D, Chauhan D, Treon SP, Richardson PG, Schlossman RL, Morgan GJ, Muller GW, Stirling DI, Anderson KC (2001) Thalidomide and immunomodulatory derivatives augment natural killer cell cytotoxicity in multiple myeloma. Blood 98:210–216

Desikan R, Barlogie B, Sawyer J, Ayers D, Tricot G, Badros A, Zangari M, Munshi NC, Anaissie E, Spoon D, Siegel D, Jagannath S, Vesole D, Epstein J, Shaughnessy J, Fassas A, Lim S, Roberson P, Crowley J (2000) Results of high-dose therapy for 1000 patients with multiple myeloma: durable complete remissions and superior survival in the absence of chromosome 13 abnormalities. Blood 95:4008–4010

Dewald GW, Kyle RA, Hicks GA, Greipp PR (1985) The clinical significance of cytogenetic studies in 100 patients with multiple myeloma, plasma cell leukemia, or amyloidosis. Blood 66:380–390

Dimopoulos MA, Palumbo A, Delasalle KB, Alexanian R (1994) Primary plasma cell leukaemia. Br J Haematol 88:754–759

Dispenzieri A, Wiseman GA, Lacy MQ, Litzow MR, Tefferi A, Inwards DJ, Gastineau DA, Ansell SM, Micallef IN, Rajkumar SV, Fonseca R, Witzig TE, Lust JA, Kyle RA, Greipp PR, Gertz MA (2000) A phase I study of a conditioning regimen for peripheral stem cell transplantation

(PBSCT) for multiple myeloma (MM): [153]Samarium ethylenediami-netetramethylenephosphonate ([153]Sm-EDMTP) and melphalan (abstract). Blood 96:558a

Drach J, Angerler J, Schuster J, Rothermundt C, Thalhammer R, Haas OA, Jager U, Fiegl M, Geissler K, Ludwig H (1995a) Interphase fluorescence in situ hybridization identifies chromosomal abnormalities in plasma cells from patients with monoclonal gammopathy of undetermined significance. Blood 86:3915–3921

Drach J, Schuster J, Nowotny H, Angerler J, Rosenthal F, Fiegl M, Rothermundt C, Gsur A, Jager U, Heinz R (1995b) Multiple myeloma: high incidence of chromosomal aneuploidy as detected by interphase fluorescence in situ hybridization. Cancer Res 55:3854–3859

Durie BG, Salmon SE (1975) A clinical staging system for multiple myeloma: correlation of measured myeloma cell mass with presenting clinical features, response to treatment, and survival. Cancer 36:842–854

Facon T, Avet-Loiseau H, Guillerm G, Moreau P, Genevieve F, Zandecki M, Lai JL, Leleu X, Jouet JP, Bauters F, Harousseau JL, Bataille R, Mary JY (2001) Chromosome 13 abnormalities identified by FISH analysis and serum β_2-microglobulin produce a powerful myeloma staging system for patients receiving high-dose therapy. Blood 97:1566–1571

Fermand JP, Ravaud P, Chevret S, Devine M, Leblond V, Belanger C, Macro M, Pertuiset E, Dreyfus F, Mariette X, Boccacio C, Brouet JC (1998) High-dose therapy and autologous peripheral blood stem cell transplantation in multiple myeloma: up-front or rescue treatment? Results of a multicenter sequential randomized clinical trial. Blood 92:3131–3136

Fonseca R, Hoyer JD, Aguayo P, Jalal SM, Ahmann GJ, Rajkumar SV, Witzig TE, Lacy MQ, Dispenzieri A, Gertz MA, Kyle RA, Greipp PR (1999) Clinical significance of the translocation (11;14)(q13;q32) in multiple myeloma. Leuk Lymphoma 35:599–605

Fonseca R, Oken MM, Greipp PR (2001a) The t(4;14)(p16.3;q32) is strongly associated with chromosome 13 abnormalities in both multiple myeloma and monoclonal gammopathy of undetermined significance. Blood 98:1271–1272

Fonseca R, Oken MM, Harrington D, Bailey RJ, Van Wier SA, Henderson KJ, Kay NE, Van Ness B, Greipp PR, Dewald GW (2001b) Deletions of chromosome 13 in multiple myeloma identified by interphase FISH usually denote large deletions of the q arm or monosomy. Leukemia 15:981–986

Garcia-Sanz R, Orfao A, Gonzalez M, Moro MJ, Hernandez JM, Ortega F, Borrego D, Carnero M, Casanova F, Jimenez R, Portero JA, San Miguel JF (1995) Prognostic implications of DNA aneuploidy in 156 untreated multiple myeloma patients. Castelano-Leones (Spain) Cooperative Group for the Study of Monoclonal Gammopathies. Br J Haematol 90:106–112

Garcia-Sanz R, Orfao A, Gonzalez M, Tabernero MD, Bladé J, Moro MJ, Fernandez-Calvo J, Sanz MA, Perez-Simon JA, Rasillo A, Miguel JF (1999) Primary plasma cell leukemia: clinical, immunophenotypic, DNA ploidy, and cytogenetic characteristics. Blood 93:1032–1037

Gertz MA, Pineda AA, Chen MG, Letendre L, Greipp PR, Solberg LA Jr, Witzig TE, Garton JP, Inwards DJ, Litzow MR, Tefferi A, Kyle RA, Noel P (1995) Refractory and relapsing multiple myeloma treated by blood stem cell transplantation. Am J Med Sci 309:152–161

Gertz MA, Lacy MQ, Inwards DJ, Gastineau DA, Tefferi A, Chen MG, Witzig TE, Greipp PR, Litzow MR (2000) Delayed stem cell transplan-

tation for the management of relapsed or refractory multiple myeloma. Bone Marrow Transplant 26:45–50

Gonzalez M, Mateos MV, Garcia-Sanz R, Balanzategui A, Lopez-Perez R, Chillon MC, Gonzalez D, Alaejos I, San Miguel JF (2000) De novo methylation of tumor suppressor gene p16/INK4a is a frequent finding in multiple myeloma patients at diagnosis. Leukemia 14:183–187

Gutierrez NC, Hernandez JM, Garcia JL, Canizo MC, Gonzalez M, Hernandez J, Gonzalez MB, Garcia-Marcos MA, San Miguel JF (2001) Differences in genetic changes between multiple myeloma and plasma cell leukemia demonstrated by comparative genomic hybridization. Leukemia 15:840–845

Hoechtlen-Vollmar W, Menzel G, Bartl R, Lamerz R, Wick M, Seidel D (2000) Amplification of cyclin D1 gene in multiple myeloma: clinical and prognostic relevance. Br J Haematol 109:30–38

Kuehl WM, Bergsagel PL (2002) Multiple myeloma: evolving genetic events and host interactions. Nature Rev/Cancer 2:175–187

Lai JL, Michaux L, Dastugue N, Vasseur F, Daudignon A, Facon T, Bauters F, Zandecki M (1998) Cytogenetics in multiple myeloma: a multicenter study of 24 patients with t(11;14)(q13;q32) or its variant. Cancer Genet Cytogenet 104:133–138

Li R, Sonik A, Stindl R, Rasnick D, Duesberg P (2000) Aneuploidy vs gene mutation hypothesis of cancer: recent study claims mutation but is found to support aneuploidy. Proc Natl Acad Sci USA 97:3236–3241

Major P, Lortholary A, Hon J, Abdi E, Mills G, Menssen HD, Yunus F, Bell R, Body J, Quebe-Fehling E, Seaman J (2001) Zoledronic acid is superior to pamidronate in the treatment of hypercalcemia of malignancy: a pooled analysis of two randomized, controlled clinical trials. J Clin Oncol 19:558–567

Malgeri U, Baldini L, Perfetti V, Fabris S, Vignarelli MC, Colombo G, Lotti V, Compasso S, Bogni S, Lombardi L, Maiolo AT, Neri A (2000) Detection of t(4;14)(p16.3;q32) chromosomal translocation in multiple myeloma by reverse transcription-polymerase chain reaction analysis of IGH-MMSET fusion transcripts. Cancer Res 60:4058–4061

Moreau P, Facon T, Attal M, Hulin C, Michallet M, Maloisel F, Sotto JJ, Guilhot F, Marit G, Doyen C, Jaubert J, Fuzibet JG, François S, Benboubker L, Monconduit M, Voillat L, Macro M, Berthou C, Dorvaux V, Pignon B, Rio B, Matthes T, Casassus P, Caillot D, Najman N, Grosbois B, Bataille R, Harousseau JL (2002) Comparison of 200 mg/m^2 melphalan and 8 Gy total body irradiation plus 140 mg/m^2 melphalan as conditioning regimens for peripheral blood stem cell transplantation in patients with newly diagnosed multiple myeloma: final analysis of the Intergroupe Francophone du Myélome 9502 randomized trial. Blood 99:731–735

Myeloma Trialists' Collaborative Group (1998) Combination chemotherapy versus melphalan plus prednisone as treatment for multiple myeloma: an overview of 6,633 patients from 27 randomized trials. J Clin Oncol 16:3832–3842

Nishida K, Tamura A, Nakazawa N, Ueda Y, Abe T, Matsuda F, Kashima K, Taniwaki M (1997) The Ig heavy chain gene is frequently involved in chromosomal translocations in multiple myeloma and plasma cell leukemia as detected by in situ hybridization. Blood 90:526–534

Noel P, Kyle RA (1987) Plasma cell leukemia: an evaluation of response to therapy. Am J Med 83:1062–1068

Osman K, Comenzo R, Rajkumar SV (2001) Deep venous thrombosis and thalidomide therapy for multiple myeloma. N Engl J Med 344:1951–1952

Pellat-Deceunynck C, Barille S, Jego G, Puthier D, Robillard N, Pineau D, Rapp MJ, Harousseau JL, Amiot M, Bataille R (1998) The absence of CD56 (NCAM) on malignant plasma cells is a hallmark of plasma cell leukemia and of a special subset of multiple myeloma. Leukemia 12:1977–1982

Perez-Simon JA, Garcia-Sanz R, Tabernero MD, Almeida J, Gonzalez M, Fernandez-Calvo J, Moro MJ, Hernandez JM, San Miguel JF, Orfao A (1998) Prognostic value of numerical chromosome aberrations in multiple myeloma: a FISH analysis of 15 different chromosomes. Blood 91:3366–3371

Portier M, Moles JP, Mazars GR, Jeanteur P, Bataille R, Klein B, Theillet C (1992) p53 and RAS gene mutations in multiple myeloma. Oncogene 7:2539–2543

Preudhomme C, Facon T, Zandecki M, Vanrumbeke M, Lai JL, Nataf E, Loucheux-Lefebvre MH, Kerckaert JP, Fenaux P (1992) Rare occurrence of p53 gene mutations in multiple myeloma. Br J Haematol 81:440–443

Rajkumar SV, Fonseca R, Lacy MQ, Witzig TE, Lust JA, Greipp PR, Therneau TM, Kyle RA, Litzow MR, Gertz MA (1999) Autologous stem cell transplantation for relapsed and primary refractory myeloma. Bone Marrow Transplant 23:1267–1272

Rajkumar SV, Gertz MA, Witzig TE (2000) Life-threatening toxic epidermal necrolysis with thalidomide therapy for myeloma. N Engl J Med 343:972–973

Rasmussen T, Knudsen LM, Johnsen HE (2001) Frequency and prognostic relevance of cyclin D1 dysregulation in multiple myeloma. Eur J Haematol 67:296–301

Riedel DA, Pottern LM, Blattner WA (1991) Epidemiology of multiple myeloma. In: Wiernik PH, Canellos GP, Kyle RA, Schiffer CA (eds) Neoplastic diseases of the blood. 2nd edn. Churchill Livingstone, New York, pp 347–372

Rosen LS, Gordon D, Antonio BS, Kaminski M, Howell A, Belch A, Mackey JA, Apffelstaedt J, Tfrin M, Hussein M, Coleman RE, Reitsma DJ, Seaman JJ, Chen BL, Ambros Y (2001) Zoledronic acid versus pamidronate in the treatment of skeletal metastases in patients with breast cancer or osteolytic lesions of multiple myeloma: a phase III, double-blind, comparative trial. Cancer J 7:377–387

San Miguel JF, Gonzalez M, Gascon A, Moro MJ, Hernandez JM, Ortega F, Jimenez R, Guerras L, Romero M, Casanova F (1991) Immunophenotypic heterogeneity of multiple myeloma: influence on the biology and clinical course of the disease. Castellano-Leones (Spain) Cooperative Group for the Study of Monoclonal Gammopathies. Br J Haematol 77:185–190

Sawyer JR, Waldron JA, Jagannath S, Barlogie B (1995) Cytogenetic findings in 200 patients with multiple myeloma. Cancer Genet Cytogenet 82:41–49

Sawyer JR, Lukacs JL, Munshi N, Desikan KR, Singhal S, Mehta J, Siegel D, Shaughnessy J, Barlogie B (1998a) Identification of new nonrandom translocations in multiple myeloma with multicolor spectral karyotyping. Blood 92:4269–4278

Sawyer JR, Tricot G, Mattox S, Jagannath S, Barlogie B (1998b) Jumping translocations of chromosome 1q in multiple myeloma: evidence for a mechanism involving decondensation of pericentromeric heterochromatin. Blood 91:1732–1741

Seong C, Delasalle K, Hayes K, Weber D, Dimopoulos M, Swantkowski J, Huh Y, Glassman A, Champlin R, Alexanian R (1998) Prognostic value of cytogenetics in multiple myeloma. Br J Haematol 101:189–194

Shaughnessy J Jr, Gabrea A, Qi Y, Brents L, Zhan F, Tian E, Sawyer J, Barlogie B, Bergsagel PL, Kuehl M (2001) Cyclin D3 at 6p21 is dysregulated by recurrent chromosomal translocations to immunoglobulin loci in multiple myeloma. Blood 98:217–223

Shou J, Martelli ML, Gabrea A, Qi Y, Brents LA, Roschke A, Dewald G, Kirsch IR, Bergsagel PL, Kuehl WM (2000) Diverse karyotypic abnormalities of the c-myc locus associated with c-myc dysregulation and tumor progression in multiple myeloma. Proc Natl Acad Sci USA 97:228–233

Singhal S, Mehta J, Desikan R, Ayers D, Roberson P, Eddlemon P, Munshi N, Anaissie E, Wilson C, Dhodapkar M, Zeddis J, Barlogie B (1999) Antitumor activity of thalidomide in refractory multiple myeloma. N Engl J Med 341:1565–1571

Smadja NV, Bastard C, Brigaudeau C, Leroux D, Fruchart C (2001) Hypodiploidy is a major prognostic factor in multiple myeloma. Blood 98:2229–2238

Taniwaki M, Nishida K, Takashima T, Nakagawa H, Fujii H, Tamaki T, Shimazaki C, Horiike S, Misawa S, Abe T (1994) Nonrandom chromosomal rearrangements of 14q32.3 and 19p13.3 and preferential deletion of 1p in 21 patients with multiple myeloma and plasma cell leukemia. Blood 84:2283–2290

Tatsumi T, Shimazaki C, Goto H, Araki S, Sudo Y, Yamagata N, Ashihara E, Inaba T, Fujita N, Nakagawa M (1996) Expression of adhesion molecules on myeloma cells. Jpn J Cancer Res 87:837–842

Teoh G, Anderson KC (1997) Interaction of tumor and host cells with adhesion and extracellular matrix molecules in the development of multiple myeloma. Hematol Oncol Clin North Am 11:27–42

Tricot G, Barlogie B, Jagannath S, Bracy D, Mattox S, Vesole DH, Naucke S, Sawyer JR (1995) Poor prognosis in multiple myeloma is associated only with partial or complete deletions of chromosome 13 or abnormalities involving 11q and not with other karyotype abnormalities. Blood 86:4250–4256

Tricot G, Alberts DS, Johnson C, Roe DJ, Dorr RT, Bracy D, Vesole DH, Jagannath S, Meyers R, Barlogie B (1996) Safety of autotransplants with high-dose melphalan in renal failure: a pharmacokinetic and toxicity study. Clin Cancer Res 2:947–952

Urashima M, Teoh G, Ogata A, Chauhan D, Treon SP, Sugimoto Y, Kaihara C, Matsuzaki M, Hoshi Y, DeCaprio JA, Anderson KC (1997) Characterization of p16(INK4A) expression in multiple myeloma and plasma cell leukemia. Clin Cancer Res 3:2173–2179

Vesole DH, Crowley JJ, Catchatourian R, Stiff PJ, Johnson DB, Cromer J, Salmon SE, Barlogie B (1999) High-dose melphalan with autotransplantation for refractory multiple myeloma: results of a Southwest Oncology Group phase II trial. J Clin Oncol 17:2173–2179

Yakoub-Agha I, Moreau P, Leyvraz S, Berthou C, Payen C, Dumontet C, Grosbois B, Beris P, Duguet C, Attal M, Harousseau JL, Facon T (2000) Thalidomide in patients with advanced multiple myeloma. Hematol J 1:186–189

Zangari M, Anaissie E, Barlogie B, Badros A, Desikan R, Gopal AV, Morris C, Toor A, Siegel E, Fink L, Tricot G (2001) Increased risk of deep-vein thrombosis in patients with multiple myeloma receiving thalidomide and chemotherapy. Blood 98:1614–1615

Zojer N, Konigsberg R, Ackermann J, Fritz E, Dallinger S, Kromer E, Kaufmann H, Riedl L, Gisslinger H, Schreiber S, Heinz R, Ludwig H, Huber H, Drach J (2000) Deletion of 13q14 remains an independent adverse prognostic variable in multiple myeloma despite its frequent detection by interphase fluorescence in situ hybridization. Blood 95:1925–1930

Heavy Chain Diseases

Dietlind L. Wahner-Roedler, M.D., Robert A. Kyle, M.D., Thomas E. Witzig, M.D.

Contents

6.1 Introduction 134

6.2 α-HCD 134
   6.2.1 Epidemiology 134
      6.2.1.1 Incidence 134
      6.2.1.2 Mortality 134
      6.2.1.3 Sex Ratio 135
      6.2.1.4 Race Ratio 135
      6.2.1.5 Age Ratio 135
      6.2.1.6 Survivorship 135
   6.2.2 Etiology 135
      6.2.2.1 Microorganisms 136
      6.2.2.2 Environmental Factors . . 136
      6.2.2.3 Immunodeficiency 136
      6.2.2.4 Genetics 136
   6.2.3 Screening and Prevention 136
   6.2.4 Molecular Biology and Genetics . . 136
   6.2.5 Clinical Presentation 138
   6.2.6 Classification and Staging 139
      6.2.6.1 Clinical 139
      6.2.6.2 Pathologic 139
   6.2.7 Diagnosis 140
      6.2.7.1 Laboratory Tests 140
      6.2.7.1.1 Hematologic and
             Metabolic Abnormalities . 140
      6.2.7.1.2 Protein Findings 140
      6.2.7.2 Cytogenetic Analysis . . . 141
      6.2.7.3 Imaging 141
      6.2.7.3.1 X-ray 141
      6.2.7.3.2 CT and Ultrasonography . 141
      6.2.7.4 Endoscopy 141
      6.2.7.5 Laparotomy 141

6.2.8 Differential Diagnosis 141
6.2.9 Therapy 142
      6.2.9.1 Diet and Lifestyle 142
      6.2.9.2 Supportive Care 142
      6.2.9.3 Pharmacologic
             Treatment 142
      6.2.9.4 Chemotherapy 142
      6.2.9.5 Surgery 142
      6.2.9.6 Radiation Therapy 142
      6.2.9.7 Stem Cell
             Transplantation 142
      6.2.9.8 Emerging Therapies 143
  6.2.10 Prognosis 143
  6.2.11 Emergencies 144

6.3 γ-HCD 144
   6.3.1 Epidemiology 144
      6.3.1.1 Incidence 144
      6.3.1.2 Mortality 144
      6.3.1.3 Sex Ratio 144
      6.3.1.4 Age Ratio 144
      6.3.1.5 Survivorship 144
   6.3.2 Etiology 144
   6.3.3 Screening 144
   6.3.4 Molecular Biology and Genetics . . 144
   6.3.5 Clinical Presentation 146
   6.3.6 Classification and Staging 147
      6.3.6.1 Clinical 147
      6.3.6.2 Pathologic 147
   6.3.7 Diagnosis 147
      6.3.7.1 Laboratory Tests 147
      6.3.7.1.1 Peripheral Blood
             and Bone Marrow 147
      6.3.7.1.2 Protein Findings 148

6.3.7.2	Cytogenetic Analysis . . .	149
6.3.7.3	Other Features	149
6.3.7.4	Imaging	149
6.3.8	Differential Diagnoses	149
6.3.9	Therapy	149
6.3.9.1	Chemotherapy	149
6.3.9.2	Surgery or Radiation Therapy	149
6.3.10	Prognosis	150
6.3.11	Emergencies	150
6.4	**μ-HCD**	**150**
6.4.1	Epidemiology	150
6.4.1.1	Incidence	150
6.4.1.2	Mortality	150
6.4.1.3	Sex Ratio	150
6.4.1.4	Race Ratio	150
6.4.1.5	Age Ratio	150
6.4.1.6	Survivorship	150
6.4.2	Etiology	150

6.4.3	Screening	150
6.4.4	Molecular Biology and Genetics . .	150
6.4.5	Clinical Presentation	151
6.4.6	Classification and Staging	152
6.4.7	Diagnosis	152
6.4.7.1	Laboratory Tests	152
6.4.7.1.1	Peripheral Blood and Bone Marrow	152
6.4.7.1.2	Protein Findings	152
6.4.7.2	Cytogenetic Analysis . . .	152
6.4.7.3	Other Features	153
6.4.7.4	Imaging	153
6.4.8	Differential Diagnosis	153
6.4.9	Therapy	153
6.4.9.1	General	153
6.4.9.2	Chemotherapy	153
6.4.10	Prognosis	153
6.4.11	Emergencies	153
References	. . . .	153

6.1 Introduction

Heavy chain diseases (HCDs) are B-cell lymphoplasma cell proliferative disorders characterized by the production of monoclonal immunoglobulins (Ig), which have the immunochemical characteristics of truncated heavy chains without associated light chains. The complex abnormalities of HCD proteins and the usual lack of normal light chains are due to several distinct gene alterations, including somatic mutations, deletions, and insertions. HCDs involving the 3 main Ig classes have been described: a-HCD is the most frequent, μ-HCD is rare, and the incidence of γ-HCD is intermediate. The diagnosis of these conditions depends on the detection of the structurally abnormal immunoglobulin molecules in the patient's serum or urine. Whereas the monoclonal proteins are always present in the serum in all HCDs and often in the urine in γ-HCD, monoclonal heavy chains are infrequent in the urine in μ-HCD and occur in small amounts in a-HCD.

HCDs can be thought of as variant types of non-Hodgkin lymphoma (NHL), with a-HCD presenting as an extranodal marginal zone lymphoma of mucosa-associated lymphoid tissue (MALT), γ-HCD as a lymphoplasmacytoid NHL, and μ-HCD as small lymphocytic NHL or chronic lymphocytic leukemia (Jaffe et al. 2001). Clinical characteristics of the HCDs are summarized in Table 6.1. Because the clinical manifestations specifically of γ-HCD vary considerably and the abnormal Ig is frequently not evident on serum electrophoresis, the HCDs are underdiagnosed.

6.2 a-HCD

6.2.1 Epidemiology

6.2.1.1 Incidence

In 1968, Seligmann et al. described an Arab woman with severe malabsorption, resulting from a lymphoplasmacytic infiltrate in the small bowel, who had a monoclonal a-heavy chain in the serum. Since this description, more than 400 cases (Seligmann 1993) have been reported in the literature.

6.2.1.2 Mortality

a-HCD usually evolves from initial benign-appearing immunoproliferative lesions of the small intestine to an often fatal highly malignant lymphoma.

Table 6.1. Summary of clinical characteristics of the heavy chain diseases

Characteristic	Finding in heavy chain disease		
	a	γ	μ
Incidence	Rare	Very rare	Very rare
Age	Young adult (< 30 years)	Older adult (60–70 years)	Older adult (50–60 years)
Demographics	Mediterranean region	Worldwide	Worldwide
Structurally abnormal monoclonal protein	IgA	IgG	IgM
MGUS phase	No	Possible	Possible
Urine light chain	No	No	Yes
Sites involved	Small intestine and mesenteric nodes	Nodes, marrow, and spleen	Nodes, marrow, liver, and spleen
Pathologic features	Extranodal marginal zone lymphoma (MALT or IPSID)	Lymphoplasmacytoid lymphoma	Small lymphocytic lymphoma or CLL
Associated diseases	Infection, malabsorption	Autoimmune diseases	–
Therapy	Antibiotics and chemotherapy	Chemotherapy	Chemotherapy

CLL, chronic lymphocytic leukemia; IPSID, immunoproliferative small intestinal disease; MALT, mucosa-associated lymphoid tissue; MGUS, monoclonal gammopathy of undetermined significance. (Modified from Witzig TE, Wahner-Roedler DL (2002) Heavy chain disease. Curr Treat Options Oncol 3:247–254. By permission of Current Science.)

6.2.1.3 Sex Ratio

The prevalence is slightly higher in males than in females.

6.2.1.4 Race Ratio

Most reports of a-HCD have been of Arab or Jewish patients from the Mediterranean area or from the Middle East, but numerous cases have been described in inhabitants of Eastern Europe; the Indian subcontinent; the Far East; Central, North, and South America; and sub-Saharan Africa. a-HCD in developed countries often occurs among immigrants from the Third World and underprivileged native populations.

6.2.1.5 Age Ratio

Unlike multiple myeloma and other HCDs, a-HCD has a predilection for young adults; most patients are in their 20s or 30s, although a-HCD has been reported in children and in persons in the 7th decade of life.

6.2.1.6 Survivorship

Long-term prognosis of patients with a-HCD remains imprecise because of the lack of large series with adequate follow-up.

6.2.2 Etiology

The cause of a-HCD is unknown. Current clinical, histologic, molecular, and immunologic data indicate that the evolutionary cause of a-HCD is a complex, multistep process. a-HCD might be considered a model showing the complex interactions of the environment with genetic factors and the complex infection-immunity-cancer interrelationships originating from the same proliferating clone. Although the mechanisms leading to the development of a clonal population synthesizing the structurally abnormal IgA are still speculative, the lymphoplasmacytic infiltration of the intestinal mucosa and regional mesenteric lymph nodes is likely a response of the alimentary tract immune system to protracted luminal antigenic stimulation.

6.2.2.1 Microorganisms

No specific microorganism has been found in bacteriologic, virologic, or parasitologic studies. However, the putative agent may be present only at the onset of the disease and absent at diagnosis. Bacterial lipopolysaccharides, dietary lectins, enterotoxins of *Vibrio* cholerae, oncogenic viruses, and asbestosis have been suspected of providing antigenic stimulation to trigger the histoimmunopathologic changes. The Epstein-Barr virus, which has been associated with B-cell lymphoproliferative disorders, was documented to have no role in the induction of B-cell proliferation in immunoproliferative small intestinal disease (IPSID) in 8 patients (Baddoura et al. 1994), whereas ultrastructural studies of lymph nodes of another patient with a-HCD described by Arista-Nasr et al. (1993) revealed viruses that resembled the Epstein-Barr virus.

6.2.2.2 Environmental Factors

A common denominator for patients with a-HCD is a low socioeconomic status and substandard hygiene, resulting in recurrent infectious diarrhea and chronic parasitic infestation. Geophagia since early infancy was almost universal in subjects at risk in Tunisia (Rambaud et al. 1990). The epidemiologic features of the disease strongly suggest that environmental factors operating since early infancy could play a major role in its pathogenesis. Support for the influence of environmental factors comes from a report of spontaneous remission of a-HCD after departure from an endemic area and a decline in the incidence rate of immunoproliferative small intestinal disease-associated primary small intestinal lymphoma among Jews born in Israel compared with Jewish immigrants with a relatively low socioeconomic standard from North Africa and Asia.

6.2.2.3 Immunodeficiency

The postulated environmental antigenic stimulation might be associated with an underlying immunodeficiency, for example, one caused by malnutrition, especially in early infancy. Defects in humoral and delayed immunity have been demonstrated in patients with a-HCD.

An increased incidence of immunoglobulin abnormalities has been found in first-degree relatives of patients with a-HCD: 23 of 129 normal family members of 8 patients with a-HCD had abnormal immunoglobulin patterns. In the same families, patients with a-HCD and normal first-degree relatives had an increase in circulating B lymphocytes and a decrease in T lymphocytes. They had decreased cellular immunity, as shown by sensitization to dinitrochlorobenzene. Tuberculin skin test reactions were negative (Alsabti et al. 1979).

6.2.2.4 Genetics

Predisposing genetic factors have not been clearly identified by the familial studies performed so far.

6.2.3 Screening and Prevention

Because of the epidemiologic features of a-HCD, screening for the disease does not appear feasible. However, awareness of the clinical features and of the incidence of the disease and increased efforts to detect the disease before the lymphomatous phase are important, because antibiotic therapy in the early stage of intestinal a-HCD can result in full clinical remission. The disease may well be eradicated and prevented without any medical intervention by improving the socioeconomic status of the underprivileged population in underdeveloped countries.

6.2.4 Molecular Biology and Genetics

Most a-HCD proteins consist of multiple polymers. The molecular weight of the basic monomeric unit varies between 29,000 and 34,000. The length of the basic polypeptide subunit differs from patient to patient and in most instances is between one-half and three-fourths that of a normal a-chain. The shortening results from an internal deletion involving most of V_H and the first constant domain. The absence of the C_H1 domain in nearly all cases of HCD probably explains the secretion of these abnormal proteins that otherwise would have been retained in the endoplasmic reticulum in the absence of light chains.

Sequence data are available for several a-HCD proteins (Def, Ait, Mal, Yao). In all instances, the normal sequence of the a1 chain constant region resumes at a valine residue in the hinge (Fig. 6.1). The NH_2 terminal of protein Def is heterogeneous and, after a short segment

Fig. 6.1. Structure of α-heavy chain disease (*HCD*) proteins compared with that of normal chain. Hatched bars correspond to hinge regions, closed bars indicate unusual sequences, and dotted lines indicate deletions. C_H, constant region; *D*, diversity; *H*, hinge region; *J*, joining; *V*, variable region. (Modified from Cogné M, Silvain C, Khamlichi AA, Preud'-homme JL [1992]. Structurally abnormal immunoglobulins in human immunoproliferative disorders. Blood 79:2181–2195. By permission of the American Society of Hematology.)

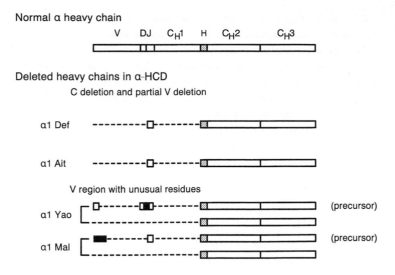

Fig. 6.2. Structure of α-heavy chain disease (*HCD*) productive gene, RNA transcript, and protein compared with their normal rearranged counterpart. C_H, constant region; *D*, diversity; *H*, hinge region; *J*, joining; *L*, leader; *S*, switch region; *V*, variable region. Solid bars represent insertions in coding (*large bar*) or noncoding (*small bar*) regions; dashed lines indicate deletion. (From Fermand and Brouet [1999]. By permission of Elsevier Science.)

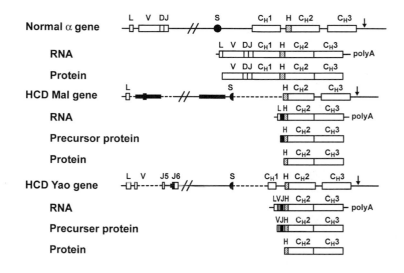

corresponding to the variable region, displays a gap that comprises the C_H1 constant domain. Attempts to determine the amino terminal sequence of protein Ait have been unsuccessful. It is not established how much of the V region is present in protein Ait. However, molecular weight determinations suggest that the V region is short, as in protein Def. Studies by Wolfenstein-Todel et al. (1975) indicated that protein Def and protein Ait are synthesized as internally deleted α chains followed by postsynthetic amino terminal proteolysis. α-HCD proteins Mal and Yao are devoid of V_H and C_H1 domains. No V-region sequence could be found (Fig. 6.1).

In a study of the nucleotide sequence of mRNA Mal and Yao and the nucleotide sequence of α-mRNA for 6 other cases of α-HCD (Ben, Arf, Mec, Lte, Har, Ayo) (Fakhfakh et al. 1992), all 8 mRNAs lacked the V_H and C_H1 sequences (Fig. 6.2). They contain in-frame inserts of unknown origin between the leader peptide and the normal C_H2 and C_H3 coding sequences. These inserts are of variable length and unrelated; thus, it is unlikely that they originate from an infectious agent. The presence of inserted sequences of unknown origin appears to be a common feature of α-HCD productive mRNA. Because the amino acid sequence of α-HCD proteins begins with the C_H2 domain, the amino terminal sequence encoded by these inserts most likely is cleaved intracellularly before secretion (Fakhfakh et al. 1992).

In studying a-HCD protein Ben, Fakhfakh et al. (1993) found 2 molecular species: 1 starting at the beginning of the hinge region and the other being 2 amino acids shorter, missing the first 2 amino acids of the hinge region. Intracellular cleavage could explain the presence of these 2 populations of a-HCD proteins; however, a limited postsecretion proteolysis also may be responsible for these findings.

Currently available molecular biologic studies indicate that genomic abnormalities such as multiple deletion or insertion processes, mutations, or duplications that are focused in the V_H–J_H and C_H1 regions are at least partly responsible for the production of a-HCD proteins (Goossens et al. 1998). Although nonsecretory a-HCD has been described, the molecular basis for nonsecretion is incompletely understood. In a case of nonsecretory a-HCD ($a1$-Sec), the productive a gene was noted to bear several noncontiguous deletions. Two deletions were accompanied by peculiar insertions containing duplications. One of the deletions located 3′ to C_H3 eliminated the polyadenylation site of secreted-form a-mRNA. As a result, only membrane-form a-mRNA was present in the tumoral plasma cells, thus explaining the nonsecretory phenotype of the disease (Cogné and Preud'homme 1990).

As a means of better understanding the molecular mechanism leading to the loss of light-chain production, a murine cell line model of a-HCD was studied (Chou and Morrison 1993). In this model, the failure of light chain synthesis was shown to result from a disruption in the normal splicing pattern caused by the insertion of a 358-nucleotide non-Ig sequence into the intron separating the leader exon from V_κ, leading to 2 mRNAs, neither of which encodes a functional light chain (Chou and Morrison 1993).

6.2.5 Clinical Presentation

In most cases, patients who have a-HCD present with an enteric disease. Nondigestive forms involving the respiratory tract, lymph nodes, or the thyroid have been described in the literature (Faux et al. 1973; Florin-Christensen et al. 1974; Itoh et al. 1991; Stoop et al. 1971; Takahashi et al. 1988; Tracy et al. 1984). The clinical picture of the digestive form is rather uniform. The onset of the

disease may be gradual or, more often, abrupt. During the early stage, diarrhea can be intermittent; progression of the disease is manifested by sustained chronic diarrhea with malabsorption, steatorrhea, weight loss, abdominal pain, and vomiting. Patients may present with abdominal surgical emergencies such as perforation or chronic small bowel obstruction, usually after a neglected or misdiagnosed period of chronic diarrhea. Tumoral signs are more often observed in the late stages of the disease. Ascites, tetany, or edema may be present. Amenorrhea, alopecia, and growth retardation in children and adolescents correlate with the duration and severity of the malabsorptive process. Clubbing of the fingers appears more frequent than in any other intestinal disease. Hepatosplenomegaly and peripheral lymphadenopathy are infrequent findings. Fever is uncommon.

In its rare respiratory form, a-HCD is confined to the respiratory tract. Two of the described patients with this form were children. An 8-year-old girl presented with pulmonary infiltrates, hilar adenopathy, skull lesions, and a pharyngeal tumor (Stoop et al. 1971). A 3-year-old boy had recurrent respiratory infections, hypogammaglobulinemia, and an a-HCD fragment (Faux et al. 1973). Another patient presented with dyspnea and had diffuse interstitial pulmonary fibrosis, pleural effusion, and mediastinal nodes (Florin-Christensen et al. 1974).

A lymphomatous form of a-HCD has been described in 3 Japanese patients (Itoh et al. 1991; Takahashi et al. 1988). A striking clinical feature in 2 of these cases was long-standing and recurring skin eruptions that developed before systemic lymphadenopathy (Takahashi et al. 1988). The 3rd patient, who had a history of rheumatoid arthritis, presented with cervical and inguinal lymphadenopathy (Itoh et al. 1991). Neither the gastrointestinal nor the respiratory tract was involved in these patients.

a-HCD has been reported in a patient with a goiter from a plasmacytoma of the thyroid (Tracy et al. 1984) and in patients with amyloidosis (Sakka et al. 1986).

Lymphomatous infiltration of the duodenum, jejunum, nasopharynx, and bone marrow was described in a Mauritian man with a-HCD (Lucidarme et al. 1993).

6.2.6 Classification and Staging

6.2.6.1 Clinical

Precise knowledge of the extent and histologic stage of the disease is important for optimal treatment. In the digestive form of α-HCD, the proliferation involves mainly the whole length or at least the proximal half of the small intestine and the mesenteric lymph nodes. In a few cases, intestinal lesions spare the duodenum and jejunum or are limited to a segment of the latter. Gastric and colorectal mucosa that belong to the IgA-secretory system may be involved. α-HCD confined to the stomach or presenting as a colonic mass has been reported. Assessment of the extent of the disease requires computed tomography (CT) of the abdomen, gastrojejunoscopy, and ileocolonoscopy, including systematic biopsies, although it is recognized that such evaluation methods may not be readily available in developing countries. In addition, because of the frequent asynchrony of the histopathologic lesions from 1 site to another, staging laparotomy should be considered, except for patients with evidence of histopathologic stage C lesions (Fermand and Brouet 1999).

6.2.6.2 Pathologic

The disease progresses in 3 histopathologic stages (Galian et al. 1977). In stage A, a mature plasmacytic or lymphoplasmacytic infiltration of the mucosal lamina propria is noted. Villous atrophy is variable and inconstant. Stage B is characterized by the presence of atypical plasmacytic or lymphoplasmacytic cells and more or less atypical immunoblastlike cells extending at least to the submucosa. Subtotal or total villous atrophy is present. Stage C corresponds to an immunoblastic lymphoma, either forming discrete ulcerated tumors or extensively infiltrating long segments and invading the whole depth of the intestinal wall (Galian et al. 1977). Equivalent to the changes described in the small intestine, 3 histologic stages (A, B, C) have been described that correspond to the cellular type of infiltrate and the degree of nodal architecture in the mesenteric lymph nodes. Involvement of liver, spleen, and peripheral lymph nodes is uncommon.

The histologic lesions may progress at any given site from stage A to stage B or from stage B to stage C. However, different stages can be found at the same time in different organs or even at different sites in the same organ. This asynchronism is important for staging.

The major lymphoma cell type in patients with α-HCD is immunoblastic lymphoma with various degrees of plasmacytoid differentiation (Rambaud et al. 1990). α-HCD associated with multiple polypoid lymphocytic lymphoma of the small intestine is rare. A patient with α-HCD associated with multiple polypoid lymphocytic lymphoma and leukemic manifestation without evidence of bone marrow involvement has been described; the findings suggest that the circulating plasmacytoid lymphocytes originated from the tumor in the small intestine. Cytogenetic analysis showed the same abnormal karyotypes of neoplastic clones in the intestinal tumor cells as in the circulating leukemic cells (Chang et al. 1992).

Spencer and Isaacson (1987) suggested that the histopathologic findings in α-HCD are in the group of lymphomas arising from MALT. Histologically, the diagnosis of MALT lymphoma is based on the existence of 4 elements: centrocyte-like cells, lymphoepithelial lesions, plasma cells, and reactive or residual follicles (Ben Rejeb et al. 1991). Spencer and Isaacson (1987) hypothesized that in α-HCD, all large cells, sometimes clustering in nodules at stage B, are neoplastic follicular center cells, although often cytologically bizarre. Similarly, the invasion, disruption, and partial destruction of intestinal crypts, sometimes found even at stage A, are part of the lymphoepithelial lesions due to centrocytic-like cells of the same clonal origin as plasma cells and are pathognomonic of all gut-associated lymphoid tissue lymphomas. Stage C tumors contain a mixture of the cytologic components (Rambaud et al. 1990).

In a few patients with typical clinical and pathologic features of α-HCD, another monoclonal Ig (γ-HCD protein), a complete monoclonal IgA, or polyclonal expression of IgA was found.

The histopathologic findings in α-HCD are characteristic of the so-called IPSID, of which α-HCD is the most frequent form. IPSIDs are part of the heterogeneous group of lymphomas, formerly called Mediterranean lymphoma, that have a common clinical pattern and a peculiar epidemiology (Rambaud et al. 1990). The term "IPSID" was suggested in 1976 by the World Health Organization (Alpha-chain disease – Bull World Health Org 1976). This term should be restricted to small intestinal lesions whose pathologic features are identical to those of α-HCD at any of its histologic stages irrespective of the type of Ig synthesized by the proliferating cells (Fine and Stone 1999). Because previously used methods to detect the protein were not sensitive, data regarding the presence of the abnormal protein vary. In the experience of Rambaud et al. (1990), among 19 consecutive patients with the epidemiologic, clinical, and pathologic features of IPSID, 16 had the a-HCD protein in their serum and 1 had it in the jejunal fluid only. In 1 case, immunofluorescence study of the small bowel mucosa showed that most of the infiltrating cells were positive for a chains and negative for other heavy or light chains (nonsecretory). The 19th patient showed a massive infiltration of the small intestine by polyclonal plasma cells.

The pathologic changes in the few cases with the respiratory form of a-HCD are poorly documented. In a case of lymph node form or lymphomatous form, lymph node biopsy showed diffuse plasmacytic lymphoma (Takahashi et al. 1988).

6.2.7 Diagnosis

6.2.7.1 Laboratory Tests

6.2.7.1.1 Hematologic and Metabolic Abnormalities

Mild to moderate anemia is often found. Because a-HCD does not usually involve the marrow, anemia occurs from malabsorption of folate, vitamin B_{12}, and iron; dietary deficiency; or bleeding. Hypokalemia, hypocalcemia, and hypomagnesemia are common. A low serum albumin concentration is nearly always present. The frequently increased serum alkaline phosphatase value is usually due to an increase in the intestinal isoenzyme fraction. Serum lipid values are low even if steatorrhea is mild.

Tests to indicate intestinal malabsorption usually have positive findings. Results of the Schilling test with intrinsic factor are low in two-thirds of patients. Results of the D-xylose test are almost always abnormal. The 24-hour fecal fat excretion has been reported to range between 6 and 15 g in 43% and was >15 g in 52% of patients studied. Heavy parasitic infestation of the intestine is a common occurrence; however, this does not appear to be significantly different from that of the population living in the same area.

6.2.7.1.2 Protein Findings

In contrast to other monoclonal gammopathies, the characteristic sharp spike of a monoclonal protein is not detected on serum protein electrophoresis in a-HCD. In about one-half of the cases, a-HCD protein may feature a broad band extending from the a_2 to the β-globulin region. This electrophoretic behavior of a-HCD protein may be related to the tendency of these chains to polymerize or to their high carbohydrate content. In the remainder of the patients, serum protein electrophoresis shows no evidence of an abnormal protein.

The diagnosis of a-HCD depends on the identification of a free a-heavy chain. Several methods may be used to document a-HCD protein in biologic fluids. A modified immunoselective technique described by Sun et al. (1994) appears to be simple, convenient, and specific. Confirming the sole presence of a heavy chain by this method is desirable for the following reasons: 1) immunofixation offers only indirect evidence of the presence of a monoclonal heavy chain without an associated light chain, 2) some light chain molecules in myeloma (particularly IgA and IgD myeloma) may not react with light chain antisera because the antigenic determinants may be hidden, 3) the possibility of a prozone effect causing absence of a light chain precipitin band, and 4) lower avidity of light chain than heavy chain antisera. This technique involves the use of combined κ- and λ-light chain antisera to precipitate all intact immunoglobulins present in the sample before electrophoresis. However, truncated heavy chains devoid of light chain counterparts are still freely mobile. They are expected to migrate further in the gel and react with their respective antisera. Therefore, the formation of a 2nd precipitin arc or rocket confirms the presence of an abnormal heavy chain.

Although 10% of normal serum Ig is of the a_2 subclass, in all cases studied so far the a-HCD protein belonged to the a_1 subclass.

In most patients, the a-HCD protein can be found in the serum but its concentration is often low. The quantity of abnormal a chains in the sera seems to be related to the nature (plasma cell type or immunoblastic type) of predominant cells in the intestinal mucosa or the mesenteric lymph nodes. During the course of the disease, the progressive diminution of mature plasma cells and their replacement by immature immunoblasts likely is followed by a progressive decrease in the serum concentration of a-HCD protein. a-HCD protein hyposecretion may also be found during the early stage of the disease.

In most cases studied, the a-HCD protein was also found in the jejunal secretions when its presence was documented in the serum. Interestingly, however, a-HCD protein was found in the intestinal or gastric fluid in a few cases when it was undetectable in the serum and urine. Whether a-HCD protein in the jejunal fluid is or is not linked to the secretory component has been disputed. The concentration of a-HCD protein in the urine is low. Bence Jones proteinuria has never been documented.

Synthesis of the a-HCD protein by the proliferating cells has been demonstrated by immunohistochemical or immunocytochemical methods and by biosynthesis studies in vitro. These techniques are not necessary when the a-HCD protein is found in the serum or intestinal fluid, but they are helpful in the recognition of nonsecreting forms of a-HCD.

6.2.7.2 Cytogenetic Analysis

Cytogenic abnormalities have been found in the lymphoid cells of patients with a-HCD. The clonal proliferation in this disease appears to be associated with frequent alterations of chromosome 14 at band q32 resulting from translocations that differ from those observed in the vast majority of other NHLs (Berger et al. 1986). Berger et al. (1986) reported abnormal karyotypes in 3 of 4 patients, 2 of whom had not reached the stage of malignant lymphoma. In 2 instances, a rearrangement of 14q32 was observed resulting from a t(9;14)(p11;q32) and a t(2;14)(p12;q32). Cloning and sequencing of the der(14) breakpoint of a chromosome translocation involving the 14q32 immunoglobulin locus suggested that the translocation originated from a local pairing of the 2 chromosomes, 9 and 14 (Pellet et al. 1990). One case showed complex rearrangements, including t(5;9). No abnormalities were found in the intestinal tumor of the 4th case with immunoblastic lymphoma. An abnormal chromosome marker (14q+) has been reported in the marrow of a patient with a-HCD (Gafter et al. 1980).

6.2.7.3 Imaging

6.2.7.3.1 X-ray

Radiographic findings in the small intestine include hypertrophic and pseudopolypoid mucosal folds in the duodenum and jejunum, sometimes associated with strictures or filling defects, suggesting extrinsic compression by hypertrophic peripancreatic or mesenteric lymph nodes. Double-contrast medium studies of the small intestine are helpful in revealing precise mucosal changes.

6.2.7.3.2 CT and Ultrasonography

The extent of the disease should be evaluated with CT of the abdomen, when available. Serial ultrasonographic evaluations are useful in following patients for development of abdominal lymphadenopathy and thickening of the small intestinal wall.

6.2.7.4 Endoscopy

Because a-HCD intestinal lesions nearly always affect the duodenum and jejunum, fiberoptic endoscopy with biopsies is a useful tool in the work-up of patients with suspected a-HCD. Five primary endoscopic patterns have been defined, occurring either alone or in various combinations. The infiltrated pattern is the most specific finding, followed by the nodular pattern. Other primary lesions (ulcerations, mosaic pattern, and mucosal fold thickening alone) are nonspecific.

6.2.7.5 Laparotomy

In all patients in whom a-HCD has been diagnosed and in whom no stage C lesions were found on peroral biopsy, a staging laparotomy to obtain adequate tissue of the bowel involved and tissue from several adjoining lymph nodes and the liver should be considered (Tabbane et al. 1988).

6.2.8 Differential Diagnosis

The digestive form of a-HCD must be differentiated from NHL, although this is an uncommon diagnosis in the age range typical of a-HCD. Other causes of small bowel malabsorption need to be considered, especially celiac disease. Enteric presentation of γ-HCD, monoclonal IgA secretion with a complete molecule, variable immunodeficiency, and acquired immunodeficiency syndrome with clinicopathologic features simulating IPSID must be excluded.

6.2.9 Therapy

6.2.9.1 Diet and Lifestyle

Efforts to improve nutrition and to decrease exposure to intestinal pathogens are of utmost importance.

6.2.9.2 Supportive Care

Administration of intravenous fluids, electrolytes, calcium and magnesium replacement, albumin, and in some cases total parenteral nutrition may be necessary.

6.2.9.3 Pharmacologic Treatment

Patients with stage A lesions limited to the bowel and to the mesenteric lymph nodes should be treated initially with oral antibiotics. For intestinal bacterial overgrowth, antibiotics selected by the sensitivity pattern should be given. In the absence of a documented parasite and intestinal bacterial overgrowth, tetracycline, metronidazole, or ampicillin is a good choice. Any documented parasite should be eradicated. Eradication of *Helicobacter pylori* has led to complete remission in 2 patients with a-HCD (Zamir et al. 1998), 1 of whom was unresponsive to prior combination chemotherapy. A minimum 6-month trial of tetracycline (1–2 g/day) is considered the prerequisite for establishing responsiveness of the lesion, although in cases in which complete remission (clinical, immunologic, and histopathologic) is obtained with antibiotics alone, the clinical improvement occurs early. Maintenance antibiotic treatment is unnecessary. Close surveillance for the early detection of overt lymphomatous transformation is advised. In 1 patient, a persistently abnormal a-chain mRNA was noted, despite an apparently complete clinical, pathologic, and immunopathologic remission after tetracycline therapy. Consistent with this finding was the subsequent rapid recurrence of a-HCD with transformation to immunoblastic lymphoma (Matuchansky et al. 1989). In patients with stage B or C disease, antiparasitic and antibiotic treatments are also useful for improving the malabsorption syndrome.

6.2.9.4 Chemotherapy

Patients with stage B or C lesions or stage A lesions without improvement after a 6-month course of antibiotic treatment should be given chemotherapy. The treatment regimens are those commonly used to treat NHL. There have been few controlled clinical trials. In a prospective randomized study, a doxorubicin-based regimen (CHOP: cyclophosphamide [Cytoxan], doxorubicin hydrochloride [Adriamycin], vincristine [Oncovin], and prednisone) provided a higher response rate than a non-doxorubicin-containing protocol (C-MOPP: cyclophosphamide, vincristine, procarbazine, prednisone) or total abdominal irradiation (Khojasteh et al. 1983). Similar results were noted in a retrospective study by Salimi and Spinelli (1996). Encouraging results were obtained in a treatment trial of cyclophosphamide, doxorubicin, teniposide, and prednisone sometimes alternating with bleomycin, vinblastine, and doxorubicin (Ben-Ayed et al. 1989). Chemotherapy with CEOP-IMVP-Dexa (cyclophosphamide, epidoxorubicin, vincristine, prednisolone, ifosfamide, methotrexate, etoposide [VP-16], dexamethasone) resulted in a complete remission in a patient with HCD associated with a high-grade malignant NHL (Hubmann et al. 1995).

6.2.9.5 Surgery

When a focal or bulky transmural lymphomatous tumor is found during staging laparotomy, surgical resection of the bowel segment bearing the tumor may significantly debulk or prevent perforation or obstruction (Tabbane et al. 1988). This approach followed by combination chemotherapy may induce complete remission (Rambaud et al. 1990). If a patient who has a-HCD presents with an extramedullary plasmacytoma, thyroidectomy can lead to a complete remission with disappearance of the a-HCD protein, as has been reported in 1 patient (Tracy et al. 1984).

6.2.9.6 Radiation Therapy

Because the disease affects multiple sites in the small intestine, radiation therapy generally is not used. Total abdominal radiation has been used in 1 trial (Khojasteh et al. 1983).

6.2.9.7 Stem Cell Transplantation

Because most patients are young, those with disseminated stage C disease who show a good response to conventional or salvage chemotherapy could be candidates for autologous bone marrow transplantation.

6.2.9.8 Emerging Therapies

Immunotherapy with rituximab, an anti-CD20 monoclonal antibody, has been a major advance in the treatment of indolent NHL. Because α-HCD is a disease of the B cells, it is likely that rituximab may be of benefit as a single agent or combined with chemotherapy. There have been no reports to date of rituximab use in patients with α-HCD.

It is difficult to evaluate the optimal treatment on the basis of the literature, partly because of the small number of cases in any 1 study, but mainly because of the poor long-term follow-up in most series. Because of the rarity of the disease, precise therapeutic protocols performed as multicenter studies are needed.

Follow-up should include a periodic search for α-heavy chain protein in serum and urine and, if negative, in the intestinal secretions. Finally, bowel radiography and esophagogastroduodenojejunal endoscopy should be performed, with multilevel biopsies studied by immunohistochemical techniques. A 2nd-look laparotomy may be necessary for accurate evaluation (Rambaud et al. 1990). Relapses, sometimes after a long disease-free interval, may occur after treatment at any stage of the disease.

6.2.10 Prognosis

The course of α-HCD is variable but generally progressive in the absence of antibiotic therapy or chemotherapy.

Long-term prognosis of patients who have α-HCD remains imprecise because of the lack of large series with prolonged follow-up. In a prospective study (Ben-Ayed et al. 1989), 20 of 21 Tunisian patients with α-HCD underwent laparotomy and were staged according to the classification by Galian et al. (1977). Six patients were classified as having stage A, 2 as stage B, and 13 as stage C. The 6 patients with stage A disease were first treated with antibiotics alone. Two had complete responses persisting 42 and 55 months, and the 4 in whom antibiotics failed received chemotherapy, with 4 subsequent failures and 2 deaths. For all 15 patients with stages B and C disease, combination therapy including doxorubicin led to 9 complete remissions with 1 early relapse, and salvage chemotherapy led to 1 more complete remission. Survival of the total group was 90% at 2 years and 67% at 3 years. All patients alive beyond 3.5 years were disease free.

Akbulut et al. (1997) reported 5-year treatment results of 23 Turkish patients with IPSID, including 5 with secretion of α chains. Seven patients had stage A disease and were treated with tetracycline for a median of 7 months, whereas the remaining 16 patients (9 stage B, 7 stage C) received combination chemotherapy (cyclophosphamide, vincristine, procarbazine, and prednisolone [COPP]). The median follow-up was 68 months. In patients with stage A disease, tetracycline yielded a 71% complete response and 43% disease-free survival rate. Eleven of the 16 patients (69%) with stage B or C disease who received the COPP regimen achieved a complete response, and only 2 patients had a recurrence (disease-free survival rate of 56%). The 5-year overall survival rate for the entire group was 70%, and the 5-year disease-free survival rate for patients with a complete response was 75%. However, the median overall survival for 3 patients with immunoblastic lymphoma was only 7 months.

Price (1990) studied 13 patients who had IPSID associated with α-HCD. Six patients, 2 with high-grade lymphoma and 4 with low-grade disease, received chemotherapy or radiation therapy or both. One of these patients died at 76 months, and 5 were alive (3 disease free) an average of 92 months after presentation. Five patients, all with low-grade disease, received conservative therapy (antibiotics and in some cases prednisone and total parenteral nutrition). All were alive an average of 40 months after presentation. Three of these 5 patients achieved histologic remission at 5, 6, and 27 months. Two of the 5 patients had persistent disease at 20 and 25 months, despite a good clinical response. Two patients died of high-grade lymphoma and were not treated.

Shih et al. (1994) described 6 patients who had α-HCD with lymphoma, mainly localized in the jejunum and mesenteric nodes. The histologic subtypes were diffuse large cell in 2 patients, immunoblastic in 3, and diffuse mixed in 1. All patients responded poorly to chemotherapy; the median duration of survival was 10.5 months.

Malik et al. (1995) studied 12 patients with IPSID. Six presented with stage A disease. Four responded to antibiotic or steroid therapy. In 2 patients, stage A disease evolved into stage C. One patient was lost to follow-up, and 1 patient was alive with disease. Three patients presented with stage B disease. Two responded completely to chemotherapy, and the 3rd refused treatment and died after 16 months. Three patients with stage C disease at diagnosis received aggressive combination chemotherapy and remained in complete remission with a median follow-up of 2.2 years.

Preliminary results suggest that flow cytometric analysis of S-phase fraction may be useful as a prognostic indicator in the clinical management of patients with IPSID (Demirer et al. 1995). Patients with a poor prognosis have a higher fraction of cells in S phase than those with a good prognosis.

6.2.11 Emergencies

A patient who has a-HCD may present with an acute abdomen owing to bowel obstruction or perforation and require immediate surgical attention.

6.3 γ-HCD

6.3.1 Epidemiology

6.3.1.1 Incidence

Since the first description of γ-HCD in 1964 (Franklin et al. 1964), approximately 100 patients have been reported in the literature (Fermand and Brouet 1999; Fermand et al. 1989; Wahner-Roedler et al. 2003).

6.3.1.2 Mortality

γ-HCD is a serologically determined entity with a great variety of clinical and histopathologic features. In the presence of a malignant lymphoproliferative disorder, mortality is high.

6.3.1.3 Sex Ratio

There is a slight predominance in males. No epidemiologic pattern has been recognized, and γ-HCD has been described throughout the world. No familial cases have been reported.

6.3.1.4 Age Ratio

The disease usually involves an older age group; 75% of patients are in the 6th decade of life or beyond. The disease can occur in children or young adults and has been noted before age 20 years in several patients.

6.3.1.5 Survivorship

Thus far, prognosis has been unfavorable, with many patients having died within months of diagnosis. However, some have survived for many years, and spontaneous disappearance of the γ-HCD protein has been reported (Fermand and Brouet 1999; Fermand et al. 1989).

6.3.2 Etiology

The etiology of γ-HCD is unknown. No viruses or chemical or physical factors have been implicated. No unique abnormalities or characteristic cytogenetic features of different lymphoma types have been found.

6.3.3 Screening

γ-HCD is probably underdiagnosed, and it is expected that immunofixation or immunoelectrophoresis done on a routine basis in patients presenting with a lymphoproliferative disorder would detect a significant number of patients with this entity. However, because the γ-HCD protein itself does not appear to influence the prognosis, routine screening of this population does not appear to be cost effective.

6.3.4 Molecular Biology and Genetics

Most γ-HCD proteins are dimers of truncated heavy chains devoid of light chains. The molecular weight of the basic monomeric unit varies between 27,000 and 49,000. The carbohydrate content of the γ-HCD proteins is high. The length of the γ-chain varies from case to case but usually is one-half to three-fourths of the length of its normal counterpart. All γ-HCD proteins show deletion of the C_H1 domain. Often the deletions are internal, with a portion of the V sequence present at the amino terminus, ruling out postsynthetic degradation. The resumption of the normal sequence occurs precisely at the beginning of a domain. On the basis of their structure, the γ-HCD proteins separate into 3 groups (Fig. 6.3).

1) Most γ-HCD proteins contain a fragment of a V region. Usually they have a normal V region amino terminus followed by an internal deletion of the V and the entire C_H1 domain. In all HCD proteins with

Fig. 6.3. Structure of various deleted γ heavy chains in γ-heavy chain disease (*HCD*) compared with that of normal chains. Hatched bars correspond to hinge regions, closed bars indicate unusual sequences, dotted bars indicate regions potentially present but not sequenced, dotted lines indicate deletions. C_H, constant region; *D*, diversity; *J*, joining; *V*, variable region. (Modified from Cogné M, Silvain C, Khamlichi AA, Preud'homme JL [1992]. Structurally abnormal immunoglobulins in human immunoproliferative disorders. Blood 79:2181–2195. By permission of the American Society of Hematology.)

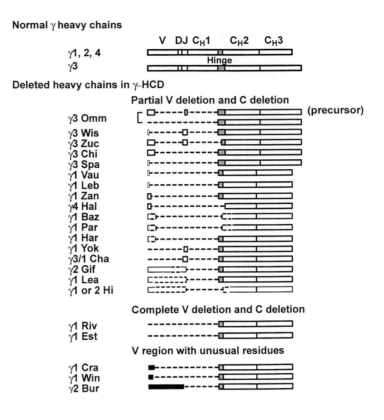

an internal V region deletion, the residues corresponding to the VDJ junction are missing. Some of these proteins contain a portion of this region and are featured by 2 noncontiguous deletions (γ3 Omm, γ3 Wis, γ3 Zuc). γ3 Omm has been shown to undergo postsynthetic degradation to yield an NH_2 terminal-deleted protein.

2) Some γ-HCD proteins lack the entire V and C_H1 domains, with the sequence starting within the hinge region (γ1 Riv, γ1 Est).

3) The 3rd group is characterized by an unusual amino acid sequence preceding the deletion. An abnormal sequence of 10 and 7 residues has been found in proteins γ1 Cra and γ1 Win, respectively. These residues are not translated from any of the known immunoglobulin heavy-chain gene sequences (Hauke et al. 1992). The complete sequence of γ2-HCD Bur has been reported (Prelli and Frangione 1992). This mutant is composed of a complete V region, hinge, and C_H2 and C_H3 domains. The unique features of this V region are the presence of methionine at position 11, 2 cysteine residues at positions 50 and 53, and 3 glycosylation sites.

γ-HCD cells usually do not secrete light chains. There are, however, a few cases in which light chains or light-chain fragments were detected as Bence Jones protein in serum and urine (Hauke et al. 1992) by immunofluorescence in the cytoplasm and at the surface of blood and bone marrow cells, or by internal labeling in cytoplasmic extract.

Gene alterations responsible for the structural abnormalities of γ-HCD proteins and the usual absence of light chain synthesis include somatic mutations, deletions, and insertions as documented for γ-heavy chain genes *Omm* and *Riv* and the light-chain genes κ *Riv* and λ *Omm*. HCD protein γ3 Omm was the product of 2 deletions – a splice correction and postsynthetic NH_2 terminal proteolysis. Sequencing of the γ1 *Riv* gene revealed that it had undergone V_H–J_H and H chain class switch recombinations. However, normal RNA splice sites had been eliminated by a DNA insertion/deletion (V_H acceptor site), mutations (J_H donor site), or a large deletion (C_H1 region). These DNA alterations resulted in aberrant mRNA processing in which the leader region was spliced directly to the hinge region, accounting for the HCD protein (Fig. 6.4).

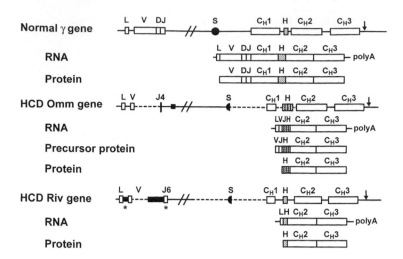

Fig. 6.4. Structure of γ-heavy chain disease (*HCD*) productive gene, RNA transcript, and protein compared with their normal rearranged counterpart. C_H, constant region; *D*, diversity; *H*, hinge; *J*, joining; *L*, leader; *S*, switch region; *V*, variable region. Asterisks indicate altered splice site; solid bars represent insertions in coding (*large bar*) or noncoding (*small bar*) regions; dashed lines indicate deletion. (From Fermand and Brouet [1999]. By permission of Elsevier Science.)

Similar to genes encoding HCD proteins, the κ-chain gene of patient Riv showed deletions, insertions, and a high rate (25%) of somatic mutations in the VJ region. Mutations of spliced sites bounding the VκJκ region resulted in exon skipping and splicing of the leader peptide exon onto the Cκ exon. A short mRNA was present and coded for a Cκ fragment devoid of the V domain (Cogné et al. 1988).

The rearranged λ-light chain gene in Omm HCD cell lines was shown to have a mutation in the splice donor site at the 3′ end of the leader J exon, resulting in direct splicing of the 3′ end of the leader to the acceptor site of the constant region. The cells contained an mRNA consisting of the leader-coding region joined directly to the constant region. The V-region exon was skipped and the shortened mRNA translated into a truncated protein containing no V-region amino acids. It was further noted that Omm cells produced an excess of heavy to light chain mRNA and protein. The excess was independent of the structural gene abnormality and thought to be due to a low level of light-chain transcription, suggesting that Omm cells either lack a transcription factor or have a functional repressor of light-chain transcription (Teng et al. 2000).

6.3.5 Clinical Presentation

Patients who have γ-HCD can present with a great variety of clinical features. Wester et al. (1982) suggested that patients with γ-HCD can be placed into 3 broad categories on the basis of the underlying pathologic process and its distribution: 1) those with disseminated lymphoproliferative disease, which occurs in approximately 67% of patients; 2) those with localized lymphoproliferative disease, occurring in approximately 25% (11% extramedullary and 14% involving the bone marrow only); and 3) those with no apparent proliferative disease. Of the patients with no proliferative disease (approximately 10%), many have autoimmune disorders (Wester et al. 1982).

γ-HCD most often presents as a lymphoproliferative disorder. Lymphadenopathy and constitutional symptoms such as fever, weakness, and fatigue are the most common initial features. Generalized peripheral lymphadenopathy with prominent cervical involvement is present at diagnosis in about two-thirds of patients, and fever is present in about one-fourth (Fermand and Brouet 1999; Fermand et al. 1989). Lymphadenopathy obstructing the vena cava has been noted. Waxing and waning of lymphadenopathy may occur. Palatal edema and swelling of the uvula related to involvement of the Waldeyer ring, which was initially thought to be a hallmark of the disease, occur in less than 15% of cases (Fermand and Brouet 1999).

Splenomegaly is present in about 60% of patients and ranges from a palpable tip to massive splenomegaly. Isolated splenomegaly may be the presenting feature of γ-HCD (Fermand et al. 1989). Spontaneous rupture of the spleen has been described (Fermand et al. 1989). Hepatomegaly is less frequent and occurs in about half of these patients (Fermand et al. 1989).

The appearance of a γ-HCD protein during the course of a treated lymphoid malignancy has also been reported, possibly indicating a mutational event or the emergence of a new clone. Several extrahematopoietic organs have been involved by tumors. Skin lesions in general have been noted to be the most frequent extrahematopoietic manifestation (Lassoued et al. 1990). Cutaneous or subcutaneous involvement, manifested by an extranodal mass or skin nodules, has been described (Fermand et al. 1989). Patients have presented with extramedullary plasmacytoma of the thyroid (Kyle et al. 1981a), parotid or submandibular swelling (Kyle et al. 1981a), or an oropharyngeal mass consisting of plasma cells. In several other cases, the initial symptoms were due to a gastric lymphoid tumor (Fermand et al. 1989).

The occurrence of autoimmune disorders, with or without associated underlying lymphoid proliferation, is frequent in patients with γ-HCD, with rheumatoid arthritis and autoimmune cytopenias (hemolytic anemia or thrombocytopenic purpura) being reported most frequently. Both may precede the discovery of the γ-HCD protein by several years (Fermand and Brouet 1999; Husby 2000). Other autoimmune or related conditions associated with γ-HCD include lupus erythematosus, Sjögren syndrome, myasthenia gravis, thyroiditis, and vasculitis.

Neurologic manifestations of uncertain mechanism have been reported in several patients with γ-HCD, as have various solid tumors diagnosed before, simultaneously with, or after the discovery of the γ-HCD protein. These diagnoses were probably fortuitous. A myeloid disorder was documented in some patients (Fermand and Brouet 1999).

A free γ-heavy chain was observed in serum and urine after high-dose chemotherapy and autologous peripheral blood stem cell transplantation in a patient with multiple myeloma. The isolated heavy chain was detected 2 months after transplantation, persisted for an additional 2 months, and was eventually replaced by an intact IgGκ monoclonal protein – as was the original Ig (Butch et al. 2001). Cases with no associated disease have been observed, and these can be thought of as monoclonal gammopathy of undetermined significance.

6.3.6 Classification and Staging

6.3.6.1 Clinical

Patients with γ-HCD presenting with a disseminated lymphoproliferative disease or an autoimmune disorder or in whom a γ-HCD protein is accidentally detected should be evaluated for the extent of their disease. The staging techniques used in patients with γ-HCD are those used in any newly diagnosed case of NHL and include CT scans of the chest, abdomen, and pelvis and bilateral bone marrow aspiration and biopsy with flow cytometry or immunocytochemistry staining of the lymphoid cells (to detect clonal B cells).

6.3.6.2 Pathologic

In contrast to α-HCD, γ-HCD has no specific histologic pattern (Fermand and Brouet 1999; Fermand et al. 1989; Wester et al. 1982). The most frequent pattern is a pleomorphic malignant lymphoplasmacytic proliferation mainly seen in bone marrow and lymph nodes. These lymphocytoid plasma cells express pan-B-cell markers and cytoplasmic γ-HC without light chain and are negative for CD5 and CD10 (Jaffe et al. 2001). In 18 of 47 patients (38%) in whom lymph nodes were examined, NHL was present without any consistent morphologic type. Lymphoplasmacytic proliferation, with or without atypia, was present in 36% of cases. There was 1 case of Hodgkin disease and 1 case of probable Hodgkin disease. Hyperplastic nodes and plasmacytoma each made up 11% of the total (Wester et al. 1982). A mainly plasmacytic infiltrate is associated with extranodal sites such as the salivary glands and thyroid (Fermand et al. 1989).

In only 6 cases reported in the literature has the lymphoma associated with γ-HCD been classified as Hodgkin disease or probable Hodgkin disease (Hudnall et al. 2001).

6.3.7 Diagnosis

6.3.7.1 Laboratory Tests

6.3.7.1.1 Peripheral Blood and Bone Marrow

Anemia is frequent. It is usually normochromic, normocytic, and moderate, except in patients with autoimmune hemolytic anemia. A Coombs-positive autoimmune hemolytic anemia has been reported in several patients and has sometimes been associated with idiopathic thrombocytopenic purpura (Evans syndrome) (Kyle et al. 1981a). The leukocyte count and differential are usually normal, but either leukopenia or leukocytosis may be present. Lymphocytosis with or without atypical lymphocytes may occur, and an occasional patient presents with chronic lymphocytic leukemia. Plasmacytoid lymphocytes or plasma cells may be found in the peripheral blood, and plasma cell leukemia has been reported in 2 patients. Eosinophilia may occur. Thrombocytopenia has been reported due to an autoimmune process, hypersplenism, or, less frequently, bone marrow failure, but thrombocytosis is not a feature of γ-HCD. The erythrocyte sedimentation rate can range from normal to >100 mm in 1 hour.

Bone marrow aspirates and biopsy specimens frequently reveal an increase in plasma cells, lymphocytes, or plasmacytoid lymphocytes, similar to the bone marrow picture of Waldenström macroglobulinemia. Typical bone marrow features of multiple myeloma or chronic lymphocytic leukemia are rare (Fermand et al. 1989; Kyle et al. 1981a). Marrow changes consistent with a myeloproliferative disorder have been noted in a few patients (Wester et al. 1982). Eosinophilia is rarely found. The presence of mast cells has been mentioned. A marked increase in erythropoiesis is present in patients with hemolytic anemia. In several instances, the bone marrow aspirate and biopsy specimens have been normal.

6.3.7.1.2 Protein Findings

The serum protein electrophoresis pattern is extremely variable. In approximately 40% of patients the abnormal protein is not detectable by electrophoresis (Fermand et al. 1989), and the pattern is normal, shows hypogammaglobulinemia, or shows hypergammaglobulinemia with a polyclonal pattern or an increase in the protein migrating in the β region without a detectable spike. If a localized band is detected, it is most commonly in the β_1 or β_2 region.

The diagnosis is established by immunofixation of the serum and a concentrated urine specimen by using specific antisera combined with immunoselection. A modified immunoselection technique for the diagnosis of HCD was described by Sun et al. (1994). Two-dimensional electrophoresis and immunoblotting also have been used for the recognition of γ-HCD. Tissot et al. (1998) showed that the combination of serum protein agarose gel electrophoresis and 2-dimensional electrophoresis can be used to characterize further abnormal protein bands detected by immunofixation. The serum level of the γ-HCD protein is usually <1 g/dL, but it can range from unmeasurable levels to 9 g/dL (Fermand

et al. 1989). The M spike was >2 g/dL in 11 of 24 cases in which it was measurable (Kyle et al. 1981b).

Analysis of the distribution of the IgG subclasses in γ-HCD shows a lower-than-expected incidence of IgG2 HCD protein. The most common subclass is IgG1, which occurs in 65% of cases. IgG3 has been identified in 27%, IgG4 in 5%, and IgG2 in 3% of patients (Fermand et al. 1989), whereas the normal distribution of IgG subclasses is IgG1, 64% to 70%; IgG2, 23% to 28%; IgG3, 4% to 7%; and IgG4, 3% to 4%.

The amount of γ-HCD protein excreted in the urine is <1 g/24 h in most instances but may reach 20 g/24 h. In many cases, careful study of adequately concentrated urine is necessary to detect the presence of the γ-HCD protein. The mobility of the monoclonal protein in the urine is the same as that in the serum, with only a rare exception. Relatively homogeneous free fragments of γ-chains unaccompanied by light chains may be found during examination of the urine with high-resolution electrophoresis and immunofixation and should not be confused with the γ-HCD protein (Charles and Valdes 1994). This urinary protein is similar to the Fc' fragment generated by the secondary action of papain on the intact Ig molecule. Differentiation from the γ-HCD protein can be accomplished by gel diffusion analysis. From a practical point of view, however, such studies are not required because the γ-HCD protein is always present in the serum and migrates in the β-γ region, whereas the free fragments of γ-chain are found only in the urine and migrate in the α_2 region. These fragments are of no known clinical significance. They probably originate from extracellular degradation of the IgG molecule (Charles and Valdes 1994). Two patients with γ-HCD and Bence Jones proteinuria have been described (Hauke et al. 1992).

Although biclonal gammopathy is reported to occur in approximately 1% to 3% of all patients with serum M components (Kyle et al. 1981b), the association between γ-HCD and another monoclonal gammopathy is much higher. The associated monoclonal immunoglobulin was of the IgM type or IgG type. No association between γ-HCD and monoclonal IgA has been described, whereas the IgG-IgA association is more frequent in series of biclonal gammopathies (Kyle et al. 1981b). One patient described by Lebreton et al. (1982) was unique in that the serum contained 2 deleted γ chains of different subclasses (IgG1 and IgG2). One of these persisted without change during the disease, and the level of the other diminished and had disappeared at the time of death. The reason for the relative predilection of γ-HCD to coexist with other unrelated paraproteins remains unclear.

6.3.7.2 Cytogenetic Analysis

Cytogenetic studies have seldom been reported. Neither unique abnormalities nor characteristic cytogenetic features of lymphoma have been found. Of 15 patients, 4 had aneuploidy (Fermand et al. 1989; Kyle et al. 1981a), and 3 others had trisomy 7, trisomy 21, and multiple chromosome abnormalities (Fermand et al. 1989). Three of these patients (Fermand et al. 1989) had received prior chemotherapy, which could have been responsible for some of the chromosome abnormalities. No chromosome abnormalities were found in 7 other patients (Fermand et al. 1989).

6.3.7.3 Other Features

Bone lesions are rare in γ-HCD. Only 4 cases with skeletal involvement have been reported (Fermand et al. 1989). γ-HCD almost never mimics multiple myeloma (Fermand and Brouet 1999). Hypercalcemia was noted in 5 patients (Fermand et al. 1989), 3 of whom had no apparent skeletal involvement. Renal insufficiency is uncommon but may occur in association with hypercalcemia. Lymphoid infiltration involving the kidneys, adrenals, lungs, and the central nervous system has been detected at postmortem examinations (Fermand et al. 1989).

6.3.7.4 Imaging

Imaging procedures consisting of CT of the chest, abdomen, and pelvis are helpful in evaluating the extent of the disease.

6.3.8 Differential Diagnoses

All patients presenting with a lymphoplasma cell proliferative disorder should be evaluated for γ-HCD. We believe that γ-HCD is underdiagnosed and urge that immunofixation of serum and urine be performed on patients with atypical lymphoplasma cell proliferative disorders.

6.3.9 Therapy

Because γ-HCD is a heterogeneous condition, the choice of therapy should rely on the underlying disorder and the pathologic findings. In an asymptomatic patient with no abnormalities other than the monoclonal gamma chain, no therapy is indicated. Any associated autoimmune disease should be managed with standard therapy without taking into account the existence of the abnormal monoclonal component.

6.3.9.1 Chemotherapy

In symptomatic patients with a low-grade lymphoplasmacytic malignancy, a trial of chlorambucil may be beneficial. Melphalan and prednisone can be used if the proliferation is predominantly plasmacytic. We recommend a trial of cyclophosphamide, vincristine, and prednisone for patients with γ-HCD and evidence of a progressive lymphoplasma cell proliferative process or high-grade NHL. If there is no response to this regimen, doxorubicin should be added. Agrawal et al. (1994) described a patient who achieved a complete remission with disappearance of the heavy chain after 6 courses of fludarabine. Successful treatment of γ-HCD with low-dose etoposide has been reported in a Japanese patient whose disease was unresponsive to combination chemotherapy (Ishikawa et al. 1997). There have been no published reports of the usefulness of rituximab in γ-HCD.

The amount of serum γ-HCD protein usually parallels the severity of the associated malignant process. Disappearance of the monoclonal component from serum and urine associated with apparent complete remission has been induced by chemotherapy (Agrawal et al. 1994; Fermand et al. 1989). In a few instances, however, relapse is not accompanied by reappearance of the pathologic protein (Fermand et al. 1989).

6.3.9.2 Surgery or Radiation Therapy

Localized extramedullary plasmacytomas have been treated successfully with radiation therapy (Fermand et al. 1989) or surgical removal of a localized process (or both) with complete clinical and serologic remission.

6.3.10 Prognosis

The clinical course of γ-HCD may range from an asymptomatic, benign, or transient process to a rapidly progressive neoplasm leading to death within a few weeks. Patients with features of a benign monoclonal gammopathy or monoclonal gammopathy of undetermined significance have remained clinically well for 2 to 7 years of follow-up after a persistent γ-heavy chain was documented (Galanti et al. 1995).

Spontaneous disappearance of the γ-HCD protein has been reported (Fermand et al. 1989). In 2 patients with rheumatoid arthritis, the γ-HCD protein disappeared (Fermand et al. 1989). One of these patients has been followed for more than 10 years and, despite slowly progressive rheumatoid arthritis, the γ-HCD protein has not reappeared and an overt lymphoproliferative disorder has not developed (Fermand et al. 1989). When an underlying lymphoid malignancy exists, the histopathologic pattern is essential for the determination of prognosis. The presence of the γ-HCD protein by itself does not seem to influence the course of the underlying disorder (Fermand et al. 1989). In general, therapeutic responses have been variable and disappointing in that responses often are incomplete or of short duration. The median duration of survival in 49 patients for whom some data were available was 12 months (range, 1 to 264 months) (Kyle et al. 1981a).

6.3.11 Emergencies

As expected from the diverse picture, there are no known medical emergencies unique to γ-HCD. Various emergencies may arise from the underlying disease.

6.4 μ-HCD

6.4.1 Epidemiology

6.4.1.1 Incidence

μ-HCD is extremely rare. It was first reported in 1969 (Forte et al. 1969) in a patient with chronic lymphocytic leukemia. Since then, only 32 additional cases have been described in the world literature (Bedu-Addo et al. 2000; Campbell and Juneja 2000; Cogné et al. 1993; Iwasaki et al. 1997; Wahner-Roedler and Kyle 1992; Witzens et al. 1998).

6.4.1.2 Mortality

Patients who have μ-HCD most commonly present with a lymphoplasma cell proliferative disorder and have high mortality.

6.4.1.3 Sex Ratio

Of 33 reported patients, 18 were male.

6.4.1.4 Race Ratio

Of the reported patients, 26 were white, 3 were African American, 2 were Asian, 1 was African, and for 1 the race was not mentioned.

6.4.1.5 Age Ratio

Most patients with μ-HCD are older than age 40 years. The median age at diagnosis in 27 patients with μ-HCD was 57.5 years (range, 15–80 years) (Wahner-Roedler and Kyle 1992).

6.4.1.6 Survivorship

The median duration of survival in patients with μ-HCD from the time of diagnosis is 24 months and ranges from <1 month to 11 years (Wahner-Roedler and Kyle 1992).

6.4.2 Etiology

The cause of μ-HCD is unknown. No viruses or chemical, physical, or genetic factors have been identified.

6.4.3 Screening

As in γ-HCD, μ-HCD is probably underdiagnosed. Immunofixation of serum and urine of patients presenting with a lymphoproliferative disorder would most certainly increase the detection rate of this disorder.

6.4.4 Molecular Biology and Genetics

The molecular weight of the μ-HCD protein has been determined in 8 patients and varied between 26,500

Fig. 6.5. Structure of 6 μ-heavy chain disease (*HCD*) proteins compared with that of normal μ chain. Closed bars indicate unusual sequences, dotted lines indicate deletions. C_H, constant region; *D*, diversity; *J*, joining; *V*, variable region. (Modified from Cogné M, Silvain C, Khamlichi AA, Preud'homme JL [1992]. Structurally abnormal immunoglobulins in human immunoproliferative disorders. Blood 79:2181–2195. By permission of the American Society of Hematology.)

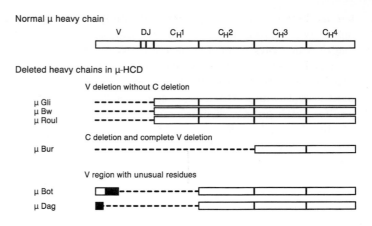

Fig. 6.6. Structure of μ-heavy chain disease (*HCD*) productive gene, RNA transcript, and protein compared with their normal rearranged counterpart. C_H, constant region; *D*, diversity; *J*, joining; *L*, leader; *S*, switch region; *V*, variable region. Asterisk indicates altered splice site; solid small bar represents insertion in noncoding region. (From Fermand and Brouet [1999]. By permission of Elsevier Science.)

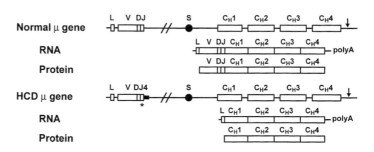

and 158,000. The higher molecular weights are believed to be due to polymerization of the μ-chain fragments. The μ-heavy chain fragments from 6 patients have been subjected to detailed chemical analysis. Figure 6.5 depicts the structure of these 6 μ-HCD proteins compared with that of the normal μ-heavy chain. The V_H domain is absent in all cases. The normal sequence begins with C_H1 in 3 cases, C_H2 in 2 cases, and C_H3 in 1 case. The deletion of protein Gli involves the first 130 residues from the amino terminus. Protein Bw is similar to protein Gli. The sequence begins at amino acid position 5 within the first constant region domain. In protein Bur, the normal amino acid sequence resumes at the beginning of C_H3.

Proteins Bot and Dag are similar in that the normal sequence resumes at the beginning of C_H2, but the deleted chain starts with an aberrant amino acid sequence (extra sequence) displaying no known homology with the protein sequences in the current databases. The extra sequence of protein Dag consists of 17 amino acids. No homology was detected when the extra sequence of protein Bot containing 42 amino acid residues was compared with the extra sequence of protein Dag.

Figure 6.6 depicts the structure of a μ-HCD gene, RNA transcript, and protein compared with the normal rearranged counterparts. The reasons for the failure to assemble a complete immunoglobulin are not understood. In studying μ-HCD protein Roul under dissociating conditions, Cogné et al. (1993) found monomers and covalent dimers of normal-sized κ chains, but no such free light chains could be detected under nondissociating conditions. Because of the lack of the V region, the interaction between the heavy and light chains might be too weak to promote the formation of the disulfide bridge.

6.4.5 Clinical Presentation

The most common presenting symptoms of patients with μ-HCD are those of lymphoproliferative malignancy. An associated lymphoplasma cell proliferative disorder was noted in 22 of 27 patients at some time during the disease and designated as chronic lymphocytic leukemia, lymphoma, Waldenström disease, or myeloma (Wahner-Roedler and Kyle 1992). μ-HCD protein has been described in 1 patient each with systemic lupus erythematosus, hepatic cirrhosis, hepatosplenomegaly with ascites, pulmonary infection, splenomegaly with pancytopenia (Wahner-Roedler and Kyle 1992), and myelodysplasia (Witzens et al. 1998). Although most patients with μ-HCD have an associated lymphoproliferative disorder, μ-chain secretion is a rare feature of chronic lymphocytic leukemia. Bonhomme et al. (1974) were unable to detect any cases when they screened more than 150 patients with chronic lymphocytic leukemia for this abnormality.

Splenomegaly and hepatomegaly are common in μ-HCD and have been noted in 21 of 22 and 15 of 21 patients, respectively (Wahner-Roedler and Kyle 1992). Peripheral lymphadenopathy is less frequent and was described in 10 of 25 patients (Wahner-Roedler and Kyle 1992). In 1 patient, massive pelvic lymphadenopathy resulted in bilateral hydronephrosis (Campbell and Juneja 2000).

6.4.6 Classification and Staging

Patients with μ-HCD should be evaluated for the presence and extent of an associated lymphoplasma cell proliferative disorder (chronic lymphocytic leukemia, lymphoma, Waldenström disease, or myeloma), including bone marrow aspiration and biopsy.

6.4.7 Diagnosis

6.4.7.1 Laboratory Tests

6.4.7.1.1 Peripheral Blood and Bone Marrow

Anemia is frequent, but lymphocytosis and thrombocytopenia are uncommon. One patient with hyperglobulinemia and anemia had a positive direct antiglobulin test; however, the anemia was not of autoimmune hemolytic origin. The eluate from the patient's red blood cells contained IgG and an immunoglobulin structure that reacted with anti-IgM in a red blood cell agglutination assay and with anti-μ antiserum in a nephelometric investigation. Whether this IgM on the patient's erythrocytes was pentameric or oligomeric, complete IgM, or the heavy chain could not be determined from these observations (Witzens et al. 1998).

Examination of the bone marrow usually shows an increase in lymphocytes, plasma cells, or plasmacytoid lymphocytes. Plasmacytosis was noted in 18 of 20 cases; in 13 of these, vacuolated plasma cells were found (Wahner-Roedler and Kyle 1992).

6.4.7.1.2 Protein Findings

A monoclonal spike was found in less than half of the patients (8 of 19) on routine serum protein electrophoresis (Wahner-Roedler and Kyle 1992). Hypogammaglobulinemia was noted in 10 of 21 patients (Wahner-Roedler and Kyle 1992). Hyperimmunoglobulinemia with polyclonal immunoglobulin expansion in the γ-globular fraction has been described in 1 case (Witzens et al. 1998).

The diagnosis of μ-HCD is made by documentation of the abnormal heavy chain. Immunofixation of both serum and urine should be done. When these procedures yield ambiguous results, 2-dimensional gel electrophoresis is a useful additional tool.

Three of the reported 33 patients had a biclonal gammopathy: IgAκ and μ (Josephson et al. 1973), IgGκ and μ (Silva-Moreno et al. 1983), and IgGκ and μ (Leach et al. 1987).

In contrast to γ- and α-HCD, in which there usually is no detectable monoclonal light chain in the serum and urine, the production of light chains (Bence Jones protein) is found in more than half of the cases of μ-HCD. Of 22 patients with μ-HCD, 14 had Bence Jones proteinuria: 11 excreted a κ chain and 2 a λ chain, and in 1 patient the type of light chain was not reported (Wahner-Roedler and Kyle 1992). μ-HCD protein was found in the urine of only 2 patients (Wahner-Roedler and Kyle 1992).

The Bence Jones proteinuria may lead to the occurrence of cast nephropathy. Preud'homme et al. (1997) described a patient with μ-HCD in whom renal failure developed after a 3-year follow-up. Kidney biopsy showed numerous tubular eosinophilic casts that stained for κ-chain determinants by immunofluorescence. Hence, this report paradoxically puts μ-HCD in the list of immunoproliferative disorders with light-chain-related visceral complications.

6.4.7.2 Cytogenetic Analysis

No cytogenetic studies have been reported on patients with μ-HCD.

6.4.7.3 Other Features

Three cases of nonsecretory μ-HCD have been described (Gordon et al. 1981; Guglielmo et al. 1982; Leglise et al. 1983). The presenting features were lymphadenopathy and splenomegaly in 1 (Gordon et al. 1981), osteoporosis and lytic lesions of the spine in 1 (Guglielmo et al. 1982), and fever and splenomegaly in 1 (Leglise et al. 1983). μ-Heavy chains were documented by immunofluorescence on the cell surface of proliferating lymphocytes in 1 patient and in bone marrow plasma cells of the 2 others.

Lytic bone lesions are rare and were described in 3 of 15 patients; osteoporosis was mentioned in 3 others (Wahner-Roedler and Kyle 1992).

6.4.7.4 Imaging

CT scan of the abdomen and chest are helpful in evaluating the extent of the disease in patients with μ-HCD.

6.4.8 Differential Diagnosis

The differential diagnosis of μ-HCD includes all lymphoplasma cell proliferative disorders (chronic lymphocytic leukemia, lymphoma, Waldenström disease, or myeloma). Without a suspicion for the disease, μ-HCD is difficult to diagnose. The finding of Bence Jones proteinuria in a patient with a lymphoproliferative disorder and vacuolated plasma cells in the bone marrow deserves further investigation for possible μ-HCD.

6.4.9 Therapy

6.4.9.1 General

There is no specific treatment of μ-HCD. Currently, the finding of μ-HCD protein in the serum of an apparently normal patient should be considered to represent a monoclonal gammopathy of undetermined significance, and the patient should be followed closely for the development of a symptomatic lymphoplasma cell proliferative disorder. If the patient presents with a non-lymphoplasma cell proliferative clinical disease, this should be treated according to current standard therapy.

6.4.9.2 Chemotherapy

Once a symptomatic lymphoplasma cell proliferative disorder develops, chemotherapy is necessary. Initially, a combination of cyclophosphamide, vincristine, and prednisone is a reasonable choice. If there is no response, either doxorubicin or carmustine or both should be added.

6.4.10 Prognosis

The median survival in μ-HCD from the time of diagnosis is 24 months and ranges from <1 month to 11 years (Wahner-Roedler and Kyle 1992). This contrasts with Waldenström macroglobulinemia, in which the median survival is 5 years. Because several of the reported patients had findings consistent with μ-HCD before recognition of the μ-HCD protein, the course is longer than indicated by the given survival. Patients who have μ-HCD can present with a benign monoclonal gammopathy for years before the development of a lymphoproliferative disorder (Wahner-Roedler and Kyle 1992). In 1 patient (Wetter et al. 1979), the hematologic data became normal and the μ-heavy chain disappeared after 2 years without specific treatment.

6.4.11 Emergencies

No particular medical emergencies have been described in patients with μ-HCD. However, emergencies similar to those observed in any lymphoplasma proliferative disorder can be anticipated.

Acknowledgment

Supported in part by National Institutes of Health grants CA62242 and CA97274.

References

Agrawal S, Abboudi Z, Matutes E, Catovsky D (1994) First report of fludarabine in gamma-heavy chain disease. Br J Haematol 88:653–655

Akbulut H, Soykan I, Yakaryilmaz F, Icii F, Aksoy F, Haznedaroglu S, Yildirim S (1997) Five-year results of the treatment of 23 patients with immunoproliferative small intestinal disease: a Turkish experience. Cancer 80:8–14

Alpha-chain disease and related small-intestinal lymphoma: a memorandum (1976) Bull World Health Org 54:615–624

Alsabti EA, Safo MH, Shaheen A (1979) Lymphocytes subpopulation in normal family members of patients with alpha-chain disease. J Surg Oncol 11:365–374

Arista-Nasr J, Armando G, Hernandez-Pando R (1993) Immunoproliferative small intestinal disease: report of a case with immunohistochemical and ultrastructural study [Spanish]. Rev Invest Clin 45:275–280

Baddoura FK, Unger ER, Mufarrij A, Nassar VH, Zaki SR (1994) Latent Epstein-Barr virus infection is an unlikely event in the pathogenesis of immunoproliferative small intestinal disease. Cancer 74:1699–1705

Bedu-Addo G, Sheldon J, Bates I (2000) Massive splenomegaly in tropical West Africa. Postgrad Med J 76:107–109

Ben-Ayed F, Halphen M, Najjar T, Boussene H, Jaafoura H, Bouguerra A, Ben Salah N, Mourali N, Ayed K, Ben Khalifa H, Garoui H, Gargouri M, Tufrali G (1989) Treatment of alpha chain disease: results of a prospective study in 21 Tunisian patients by the Tunisian-French Intestinal Lymphoma Study Group. Cancer 63:1251–1256

Ben Rejeb A, Khediri F, Souissi H, Machghoul S, Ben Othman M, Gamoudi A, Bahri M, Chouikha M, Ben Ayed F (1991) Malt digestive system lymphomas and alpha heavy chain diseases: histological and immunohistochemical study; apropos of 3 cases [French]. Arch Anat Cytol Pathol 39:27–33

Berger R, Bernheim A, Tsapis A, Brouet JC, Seligmann M (1986) Cytogenetic studies in four cases of alpha chain disease. Cancer Genet Cytogenet 22:219–223

Bonhomme J, Seligmann M, Mihaesco C, Clauvel JP, Danon F, Brouet JC, Bouvry P, Martine J, Clerc M (1974) Mu-chain disease in an African patient. Blood 43:485–492

Butch AW, Badros A, Desikan KR, Munshi NC (2001) Expression of a free gamma heavy chain in serum following autologous stem cell transplantation for IgG kappa multiple myeloma. Bone Marrow Transplant 27:663–666

Campbell JK, Juneja SK (2000) Test and teach: number one hundred and four; mu heavy chain disease (mu-HCD). Pathology 32:202–203; 227

Chang CS, Lin SF, Chen TP, Liu HW, Liu TC, Li CY, Chao MC, Wu PL (1992) Leukemic manifestation in a case of alpha-chain disease with multiple polypoid intestinal lymphocytic lymphoma. Am J Hematol 41:209–214

Charles EZ, Valdes AJ (1994) Free fragments of gamma chain in the urine: a possible source of confusion with gamma heavy-chain disease. Am J Clin Pathol 101:462–464

Chou CL, Morrison SL (1993) An insertion-deletion event in murine immunoglobulin kappa gene resembles mutations at heavy-chain disease loci. Somat Cell Mol Genet 19:131–139

Cogné M, Preud'homme JL (1990) Gene deletions force nonsecretory alpha-chain disease plasma cells to produce membrane-form alpha-chain only. J Immunol 145:2455–2458

Cogné M, Bakhshi A, Korsmeyer SJ, Guglielmi P (1988) Gene mutations and alternate RNA splicing result in truncated Ig L chains in human gamma H chain disease. J Immunol 141:1738–1744

Cogné M, Aucouturier P, Brizard A, Dreyfus B, Duarte F, Preud'homme JL (1993) Complete variable region deletion in a mu heavy chain disease protein (ROUL): correlation with light chain secretion. Leuk Res 17:527–532

Demirer T, Uzunalimoglu O, Anderson T, Koethe SM, McFadden PW, Demirer S, Uzunalimoglu B, Kucuk O (1995) Flow cytometric measurement of proliferation-associated nuclear antigen P105 and DNA content in immuno-proliferative small intestinal disease (IPSID). J Surg Oncol 58:25–30

Fakhfakh F, Dellagi K, Ayadi H, Bouguerra A, Fourati R, Ben Ayed F, Brouet JC, Tsapis A (1992) Alpha heavy chain disease alpha mRNA contain nucleotide sequences of unknown origins. Eur J Immunol 22:3037–3040

Fakhfakh F, Mihaesco E, Ayadi H, Brouet JC, Tsapis A (1993) Alpha heavy chain disease: molecular analysis of a new case [French]. Presse Med 22:1047–1051

Faux JA, Crain JD, Rosen FS, Merler E (1973) An alpha heavy chain abnormality in a child with hypogammaglobulinemia. Clin Immunol Immunopathol 1:282–290

Fermand JP, Brouet JC (1999) Heavy-chain diseases. Hematol Oncol Clin North Am 13:1281–1294

Fermand JP, Brouet JC, Danon F, Seligmann M (1989) Gamma heavy chain "disease": heterogeneity of the clinicopathologic features; report of 16 cases and review of the literature. Medicine (Baltimore) 68:321–335

Fine KD, Stone MJ (1999) Alpha-heavy chain disease, Mediterranean lymphoma, and immunoproliferative small intestinal disease: a review of clinicopathological features, pathogenesis, and differential diagnosis. Am J Gastroenterol 94:1139–1152

Florin-Christensen A, Doniach D, Newcomb PB (1974) Alpha-chain disease with pulmonary manifestations. Br Med J 2:413–415

Forte FA, Prelli F, Yount W, Kochwa S, Franklin EC, Kunkel H (1969) Heavy chain disease of the μ type: report of the first case (abstract). Blood 34:831

Franklin EC, Lowenstein J, Bigelow B, Meltzer M (1964) Heavy chain disease – a new disorder of serum γ-globulins: report of the first case. Am J Med 37:332–350

Gafter U, Kessler E, Shabtay F, Shaked P, Djaldetti M (1980) Abnormal chromosomal marker (D14 q+) in a patient with alpha heavy chain disease. J Clin Pathol 33:136–144

Galanti LM, Doyen C, Vander Maelen C, Dapare N, Bosly A, Pouthier F, Vaerman JP (1995) Biological diagnosis of a gamma-1-heavy chain disease in an asymptomatic patient. Eur J Haematol 54:202–204

Galian A, Lecestre MJ, Scotto J, Bognel C, Matuchansky C, Rambaud JC (1977) Pathological study of alpha-chain disease, with special emphasis on evolution. Cancer 39:2081–2101

Goossens T, Klein U, Kuppers R (1998) Frequent occurrence of deletions and duplications during somatic hypermutation: implications for oncogene translocations and heavy chain disease. Proc Natl Acad Sci U S A 95:2463–2468

Gordon J, Hamblin TJ, Smith JL, Stevenson FK, Stevenson GT (1981) A human B-cell lymphoma synthesizing and expressing surface mu-chain in the absence of detectable light chain. Blood 58:552–556

Guglielmo P, Granata P, Di Raimondo F, Lombardo T, Giustolisi R, Cacciola E (1982) 'Mu' heavy chain type 'non-excretory' myeloma. Scand J Haematol 29:36–40

Hauke G, Schiltz E, Bross KJ, Hollmann A, Peter HH, Krawinkel U (1992) Unusual sequence of immunoglobulin L-chain rearrangements in a gamma heavy chain disease patient. Scand J Immunol 36:463–468

Hubmann R, Kaiser W, Radaszkiewicz T, Fridrik M, Zazgornik I (1995) Malabsorption associated with a high-grade-malignant non-Hodgkin's lymphoma, alpha-heavy-chain disease and immunoproliferative small intestinal disease. Z Gastroenterol 33:209–213

Hudnall SD, Alperin JB, Petersen JR (2001) Composite nodular lymphocyte-predominance Hodgkin disease and gamma-heavy-chain disease: a case report and review of the literature. Arch Pathol Lab Med 125:803–807

Husby G (2000) Is there a pathogenic link between gamma heavy chain disease and chronic arthritis? Curr Opin Rheumatol 12:65–70

Ishikawa K, Hirai M, Tsutsumi H, Kumakawa T, Mori M, Masami M (1997) Successful treatment of heavy-chain disease with etoposide [Japanese]. Nippon Ronen Igakkai Zasshi 34:221–225

Itoh Y, Ohtaki H, Ono T, Mori N, Kawaoi A, Kawai T (1991) A case of lymphoma-type alpha-chain disease. Acta Haematol 86:107–110

Iwasaki T, Hamano T, Kobayashi K, Kakishita E (1997) A case of mu-heavy chain disease: combined features of mu-chain disease and macroglobulinemia. Int J Hematol 66:359–365

Jaffe ES, Harris NL, Stein H, Vardiman JW (eds) (2001) World Health Organization Classification of Tumours. Pathology and genetics of tumours of haematopoietic and lymphoid tissues. IARC Press, Lyon, p 154

Josephson AS, Nicastri A, Price E, Biro L (1973) H chain fragment and monoclonal IgA in a lymphoproliferative disorder. Am J Med 54:127–135

Khojasteh A, Haghshenass M, Haghighi P (1983) Current concepts immunoproliferative small intestinal disease: a "Third-World lesion." N Engl J Med 308:1401–1405

Kyle RA, Greipp PR, Banks PM (1981a) The diverse picture of gamma heavy-chain disease: report of seven cases and review of literature. Mayo Clin Proc 56:439–451

Kyle RA, Robinson RA, Katzmann JA (1981b) The clinical aspects of biclonal gammopathies: review of 57 cases. Am J Med 71:999–1008

Lassoued K, Picard C, Danon F, Pocidalo M, Grossin M, Crickx B, Belaich S (1990) Cutaneous manifestations associated with gamma heavy chain disease: report of an unusual case and review of literature. J Am Acad Dermatol 23:988–991

Leach IH, Jenkins JS, Murray-Leslie CF, Powell RJ (1987) Mu-heavy chain and monoclonal IgG K paraproteinaemia in systemic lupus erythematosus. Br J Rheumatol 26:460–462

Lebreton JP, Fontaine M, Rousseaux J, Youinou P, Hurez D, Rivat-Peran L, Bernards JP (1982) Deleted IgG1 and IgG2 H chains in a patient with an IgG subclass imbalance. Clin Exp Immunol 47:206–216

Leglise MC, Briere J, Abgrall JF, Hurez D (1983) Non-secretory myeloma of heavy mu-chain type [French]. Nouv Rev Fr Hematol 25:103–106

Lucidarme D, Colombel JF, Brandtzaeg P, Tulliez M, Chaussade S, Marteau P, Dehennin JP, Vaerman JP, Rambaud JC (1993) Alpha-chain disease: analysis of alpha-chain protein and secretory component in jejunal fluid. Gastroenterology 104:278–285

Malik IA, Shamsi Z, Shafquat A, Aziz Z, Shaikh H, Jafri W, Khan MA, Khan AH (1995) Clinicopathological features and management of immunoproliferative small intestinal disease and primary small intestinal lymphoma in Pakistan. Med Pediatr Oncol 25:400–406

Matuchansky C, Cogné M, Lemaire M, Babin P, Touhard G, Chamaret S, Preud'homme JL (1989) Nonsecretory alpha-chain disease with immunoproliferative small-intestinal disease. N Engl J Med 320:1534–1539

Pellet P, Tsapis A, Brouet JC (1990) Alpha heavy chain disease of patient MAL: structure of the non-functional rearranged alpha gene translocated on chromosome 9. Eur J Immunol 20:2731–2735

Prelli F, Frangione B (1992) Franklin's disease: Ig gamma 2 H chain mutant BUR. J Immunol 148:949–952

Preud'homme JL, Bauwens M, Dumont G, Goujon JM, Dreyfus B, Touchard G (1997) Cast nephropathy in mu heavy chain disease. Clin Nephrol 48:118–121

Price SK (1990) Immunoproliferative small intestinal disease: a study of 13 cases with alpha heavy-chain disease. Histopathology 17:7–17

Rambaud JC, Halphen M, Galian A, Tsapis A (1990) Immunoproliferative small intestinal disease (IPSID): relationships with alpha-chain disease and "Mediterranean" lymphomas. Springer Semin Immunopathol 12:239–250

Sakka T, Meknini B, Ayed K, Ben Jilani S, Ben Maiz H, Ben Moussa F, Ben Mami N, Derouiche N (1986) An unusual case of heavy alpha chain disease associated with amyloidosis. Tunis Med 64:161–164

Salimi M, Spinelli JJ (1996) Chemotherapy of Mediterranean abdominal lymphoma: retrospective comparison of chemotherapy protocols in Iranian patients. Am J Clin Oncol 19:18–22

Seligmann M (1993) Heavy chain diseases [French]. Rev Prat 43:317–320

Seligmann M, Danon F, Hurez D, Mihaesco E, Preud'homme JL (1968) Alpha-chain disease: a new immunoglobulin abnormality. Science 162:1396–1397

Shih LY, Liaw SJ, Dunn P, Kuo TT (1994) Primary small-intestinal lymphomas in Taiwan: immunoproliferative small-intestinal disease and nonimmunoproliferative small-intestinal disease. J Clin Oncol 12:1375–1382

Silva-Moreno M, Ruiz-Arguelles GJ, Lopez-Karpovitch X, Labardini-Mendez J (1983) Heavy chain disease: report of four cases [Spanish]. Sangre 28:89–98

Spencer J, Isaacson PG (1987) Immunology of gastrointestinal lymphoma. Baillieres Clin Gastroenterol 1:605–621

Stoop JW, Ballieux RE, Hijmans W, Zegers BJ (1971) Alpha-chain disease with involvement of the respiratory tract in a Dutch child. Clin Exp Immunol 9:625–635

Sun T, Peng S, Narurkar L (1994) Modified immunoselection technique for definitive diagnosis of heavy-chain disease. Clin Chem 40:664

Tabbane F, Mourali N, Cammoun M, Najjar T (1988) Results of laparotomy in immunoproliferative small intestinal disease. Cancer 61:1699–1706

Takahashi K, Naito M, Matsuoka Y, Takatsuki K (1988) A new form of alpha-chain disease with generalized lymph node involvement. Pathol Res Pract 183:717–723

Teng MH, Rosen S, Gorny MK, Alexander A, Buxbaum J (2000) Gamma heavy chain disease in man: independent structural abnormalities and reduced transcription of a functionally rearranged lambda L-chain gene result in the absence of L-chains. Blood Cells Mol Dis 26:177–185

Tissot JD, Tridon A, Ruivard M, Layer A, Henry H, Philippe P, Schneider P (1998) Electrophoretic analyses in a case of monoclonal gamma chain disease. Electrophoresis 19:1771–1773

Tracy RP, Kyle RA, Leitch JM (1984) Alpha heavy-chain disease presenting as goiter. Am J Clin Pathol 82:336–339

Wahner-Roedler DL, Kyle RA (1992) Mu-heavy chain disease: presentation as a benign monoclonal gammopathy. Am J Hematol 40:56–60

Wahner-Roedler DL, Witzig TE, Loehrer LL, Kyle RA (2003) γ-Heavy chain disease: review of 23 cases. Medicine (Baltimore) 82:236–250

Wester SM, Banks PM, Li CY (1982) The histopathology of gamma heavy-chain disease. Am J Clin Pathol 78:427–436

Wetter O, Schmidt CG, Linder KH, Leene W (1979) Heavy chain disease: humoral and cellular findings in six patients with mu chain disease (author's transl) [German]. J Cancer Res Clin Oncol 94:207–223

Witzens M, Egerer G, Stahl D, Werle E, Goldschmidt H, Haas R (1998) A case of mu heavy-chain disease associated with hyperglobuline-mia, anemia, and a positive Coombs test. Ann Hematol 77:231–234

Wolfenstein-Todel C, Mihaesco E, Frangione B (1975) Variant of a human immunoglobulin: "alpha chain disease" protein AIT. Biochem Biophys Res Commun 65:47–53

Zamir A, Parasher G, Moukarzel AA, Guarini L, Zeien L, Feldman F (1998) Immunoproliferative small intestinal disease in a 16-year-old boy presenting as severe malabsorption with excellent response to tetracycline treatment. J Clin Gastroenterol 27:85–89

Immunoglobulin Light Chain Amyloidosis (Primary Amyloidosis, AL)

Morie A. Gertz, M.D., Martha Q. Lacy, M.D., Angela Dispenzieri, M.D.*

Contents

7.1   History   157

7.2   Ultrastructure and Classification   158

7.3   When Should Amyloidosis
      Be Suspected?   160

7.4   Making a Diagnosis of Amyloidosis . .   162

7.5   Differentiating AL From Other Forms
      of Amyloidosis   166

7.6   Clinical Presentation
      and Clinical Features   169
      7.6.1 Heart   170
      7.6.2 Kidney   172
      7.6.3 Liver   174
      7.6.4 Gastrointestinal Tract   175
      7.6.5 Nervous System   176
      7.6.6 Respiratory Tract   177
      7.6.7 Coagulation System   178

7.7   Prognosis   179

7.8   Therapy   181
      7.8.1 Adjunctive and Supportive Therapy
            for Systemic Amyloid   181
            7.8.1.1 Cardiac Amyloid   181
            7.8.1.2 Renal Amyloid   182
            7.8.1.3 Gastrointestinal Tract
                    Amyloid   183
      7.8.2 Nonchemotherapy Treatment of AL   183
            7.8.2.1 DMSO (Dimethyl Sulfoxide) .   183
            7.8.2.2 Colchicine   184
      7.8.3 Defining Responses in Amyloidosis   184
      7.8.4 Cytotoxic Chemotherapy in the
            Treatment of AL   185
      7.8.5 Stem Cell Transplantation for AL . .   187
            7.8.5.1 Autologous Peripheral Blood
                    Stem Cell Transplantation . .   188

7.9   Conclusion   193

References   193

7.1 History

The term lardaceous change has ... come more into use chiefly through the instrumentality of the Vienna School. ... The term, lardaceous changes ... has but very little to do with these tumours, and rather refers to things, upon which the old writers ... who were better connoisseurs in bacon than our friends in Vienna, would hardly have bestowed such a name. ... The appearance of such organs ... are said to look like bacon, bears ... a much greater resemblance to wax, and I have therefore now for a long time ... made use of the term waxy change. ... These structures ... by the simple action of iodine ... assume just as blue a colour as vegetable starch. ...

This quotation is from a lecture entitled "Amyloid Degeneration" that was delivered by Rudolph Virchow on April 17, 1858. In it, Virchow defined the waxy change of amyloidosis and described its reaction with iodine

* Partial support provided by the Hematologic Malignancies Fund, Mayo Clinic.

and sulfuric acid, which at the time was a marker for starch – hence the term "amyloid" or starchlike (Cohen 1992). At the same time, Virchow took a backhanded slap at his main competitor of the day, Rokitansky. Virchow was the chief prosector in Berlin, whereas Rokitansky headed the pathology department in Vienna. Rokitansky had described lardaceous change in 1842 in persons suffering from malaria, tuberculosis, or syphilis. The amyloid deposits were glistening and white and therefore resembled lard. Virchow took strong issue, believing that amyloid was made of starch because of the iodine-sulfuric acid reaction that commonly turns starchlike substances blue (Cohen and Calkins 2000). The term "amyloid" was actually coined in 1838 by Matthias Schleiden, a German botanist, to describe a normal constituent of plants. In 1859, Friedreich, Nikolau, and Kekule (the first known for the description of ataxia that bears his name and the last who dreamt of a serpent biting its own tail, leading to his description of the structure of benzene), recognized that the waxy spleen described by Virchow contained no material that corresponded to cellulose and concluded it was probably albuminoid (proteinaceous) material that had been modified.

George Budd (1808–1882), who had made important contributions in the descriptions of rickets and scurvy, analyzed the liver of a patient with amyloidosis and found a low fat content. He concluded that the liver was not of lardaceous origin. Sir Samuel Wilks, who had first achieved fame for his descriptions of myasthenia gravis and for the use of bromide in the treatment of epilepsy, reported on a 52-year-old patient with lardaceous change that was unrelated to any obvious cause because no precipitating feature was found. This may have been the first reported case of primary amyloidosis (AL) (idiopathic or unassociated with a precipitating cause, based on the terminology of the day). In 1920, Schmiedeberg reported that the amino acid composition of amyloid strongly resembled that of serum globulin and was therefore protein and neither fat nor carbohydrate. In 1922, Hermann Bennhold introduced the use of Congo red as a specific stain for the detection of amyloid. Five years later, Divry and Florkin described green birefringence of amyloid-laden material when viewed under polarized light. Importantly, the tissues were from the brain of a patient with Alzheimer disease. This was one of the first recognitions that the neurodegeneration of Alzheimer disease was associated with amyloid. In 1931, Magnus-Levy noted that there was a relationship

between the Bence Jones protein and amyloid and between multiple myeloma and amyloid. He postulated that Bence Jones protein was the origin of amyloidosis.

In 1959, Cohen and Calkins observed with the newly developed electron microscope that all forms of amyloid demonstrated a nonbranching fibrillar structure. Fibril length varied. Fibril width was 9.5 nm. Apitz, who coined the term "paraprotein" to describe immunoglobulin proteins, claimed that amyloid in the tissues was analogous to the excretion of immunoglobulin light chain proteins by the kidneys. In 1964, Elliott Osserman (Isobe and Osserman 1974) first recognized that the Bence Jones proteins played a direct role in the pathogenesis of AL. In 1968, Eanes and Glenner reported that the x-ray defraction properties of amyloid did not resemble those of normal proteins, which were those of an α helix, but formed the alternate configuration of a β-pleated sheet, a configuration found in nature in silk, a material highly impervious to the action of acids and alkalis. In fact, amyloid is so resistant to solubilization that this fact was used to purify the substance for the first time. Repeated homogenizations of amyloid in saline result in the removal of all soluble components that can be discarded in the supernatant. The residual nonsoluble material represents amyloid and forms a suspension in distilled water. This purification, first described by Pras et al. in 1968, allowed Levin et al. (1972) to sequence the first amyloid fibril protein, calling it amyloid A. This was described independently by Earl Benditt. The first amyloid light chain protein was sequenced in 1970 by Glenner et al., who recognized it as the N-terminus of an immunoglobulin light chain and not the intact 25-kilodalton light chain.

7.2 Ultrastructure and Classification

All forms of amyloid are characterized by positive histologic staining with Congo red, and this remains a requirement for a diagnosis of the disease. Under a light microscope, amyloid deposits are amorphous extracellular deposits when stained with hematoxylin and eosin; they are often referred to as hyaline. Under polarized light, the classic apple green birefringence can be recognized. The Congo red stain is not a particularly easy stain to use and many false-positive results can occur if the stain is not regularly used in a diagnostic laboratory. All forms of amyloid are fibrillar and are rigid and nonbranching. Under the electron microscope, however,

Table 7.1. Nomenclature of amyloidosis

Protein	Precursor	Clinical
AL or AH	Immunoglobulin light or heavy chain	Primary or localized; myeloma or macroglobulinemia association
AA	SAA	Secondary or familial Mediterranean fever
ATTR	Transthyretin	Familial and senile
A fibrinogen	Fibrinogen	Familial renal amyloidosis (Ostertag)
A β_2M	β_2-Microglobulin	Dialysis-associated carpal tunnel syndrome
Aβ	ABPP	Alzheimer disease
ApoAI, AII	Apolipoprotein	Renal, nephrotic syndrome
Lysozyme	Lysozyme	Renal, hepatic rupture

ABPP, amyloid β protein precursor; ATTR, amyloid transthyretin; SAA, serum amyloid A.

all fibrils are not amyloid. Therefore, the finding of fibrils in the absence of a positive Congo red stain must be considered tentative.

Historically, amyloid was classified by its anatomic distribution. Initially, involvement of the liver, spleen, and kidneys was thought to be diagnostic of secondary amyloidosis (AA), whereas involvement of the heart, tongue, and peripheral nerves was most consistent with AL. Subsequently, amyloid was classified by the anatomic site of first deposition and was referred to as either perireticular or pericollagenous. Before the recognition of the amino acid sequence of the amyloid subunit protein, amyloid was assigned to 3 clinical categories. The familial type was recognized by its presentation, which usually was that of a progressive or painful peripheral neuropathy with autosomal dominant inheritance pattern. Early in the 20th century, families with inherited renal amyloidosis had been described. The secondary form of amyloidosis was characterized by its associated long-standing inflammatory disorder. In the 19th century this was tuberculosis, leprosy, syphilis, and chronic infected sinuses. With the advent of antibiotic therapy, amyloidosis became associated with chronic inflammatory polyarthritis, particularly ankylosing spondylitis and juvenile rheumatoid arthritis. Other associated inflammatory processes included Crohn disease and chronic osteomyelitis (Kyle and Rajkumar 1999). All other forms of amyloidosis that were not secondary or familial were relegated to the category primary. In the 20th century, primary actually meant idiopathic amyloidosis, and this certainly consisted of a heterogeneous combination of unrecognized familial, secondary amyloid without an apparent cause, some

forms of localized amyloidosis, and, of course, true immunoglobulin light chain amyloidosis.

Today, the term "primary amyloidosis" actually refers to amyloidosis derived from immunoglobulin light chains and always is associated with a clonal plasma cell disorder. The clonal plasma cell disorder may represent multiple myeloma (Rajkumar et al. 1998a) or may not have any of the characteristics of a malignant plasma cell dyscrasia. Table 7.1 contains a modified classification of the various forms of amyloid that have been described. The designation "AL" indicates amyloid of immunoglobulin light chain origin.

Amyloid fibrils have been produced in vitro by peptic digestion of purified monoclonal human immunoglobulin light chains. By use of reducing agents that break the disulfide bonds of intact immunoglobulin, amyloid fibrils have also been produced in vitro. Immunoglobulin heavy chains also are involved in the structure of amyloid fibrils and are designated AH. The immunoglobulin light chains of patients with amyloid have an abnormal sequence and an abnormal tertiary structure. They have a greater tendency to configure as a β-pleated sheet as opposed to an α helix. Injections of immunoglobulin light chains purified from the urine of patients with AL produce AL deposits in mice. Control mice injected with the light chain from a patient with myeloma who does not have amyloid do not produce a similar lesion (Solomon et al. 1992). In addition, most human light chains (two-thirds) are of the κ immunoglobulin group (Kyle and Rajkumar 1999). In amyloidosis, however, nearly three-fourths are of the λ group, suggesting that λ immunoglobulin light chains have more of a tendency toward forming a β-pleated sheet structure. The λ_{VI} subgroup of light chain is virtually always associated with amyloid, reinforcing the hypothesis that there is a unique amino acid structure that renders these proteins amyloidogenic.

The classification of patients with light chain amyloidosis into those with and without myeloma is often made on clinical criteria alone, and significant overlap exists. Myeloma-associated amyloid with lytic bone disease or multiple lumbar spine compression or rib fractures is rare. Most patients with amyloid and renal insufficiency do not have evidence of myeloma cast nephropathy; rather, the renal failure is due to tubular atrophy associated with long-standing albuminuria, a consequence of glomerular amyloid deposition. It is naive to believe that patients who have greater than 10% plasma cells have multiple myeloma and those with less than 10% do not (Kyle and Bayrd 1975). Serial bone marrow biopsies in patients with amyloid do not show a progressive increase in the percentage of plasma cells over time. This suggests that the process is clonal but not malignant because the characteristic of unrestrained growth is not met. Amyloidosis patients with between 10% and 30% plasma cells virtually never go on to develop multiple myeloma if it was not present at diagnosis. In our review of 1,600 patients with AL, multiple myeloma developed in less than one-half of 1% (Rajkumar et al. 1998a). For descriptive purposes, we do arbitrarily label patients with greater than 30% plasma cells in the bone marrow as having multiple myeloma. The clinical course of these patients is generally dominated by the amyloid and not by myeloma, bone disease, or anemia.

The incidence of amyloidosis is 8 per million per year and has not changed since 1950 (Kyle et al. 1992b). Amyloidosis is approximately one-fourth as common as multiple myeloma (Kyle et al. 1994) and has an incidence similar to Hodgkin disease, chronic granulocytic leukemia, and polycythemia rubra vera.

Chromosomal abnormalities are commonly seen in the bone marrow plasma cells from patients with amyloidosis (Fonseca et al. 2000). Bone marrow samples from 21 patients with AL were studied by standard cytogenetics and fluorescence in situ hybridization probes for 6 chromosomes. Trisomies of chromosomes 7, 9, 11, 15, and 18 were seen in 42%, 52%, 47%, 39%, and 33%, respectively (Fonseca et al. 1998). Trisomy X was seen in 13% of women and 54% of men. Monosomy of chromosome 18 was seen in 72% of patients. The aneuploidy seen in these monoclonal plasma cells supports

the neoplastic nature of the disorder, even when the percentage of plasma cells in the bone marrow is 5% or less. Translocations at the immunoglobulin heavy chain locus (IgH)-band 14q32 represent early pathogenetic events in the development of multiple myeloma. When FISH analysis was performed on the plasma cells of amyloidosis patients, 16 of 29 had a definite IgH translocation (55%) and 5 additional patients (17%) had a pattern compatible with a possible IgH translocation (Hayman et al. 2001a). In total, 21 of 29 patients had evidence of an IgH translocation. Sixteen of the 21 were confirmed to have a t(11;14)(q13;q32), accounting for 76% of all IgH translocations. Fifteen of the 16 patients with 11;14 translocation displayed cyclin D1 overexpression.

In summary, immunoglobulin light chain amyloidosis is a monoclonal plasma cell disorder. This fact serves as the key for diagnostic recognition and for the diagnostic algorithm. Occasionally, amyloid is misdiagnosed as multiple myeloma because of the presence of a serum monoclonal immunoglobulin, the high prevalence of proteinuria, and the plasmacytosis of the bone marrow.

7.3 When Should Amyloidosis Be Suspected?

The most common presenting symptoms of amyloidosis are fatigue, dyspnea, edema, paresthesias, and weight loss (Fig. 7.1) (Kyle and Greipp 1983). These symptoms provide little guidance to a clinician trying to formulate a differential diagnosis in evaluation of these highly nonspecific complaints. Many patients with unexplained weight loss will undergo an in-depth investigation to detect an underlying occult malignancy. The fatigue, which is generally caused by cardiac involvement in the absence of overt congestive heart failure, is frequently misdiagnosed as functional or stress related. We have seen many patients undergo coronary angiography, inevitably normal, and the patient evaluation is stopped at that point. Light-headedness is commonly seen. The light-headedness is nonspecific because it is such a common complaint in the primary care setting. Light-headedness in amyloidosis is multifactorial. It occurs in patients with nephrotic syndrome, because hypoalbuminemia leads to significant contraction of the plasma volume, which leads to orthostatic hypotension even in the absence of autonomic failure. In patients with cardiac amyloidosis who have poor diastolic fill-

Fig. 7.1. Prevalence of symptoms in patients with primary amyloidosis evaluated within 1 month before or after diagnosis (1981–1992). (From Kyle and Gertz [1995]. By permission of Elsevier.)

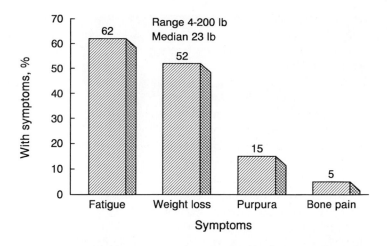

Fig. 7.2. Classic truncal purpura in primary amyloidosis. (From Gertz MA, Lacy MQ, Dispenzieri A [1999] Amyloidosis. Hematol Oncol Clin North Am 13:1211–1233. By permission of WB Saunders Company.)

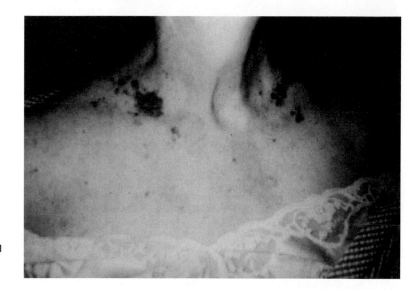

ing, the stroke volume is decreased as a result of the low end-diastolic volume. This produces a low cardiac output in the presence of a normal ejection fraction and can be overlooked during an evaluation of the lightheadedness. Patients who have autonomic neuropathy develop orthostatic hypotension that results in lightheadedness and occasionally syncope.

The physical findings of amyloidosis are present infrequently (15% of patients) and are easily overlooked. When they are seen, they may be specific and diagnostic. The classic amyloid purpura is seen in only approximately 1 patient in 6 (Fig. 7.2). The purpura occurs above the nipple line, most frequently in the webbing of the neck, the face, and the eyelids. Purpura on the dorsa of the arms is not characteristic of amyloid and most commonly represents purpura simplex. Occasionally, only petechial lesions are seen on the eyelids, and without inspection with the eyes fully closed, the purpura may be missed. Because of the age of these patients, the purpura can be misdiagnosed as senile purpura.

Hepatosplenomegaly is present in a substantial proportion of patients with amyloid, as many as one-fourth. The liver edge is palpable greater than 5 cm below the right costal margin in only 10% of patients, and splenomegaly rarely exceeds a palpable tip.

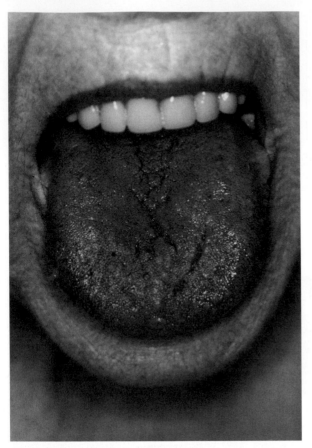

Fig. 7.3. Tongue enlargement in primary amyloidosis. (From Gertz MA, Lacy MQ, Dispenzieri A [1999] Amyloidosis. Hematol Oncol Clin North Am 13:1211–1233. By permission of WB Saunders Company.)

become palpable and are frequently misdiagnosed as submandibular lymph nodes. In addition, the tongue may become so large it will force the submandibular salivary glands inferiorly so that they become palpable even when they are not actually enlarged. The infiltration of the salivary glands with amyloid is responsible for the sicca syndrome these patients frequently present with and may be misdiagnosed as Sjögren syndrome.

Occasionally, patients present because of diffuse vascular involvement with amyloid without visceral disease. There are at least a score of reports wherein the temporal arteries are involved with amyloid and produce vascular occlusion and ischemic symptoms, including jaw claudication (Gertz et al. 1986). Many of these patients also have calf and limb claudication due to peripheral microvascular involvement. To add to the confusion, the presence of a serum monoclonal protein raises the erythrocyte sedimentation rate. The presence of an increased sedimentation rate in this age group with jaw claudication has led to the diagnosis of polymyalgia rheumatica with temporal arteritis. Frequently, a biopsy is not performed, which would have shown amyloid deposits in the temporal artery, and these patients are treated empirically with corticosteroids. This provides no benefit to these patients and of course delays the diagnosis further. A rare patient presents because of muscle infiltration with amyloid. Skeletal muscle pseudohypertrophy, the so-called shoulder pad sign, is a manifestation of this. However, the majority of patients with muscular infiltration actually have diffuse muscular weakness related to muscular atrophy, a consequence of chronic vascular occlusion.

The most specific and diagnostic physical finding in AL is macroglossia. Enlargement of the tongue is not found in familial, secondary, or senile systemic amyloidosis, and amyloidosis is far more common than other causes of tongue enlargement such as tongue tumors or acromegaly. Therefore, macroglossia is highly specific for AL (Fig. 7.3). Unfortunately, only 9% of AL patients have enlargement of the tongue, and because it is the base of the tongue that preferentially enlarges, it would be easy to overlook unless one inspects for the presence of dental indentations on the underside of the tongue (Fig. 7.3). The tongue is certainly not an area that an internist typically examines thoroughly in a patient presenting with proteinuria and cardiac failure. Confirmation of the presence of an enlarged tongue can be sought by examining the submandibular salivary glands. These glands are frequently involved with amyloid and they

7.4 Making a Diagnosis of Amyloidosis

Because the subjective symptoms and the physical findings associated with amyloidosis are nonspecific, when should a clinician suspect this rare problem and begin diagnostic procedures to confirm the diagnosis? Because the history and physical are so frequently not helpful, recognition of the specific clinical syndromes associated with amyloidosis is essential. The 7 most common presentations of patients who have immunoglobulin light chain amyloidosis are: 1) infiltrative cardiomyopathy with restrictive hemodynamics, 2) nephrotic-range proteinuria with or without renal insufficiency, 3) idiopathic peripheral neuropathy, 4) unexplained hepatomegaly, 5) carpal tunnel syndrome, 6)

Table 7.2. Syndromes in primary amyloidosis

Syndrome	Patients, %
Nephrotic or nephrotic and renal failure	30
Hepatomegaly	24
Congestive heart failure	22
Carpal tunnel	21
Neuropathy	17
Orthostatic hypotension	12

tongue enlargement, and 7) gastrointestinal tract symptoms of pseudo-obstruction or steatorrhea. When any one of these symptoms is seen in an adult, the diagnosis of AL must be considered (Table 7.2). Many patients who have AL are evaluated for weight loss and fatigue and have a monoclonal gammopathy. An aggressive evaluation for multiple myeloma may frequently be conducted. These patients have only a few percent clonal plasma cells in the bone marrow, and the clinical presentation does not "fit" multiple myeloma. These patients remain without a diagnosis until the syndrome is correctly associated with the monoclonal protein and a biopsy is performed.

When a clinician evaluates a patient with proteinuria, cardiomyopathy, hepatomegaly, or neuropathy, the first and most important noninvasive screening test is **immunofixation of the serum and urine**. All patients

with amyloidosis have a clonal population of plasma cells detectable (Gertz et al. 1991a). These plasma cells are responsible for the production of the monoclonal immunoglobulin light chains that are ultimately deposited as the insoluble fibrillar β-pleated sheet of amyloid. The finding of a monoclonal protein in a patient with a compatible syndrome is compelling evidence for pursuing a diagnosis further to confirm or exclude AL. Often, a screening serum protein electrophoresis is performed in these patients, but this is inadequate. Immunofixation of serum and urine is required. One-fourth of patients with AL lack a monoclonal protein in the serum (Fig. 7.4), and urine evaluation is required because it detects nearly one-fourth of the patients. In addition, the monoclonal proteins seen in AL are frequently small, in large part the result of the high prevalence of Bence Jones proteinemia or Bence Jones proteinuria, neither of which produces a measurable peak in the electrophoretic pattern. Moreover, the high prevalence of proteinuria in these patients frequently obscures small monoclonal proteins in the urine (Fig. 7.5). Inspection of the electrophoretic pattern is insufficient and immunofixation is mandatory if amyloid is really in the differential diagnosis.

When immunofixation is performed in the serum or in the urine, a monoclonal light chain is detected successfully in 90% of patients with AL. Immunofixation of serum and urine is the single best noninvasive screening test when a patient is seen with a suggestive

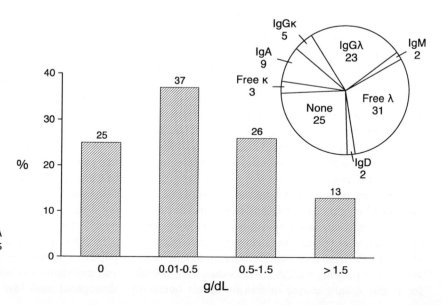

Fig. 7.4. Amount of serum monoclonal protein in patients with primary amyloidosis and immunofixation results. (From Gertz MA, Lacy MQ, Dispenzieri A [2002] Amyloidosis. In Mehta J, Singhal S [eds] Myeloma. Martin Dunitz, London, pp 445–463. By permission of the publisher.)

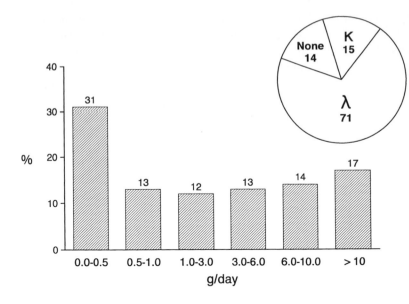

Fig. 7.5. Distribution of 24-hour urine total protein and immunofixation results in primary amyloidosis. (From Gertz MA, Lacy MQ, Dispenzieri A [2002] Amyloidosis. In Mehta J, Singhal S [eds] Myeloma. Martin Dunitz, London, pp 445–463. By permission of the publisher.)

clinical syndrome (Gertz et al. 1999). In patients who do not have a detectable light chain in the serum or urine, a bone marrow specimen almost always demonstrates a clonal population of plasma cells by immunohistochemistry, immunofluorescence, or flow cytometry. This is not unexpected because this is the clinical counterpart of nonsecretory multiple myeloma, which we refer to as nonsecretory light chain amyloidosis. Presumably, light chains are present but the concentrations are below the level of detection by conventional techniques because the amyloid protein precursor is being removed from the plasma rapidly and deposited as amyloid deposits or because available antisera are unable to recognize expressed epitopes on the circulating light chain fragments. Of the first 16 patients we saw without a detectable monoclonal protein by serum or urine immunofixation, 15 had a clear clonal population of plasma cells in their bone marrow. A combination of serum and urine immunofixation and clonal analysis for plasma cells detects virtually all patients with AL. Lacking 1 of these 3, AL is not the likely diagnosis and these patients have amyloidosis that is not immunoglobulin light chain derived.

A new technique for the analysis of serum immunoglobulin free light chains is likely to enhance the sensitivity of light chain detection. Antisera have been developed capable of recognizing epitopes of free immunoglobulin light chains. We applied this technique to the sera of 100 patients with AL. Antibodies were specific for κ and λ light chains in free form, not bound to the heavy chain. In the group with κ monoclonal free light chains detected in serum or urine by immunofixation, this simple nephelometric analysis for free light chain had a sensitivity of 90%. A similar profile was obtained in the group with λ monoclonal free light chains. In patients who had a positive result of urine immunofixation but a negative result of serum immunofixation, the free light chain technique detected serum free light chains in 85% of patients with κ and 80% of patients with λ. In the group of patients with AL who had no detectable monoclonal protein in serum or urine by immunofixation, a free κ light chain was found in 86% and a free λ light chain in 30%. The detection of free light chains in serum by nephelometry provides a more convenient assay system for detecting monoclonal light chains in AL and is particularly important in those patients who do not have light chains detected by immunofixation. This screening will decrease the number of biopsies that are performed to diagnose AL when the likelihood of finding it is small.

Amyloid P component is a pentagonal glycoprotein that can comprise as much as 10% of the amyloid fibril by weight. All forms of amyloid contain P component. P component is structurally related to C-reactive protein but is not an acute-phase reactant in humans. P component is not irreversibly bound to the amyloid fibril and is in dynamic equilibrium with plasma amyloid P component. Plasma P component is found in all humans and maintains a relatively stable plasma concentration throughout one's life.

Human amyloid P component has been radiolabeled, usually with a radioisotope of iodine. This tracer has been used successfully as a radionuclide imaging technique to visually demonstrate amyloid deposits. The serum concentration of the radioactive tracer and its clearance from the plasma can also be used to estimate the total body burden of amyloid and to assess the various impacts of therapy. Patients with high burdens of amyloid have rapid plasma clearance of radiolabeled P component. Patients with small amounts have clearance of the plasma akin to normal patients. Serial studies using amyloid P scanning can determine whether patients are having progressive organ deposition or resolution of amyloid deposits. This technique does not distinguish AL amyloid from the other forms of amyloid. In large numbers of patients, imaging demonstrates deposits in the spleen (87%), the liver (60%), and the kidneys (25%). This technique is not sensitive in detecting myocardial amyloid deposits and is generally used in conjunction with echocardiography (Hawkins et al. 1998). Plasma clearance of amyloid has been correlated with survival, with rapid plasma clearance associated with a shorter survival. Imaging using radiolabeled P component does not demonstrate deposits in the gastrointestinal tract or carpal tunnel and is severely limited in recognizing renal deposits. The total blood and extravascular fluid contain just 50 to 100 mg of amyloid P component, whereas amyloid deposits can contain as much as 20,000 mg. Iodine-123 is used for imaging (Hawkins et al. 1990), and iodine-125 is used for clearance studies. These scans have demonstrated that the distribution of amyloid within individual organs can be nonhomogeneous, and there is a poor correlation between the imaging studies and the degree of organ dysfunction seen clinically. This technique is not widely available, in part due to the expense of iodine-123, the difficulty of obtaining human serum amyloid P that would be a viral-free preparation, and the possibility that radiolabeling with iodine may denature the P component.

Although patients with amyloid demonstrate uptake of tracer, a positive scan is not a substitute for the histologic confirmation of this disease. Given the life-threatening prognosis, a diagnosis of amyloidosis must be confirmed by biopsy, as for patients with suspected malignancy. In patients who have renal, cardiac, hepatic, or neural amyloid, the diagnosis could be established by direct biopsy of those tissues; however, biopsies of viscera are generally not required to establish a diagnosis. By its nature, amyloid is widespread in blood vessels at presentation, and biopsies that are less invasive generally establish the diagnosis and have a lower morbidity.

At Mayo Clinic, when a patient with a compatible syndrome is evaluated, and our suspicion is heightened by the finding of a monoclonal immunoglobulin light chain, we begin histologic confirmation by performing a subcutaneous fat aspiration and a bone marrow biopsy. The subcutaneous fat aspiration can be done by skilled technical personnel and is a risk-free procedure. Results are available in 24 hours and are positive in 70% to 80% of patients with amyloid (Fig. 7.6). The bone marrow biopsy demonstrates amyloid deposits in half of patients in the vessels of the biopsy specimen. A bone marrow biopsy is generally required in any case because once a monoclonal immunoglobulin light chain is detected, evaluation to exclude the diagnosis of multiple myeloma is required, and the percentage of plasma cells in the bone marrow is quite useful. When subcutaneous fat aspiration and bone marrow biopsy are combined, 87% of patients with AL have a positive result (Table 7.3). In the remaining 13%, biopsies of the affected organ can be performed.

Other sites can undergo less invasive biopsy. The high incidence of xerostomia in amyloidosis results in a high prevalence of positive minor salivary gland biopsy specimens taken from the lip. This was reported in 1 study as being positive in 26 of 30 patients. Skin biopsies including uninvolved skin demonstrate subcutaneous blood vessel positivity in the majority of patients. For decades, the rectal biopsy was a preferred technique for the confirmation of amyloid (Kyle et al. 1966). This could be performed as an outpatient procedure at minimal risk. Occasionally, rectal bleeding did occur after a biopsy, and a deep biopsy is required because endoscopic biopsies regularly provide only mucosal samples. A common clinical scenario would be that a patient would see a nephrologist for the diagnosis of nephrotic syndrome. Our nephrologists do an immunofixation of serum and urine on all patients with nephrotic syndrome and, when positive, order a fat aspiration. This eliminates the need for renal biopsy in 70% of patients, reducing cost, hospitalization, and the risk of renal biopsy-associated complications.

The Congo red stain, although the standard for confirming the diagnosis, is not the simplest staining procedure. Overstaining of subcutaneous fat with Congo red can result in the dye's precipitation in the tissue,

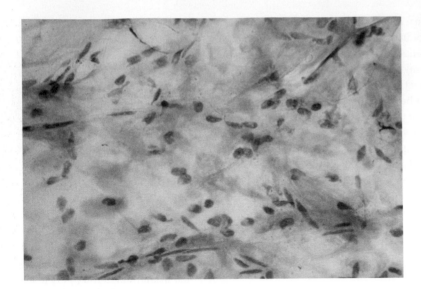

Fig. 7.6. Subcutaneous fat aspirate demonstrates amyloid. (x100.) (From Gertz MA, Lacy MQ, Dispenzieri A [2002] Amyloidosis. In Mehta J, Singhal S [eds] Myeloma. Martin Dunitz, London, pp 445–463. By permission of the publisher.)

Table 7.3. Noninvasive biopsies in primary amyloidosis

Finding		Patients , %
Fat +	Marrow +	55
Fat +	Marrow –	22
Fat –	Marrow +	10
Fat –	Marrow –	13

Modified from Gertz MA, Lacy MQ, Lust JA, Greipp PR, Witzig TE, Kyle RA (1999) Prospective randomized trial of melphalan and prednisone versus vincristine, carmustine, melphalan, cyclophosphamide, and prednisone in the treatment of primary systemic amyloidosis. J Clin Oncol 17:262–267. By permission of the American Society of Clinical Oncology.

which can be interpreted as being a positive result. Fibers of elastin and Type I collagen typically found in skin and subcutaneous fat bind Congo red and can be misinterpreted as a false-positive result. Conversely, we have seen rectal biopsy specimens containing amyloid misinterpreted as collagenous colitis. Occasionally, amyloid deposits in the kidney can be misinterpreted as hyalinization of the glomerulus. In routine clinical practice, our cardiac pathologists prefer sulfated alcian blue for the recognition of amyloid deposits in the myocardium, and our peripheral nerve pathologists use crystal violet to screen sural nerve biopsy specimens and confirm positive reactions with Congo red staining.

7.5 Differentiating AL From Other Forms of Amyloidosis

Once a diagnosis of amyloidosis has been established histologically, it is imperative that one is certain that amyloidosis is of the immunoglobulin light chain type because the therapy for AL is distinct from the therapy for all other forms of amyloidosis. In addition to immunoglobulin light chain amyloidosis, there are localized, familial, secondary (Gillmore et al. 2001), and senile systemic forms. One must remember that only AL is associated with a plasma cell dyscrasia. Only AL will have a monoclonal light chain in the serum or urine and a clonal population of plasma cells in the bone marrow. Localized forms of amyloidosis can be confused with systemic forms because patients can present with important clinical problems such as hematuria, respiratory difficulties, and visual disturbances. The amyloid with one of the localized amyloid syndromes (eg, skin, laryngeal, urogenital) does not ever become systemic. In localized amyloid, the fibrils themselves frequently will be immunoglobulin light chain derived, but no plasma cell dyscrasia is seen; this represents localized plasma cell production of fibrillar material.

An important clue to recognize localized amyloidosis is its location, because many of these organs are not typically involved in systemic AL. Most localized amyloidosis is seen in the respiratory tract, genitourinary tract, and skin. Amyloidosis involving the lung can be divided into tracheobronchial, nodular, or diffuse interstitial. The first 2 of these are forms of localized amyloidosis. The third is a pulmonary manifestation of systemic AL (Utz et al. 1996). In the tracheobronchial form, submucosal deposits can produce obstruction, cough, dyspnea, wheezing, and hemoptysis. The diagnosis is usually made via bronchoscopy, and the treatment is usually yttrium-aluminum-garnet (YAG) laser resection of the tissue. These deposits are immunoglobulin light chain derived. Localized pulmonary amyloid may also manifest as solitary pulmonary nodules and is referred to as nodular amyloid of the lung. Patients can have multiple nodules, and this still does not represent systemic AL. These diagnoses are usually made at thoracotomy or video thoracoscopic surgical procedures, because these nodules are noncalcified and are often resected to exclude a diagnosis of pulmonary malignancy. Amyloid can also be confined to the larynx and involve the vocal cords and false vocal cords, causing traction on these structures and leading to hoarseness.

Amyloid, when seen in the urinary bladder, is generally localized. Cystoscopically, these patients usually evaluated for hematuria are initially thought to have bladder cancer. Hematuria is seen in 85% of these patients. Treatment consists of transurethral resection, fulguration, or partial cystectomy. Intravesical dimethyl sulfoxide was reported to produce regression of these deposits. Oral colchicine also was reported to be beneficial.

Amyloid may also be localized to both the ureter and the renal pelvis. This is generally diagnosed because of hematuria or obstruction, producing colic symptoms. These deposits are generally found at surgical intervention. Recognition of amyloid preoperatively often avoids a nephrectomy. Urethral amyloidosis is always a localized process when the patient presents with hematuria. Again, the preoperative diagnosis is usually a urethral malignancy, and transurethral resection is generally successful.

Amyloidosis of the skin can be classified into lichen, macular, or nodular amyloidosis. The lichen and macular forms are localized. The nodular form is associated with AL. The deposits of macular and papular amyloidosis appear to be derived from keratin. Local therapy suffices. Dermabrasion is beneficial. Skin inflammation is usually found as a precursor to lichen or macular amyloid. It is important to make the distinction between these forms of amyloid because macular and lichen amyloid are benign conditions, whereas the nodular

form may be a clue to an underlying life-threatening process.

Amyloid is found in the carpal tunnel in localized amyloid and systemic AL. When patients had symptoms of only carpal tunnel syndrome, the median survival of 124 patients was 12 years. Systemic amyloid developed in only 2 patients (Kyle et al. 1992 a). The amyloid deposits in localized carpal tunnel amyloid are transthyretin derived.

Amyloid can be localized to the conjunctiva or orbits. Conjunctival amyloid is best treated by surgical excision. Other sites where amyloid has been localized include the breast, mesenteric lymph nodes, polyps in the bowel, thyroid, ovary, and retroperitoneum. Localized deposits of amyloid are seen frequently in degenerative joint disease. It is a common finding in resected specimens after a total hip arthroplasty – in trace amounts in the cartilage and on the hip surface. It can be found in the knee joint. These are never associated with systemic disease.

AA is a form of systemic amyloidosis that must be distinguished from AL. AA is not associated with the presence of immunoglobulin light chains or clonal bone marrow plasma cells. AA is a consequence of longstanding uncontrolled systemic inflammation. In underdeveloped countries, AA remains prevalent because it can be seen after tuberculosis, lepromatous leprosy, malaria, and syphilis. The most common clinical manifestation of AA is nephrotic-range proteinuria (Gertz and Kyle 1991). Therefore, from a syndrome standpoint, it is not easily differentiated from AL.

In the Western world, AA is quite rare and comprises only 2% of patients seen with amyloid at Mayo Clinic. The most common cause is poorly controlled symmetric inflammatory polyarthropathies, which include ankylosing spondylitis, juvenile rheumatoid arthritis, psoriatic arthritis, and rheumatoid arthritis. The median duration of the arthritis is 15 years before the diagnosis of amyloid, so the underlying cause is generally obvious (Gertz 1992). In a 10-year study of 1,000 patients with rheumatoid arthritis, 3.1% died of AA. Amyloidosis can also be seen in Crohn disease, long-standing bronchiectasis, or chronic osteomyelitis not amenable to surgical excision and poorly controlled with antibiotics. The clinical manifestation of AA in this setting is proteinuria. In these patients, the bowel disorder or infection is generally present for many years and is easily recognized. These patients do not have detectable immunoglobulin light chains or a clonal plasma cell disorder. AA was described in drug users who injected drugs subcutaneously. These individuals frequently develop skin abscesses at multiple sites that produce the sustained inflammation characteristic of AA. Rare instances of AA have been described in patients with Hodgkin disease and renal cell cancer. Rarely, AA has been seen in patients who are paraplegic due to chronic infected decubitus ulcers or chronic infection of the urinary tract. At autopsy, amyloidosis is found in more than half of patients who have had spinal cord injuries for more than 10 years.

In our practice, inherited forms of amyloid are now more common than secondary amyloid. These patients can present with cardiomyopathy (Ranlov et al. 1992), peripheral neuropathy, or nephrotic syndrome and can be difficult to distinguish from patients with AL. Patients with familial amyloid do not have evidence of a plasma cell dyscrasia or of a monoclonal gammopathy. The most common forms of familial amyloid are due to mutations of the transthyretin (TTR) molecule. To date, more than 60 mutations in the *TTR* gene have been described and associated with the development of amyloid neuropathy (Connors et al. 2000). Half of the patients seen at Mayo Clinic with amyloid neuropathy on a familial basis do not have a positive family history of peripheral neuropathy and, therefore, this is not sufficient in making the distinction (Gertz et al. 1992b). The presence of amyloid neuropathy, either sensorimotor or autonomic, in the absence of a monoclonal protein or clonal plasma cell disorder should raise the suspicion of familial amyloid.

Cardiac amyloid is seen in mutations in *TTR* and in wild-type TTR (Olson et al. 1987). Cardiac amyloidosis in the elderly due to the deposition of normal TTR occurs in 8% to 25% of people older than age 80 years (Gertz et al. 1989a). These deposits, although widespread, generally cause dysfunction of only the heart. Familial amyloid cardiomyopathy without neuropathy was first recognized 40 years ago in a Danish kindred, but has been detected subsequently in pedigrees throughout the United States and Ireland. Symptoms typically begin after age 60 years. The clinical picture of patients with senile cardiac amyloidosis is similar to that of familial amyloid cardiomyopathy with congestive heart failure or arrhythmias. In an autopsy series in patients older than age 90 years, 21% had amyloid deposits due to normal sequence TTR (Smith et al. 1984). Fifteen years ago, a *TTR* I1e122 mutation was first described in a black man (age 68 years). Studies of

5,000 DNA samples revealed that this allele is carried by 3.9% of African Americans. This variant, therefore, is carried by 1.3 million people in the United States. This allele is a major cause of cardiac amyloidosis among African Americans. Therefore, the finding of cardiac amyloidosis in the absence of a monoclonal gammopathy should raise the possibility that this is not straightforward AL but may represent familial amyloid cardiomyopathy with or without a family history (Jacobson et al. 1997).

Familial types of renal amyloidosis have been described. In these instances, the amyloid is composed of a mutant fibrinogen, lysozyme (Pepys et al. 1993), or apolipoprotein A-I. These patients present with a clinical course that is far more indolent than amyloid nephrotic syndrome associated with AL. Patients may have proteinuria for more than a decade without renal insufficiency. There are no other clinical distinguishing features, although extrarenal involvement is uncommon. Again, the presentation is clinically indistinguishable from AL; the only difference is the lack of a monoclonal immunoglobulin disorder.

The distinction between familial and AL amyloid is important because liver transplantation has been applied successfully for the treatment of TTR-derived familial amyloid. TTR is produced in the liver only, and liver transplantation before the development of severe peripheral or autonomic neuropathy or advanced cardiac disease produced regression of amyloid deposits. The outcome of transplantation appears to be best for patients with a Val30Met mutation. Patients with other mutations in TTR who have had liver transplantation have been reported to develop progressive cardiac disease posttransplantation. Analysis of amyloid deposits in the heart of patients who have undergone liver transplantation demonstrates wild-type TTR and mutant TTR (Stangou et al. 1998). It has been suggested that once mutant TTR is deposited in the myocardium, it serves as a nidus for further deposition of native TTR produced by the transplanted liver (Dubrey et al. 1997). In summary, any patient with diagnosed amyloidosis who lacks a monoclonal protein in the serum and urine and has no monoclonal population of bone marrow plasma cells should be evaluated for localized, AA, or familial amyloidosis.

7.6 Clinical Presentation and Clinical Features

We reviewed all patients diagnosed with AL from June 1, 1988, through June 30, 1998, at Mayo Clinic. All had a histologic diagnosis of amyloidosis and evidence of a clonal plasma cell dyscrasia. Patients who had overt multiple myeloma were excluded. Males outnumbered females 2 to 1 (67.3%). This male preponderance has remained constant for the past 40 years. The reason there is an excess of men with AL remains unknown since the frequency of multiple myeloma in men is only 55%. The median patient age is 67 years (range, 39 to 89; standard deviation, 10 years). There are a significant number of patients being seen younger than age 45 years. The median age of patients with AL seen in Olmsted County is 73 years (Kyle et al. 1992b). This difference of 6 years suggests the presence of referral bias such that patients who are younger are more likely to seek a second opinion regarding their amyloidosis.

When patients are classified by a single dominant organ manifestation, cardiac amyloid dominates and is found in 37.4% of patients. Only half of these patients actually have symptoms of congestive heart failure. The other half have cardiac manifestations that include progressive fatigue due to poor cardiac filling but with a preserved ejection fraction, arrhythmias, or syncope. The widespread use of echocardiography led to a sharp increase in the recognition of cardiac amyloidosis (Cueto-Garcia et al. 1984, 1985).

The second most common presentation is renal amyloid, seen in 30%. Virtually all of these patients had nephrotic-range proteinuria leading to evaluation. Amyloid peripheral neuropathy, usually sensorimotor, symmetric, ascending, and associated with paresthesias, was seen in 15.3%. Hepatomegaly was found in 17.7% of patients, but liver amyloid presenting as the dominant syndrome was seen in only 4.6% of patients. Gastrointestinal tract amyloid, manifested by intestinal bleeding, pseudo-obstruction, or diarrhea, was seen in 7.1% of patients, and in the remainder, a heterogeneous mix of soft tissue, tongue, interstitial pulmonary, and joint amyloid comprised 7.8% of the group.

The definition of a "dominant" amyloid syndrome is not always clear. In our patient population, 36.3% of patients presented with 2 or more organs involved. Often, the distinction of the dominant amyloid syndrome is arbitrary, and it may be difficult to know which of the organs involved are responsible for the patients' symptoms. In Mayo patients, 29.9% had 2 organs involved;

6%, 3 organs involved; and 0.5%, 4 or more organs involved. The liver was the organ most likely to be associated with involvement of an additional organ.

Although reported to be more prevalent, in our population, only 2.3% presented with significant bleeding (purpura excluded). Of our patients, 16.4% had carpal tunnel syndrome and 19.6% had congestive heart failure, even though more than double that number had cardiac involvement by echocardiography. Symptoms included edema in 44.8% and fatigue in 46.4%. Twenty-one percent had nephrotic-range proteinuria, and 12.5% had orthostatic hypotension. Lower extremity paresthesias were reported by 34.9% and weight loss was seen in 51.7%.

Anemia is uncommon in amyloidosis; 64.4% of patients had a hemoglobin value greater than 12 g/dL and 90%, greater than 10 g/dL. A hemoglobin value less than 9 g/dL was seen in only 1.5% and was generally associated with active gastrointestinal tract hemorrhage or advanced renal failure. The median platelet count for all patients was 257×10^9/L, ranging from 46×10^9/L to 809×10^9/L. Only 5.5% had a platelet count greater than 500×10^9/L, and these patients generally had hepatic amyloidosis with associated hyposplenism causing the thrombocytosis. The serum creatinine concentration was greater than or equal to 2 mg/dL in 13.6% of patients. An alkaline phosphatase concentration greater than twice our institutional normal value was seen in 6.7%, correlating well with the percentage of patients with hepatic involvement. The median number of bone marrow plasma cells was 7%, ranging from 1% to 30% (Fig. 7.7). All patients whose bone marrow plasma cells were greater than 30% were excluded and were diagnosed as having myeloma-associated amyloid. Of pa-

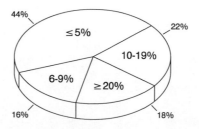

Median plasma cells 7%

Fig. 7.7. Distribution of bone marrow plasma cells in patients with primary amyloidosis. (From Gertz MA, Lacy MQ, Dispenzieri A [1999] Amyloidosis. Hematol Oncol Clin North Am 13:1211–1233. By permission of WB Saunders Company.)

tients with amyloidosis, 11.3% have greater than 20% plasma cells in the bone marrow with no other signs of multiple myeloma. The median 24-hour urine protein loss in all patients was 790 mg/24 hours. The monoclonal light chain type found in the serum or urine was λ in 70.1%, κ in 18.9%, and absent in 11%. In the patients who had a detectable immunoglobulin heavy chain that was IgG in 58%, IgA in 10%, and IgM in 8.2%, the presence of IgM amyloidosis is important to recognize because we have seen many patients misdiagnosed with Waldenström macroglobulinemia by virtue of the presence of the IgM protein alone (Gertz et al. 1993). On echocardiography, the median septal thickness of the entire group was 14 mm; the septal thickness was less than 15 mm in 52.9% and greater than or equal to 15 mm in 47.1%, reflecting the high proportion of cardiac amyloidosis in this group.

The median survival of the entire cohort was 12 months. The 2-year survival rate was 33.6%, and the 5-year survival rate was 14.9%. In a Cox multivariate analysis, variables that were significant in predicting survival were age, Eastern Cooperative Oncology Group performance status, heart involvement as the dominant syndrome, and 2 or more organs involved.

7.6.1 Heart

The heart is the organ most frequently involved in patients seen at Mayo Clinic and is prognostically the most important because the extent of involvement is directly associated with an adverse outcome and shortened survival (Klein et al. 1989, 1990, 1991). Amyloid deposits in the myocardium are extracellular and result in a noncompliant, thickened left ventricle. Patients present because of progressive infiltrative cardiomyopathy that leads to restriction in ventricular filling (Fig. 7.8). The diagnosis of a cardiac syndrome in AL is generally subtle. Patients may present with disabling fatigue and unexplained weight loss as their only symptom. The nature of restrictive cardiomyopathy is to produce early diastolic dysfunction and no systolic dysfunction (Klein et al. 1999). In these instances, the chest radiograph will not show cardiomegaly or pulmonary vascular redistribution. On echocardiography, the ejection fraction is preserved. The low stroke volume frequently results in a hyperdynamic myocardium with ejection fractions as high as 70%. These patients have poor diastolic filling, but contractility is normal, and they will pump a normal percentage of a reduced end-diastolic volume, resulting in reduced cardiac output. Silent ischemia is frequently postulated and leads to coronary arteriography, which is invariably normal. The echocardiogram shows wall thickening (Fig. 7.9). This is easily misinterpreted as concentric left ventricular hypertrophy or asymmetric septal hypertrophy rather than infiltrative cardiomyopathy. When the measurements of the septum and free wall are identical, this is read as concentric left ventricular hypertrophy. Frequently, the septum is thicker than the free wall, and this is interpreted as

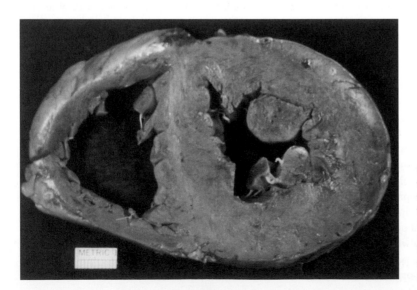

Fig. 7.8. Myocardial wall diffusely thickened with amyloid. The whitish deposits represent the amyloid and are the lardaceous changes first recognized by Rokitansky. (From Gertz MA, Kyle RA [2003] Amyloidosis [AL]. In Wiernik PH, Goldman JM, Dutcher JP, Kyle RA [eds] Neoplastic diseases of the blood, 4th edn. Cambridge University Press, Cambridge, pp 595–618. By permission of the publisher.)

Fig. 7.9. Echocardiographic demonstration of concentric thickening of the left ventricular (*LV*) wall from amyloid. *RV*, right ventricle. (From Gertz MA, Kyle RA [2003] Amyloidosis [AL]. In Wiernik PH, Goldman J, Dutcher JP, Kyle RA [eds] Neoplastic diseases of the blood, 4th edn. Cambridge University Press, Cambridge. By permission of the publisher.)

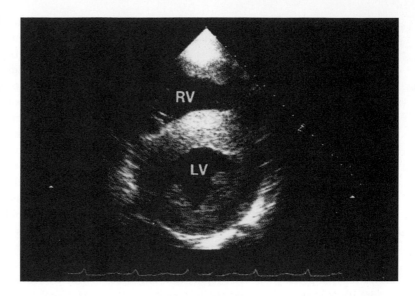

asymmetric septal hypertrophy. In virtually all cases, the electrocardiogram does not show the voltage change consistent with ventricular hypertrophy and shows the pseudoinfarction pattern or low voltage typical of amyloid. Any patient with diastolic heart failure, restrictive hemodynamics, or wall thickening needs to have a monoclonal protein screen in the serum or in the urine.

Doppler studies are required to assess myocardial function accurately in amyloid patients because these are best designed to demonstrate the restriction of blood inflow that characterizes this disease. Doppler filling patterns are closely related to the degree of amyloid infiltration. Early cardiac amyloidosis shows abnormal relaxation. In contrast, advanced cardiac amyloidosis shows a short deceleration time consistent with restrictive physiology. Increased ventricular wall thickness and decreased fractional shortening is the best predictor of poor outcome in cardiac amyloidosis. The combination of decreased fractional shortening of less than 20% and a mean left ventricular wall thickness of 15 mm has been associated with a median survival of only 4 months. The deceleration time is an important measurement. A short deceleration time by Doppler study is indicative of restrictive physiology, and these patients have adverse outcomes compared with patients who have a deceleration time of greater than 150 ms.

In 204 patients with AL evaluated at Mayo Clinic, the median septal thickness was 14 mm: 108 (53%) had a septal thickness less than 15 mm and 47% had a septal thickness greater than or equal to 15 mm (Cueto-Garcia

et al. 1985). The normal thickness of the ventricular septum is 9 to 12 mm. The most common echocardiographic features are thickening of the right ventricular wall, septum, and left ventricular free wall. The left ventricular cavity size is reduced. Cardiac involvement is seen in 41% of our population, but overt congestive heart failure is seen in approximately 20%. There is a high proportion of patients who have cardiac amyloid manifested by mild symptoms such as fatigue and dyspnea on exertion, but who would not fulfill the clinical criteria of congestive heart failure. In patients who have a ventricular septal thickness greater than or equal to 15 mm, the median survival is less than 1 year. If the septal thickness is less than 15 mm at diagnosis, the median survival is approximately 4 years. In some series, almost one-third of patients with cardiac amyloid experience syncope with exercise. Exercise-induced syncope has been associated with a median survival of only 2 months.

Early recognition of cardiac amyloidosis depends on the clinician performing immunofixation of the serum and urine in any patient presenting with symptoms of cardiomyopathy or heart failure that does not have an obvious ischemic origin. The standard for the diagnosis of amyloid cardiomyopathy is the echocardiogram. Occasionally, a patient has an echocardiogram that is nondiagnostic but has histologically proven amyloid. These are uncommon instances (Gertz et al. 1997). Because the electrocardiogram in amyloidosis may show loss of anteroseptal forces (pseudoinfarction pattern), the patient may be incorrectly diagnosed as having silent isch-emia. Low voltage, although seen in nearly two-thirds of patients with cardiac amyloidosis, is frequently over-looked. Cardiac amyloidosis can produce atrial systolic failure and dilatation of the right ventricle, both of which are associated with a poor prognosis. Thickening of the mitral and tricuspid valves is common in amyloi-dosis and is an important clue in a patient initially thought to have ventricular hypertrophy. Doppler exam-ination regularly demonstrates valvular regurgitation, but this does not appear to be a clinically significant ab-normality. It does not appear that atrioventricular se-quential pacing is useful in improving cardiac hemody-namics.

The presence of a restrictive cardiomyopathy can be confused with pericardial disease causing restriction. Pericardial tamponade has been reported in amyloido-sis, but it would be rare for a pericardiectomy to produce clinical benefit, and the hazards of the surgical proce-dure are substantial. The diagnosis of amyloidosis is generally made noninvasively, but when infiltrative car-diomyopathy is recognized, endomyocardial biopsy pro-vides a correct diagnosis 100% of the time when at least 3 biopsy specimens are obtained (Pellikka et al. 1988).

Stasis of blood commonly occurs within the cardiac chambers. This results in the development of thrombi in both ventricles. These thrombi become sources of cardi-ac embolism, and patients can present with a stroke as the first manifestation of amyloid. Atrial thrombi have also been demonstrated in amyloidosis patients in sinus rhythm. Atrial standstill is well recognized in amyloido-sis and is an indication for anticoagulation therapy. Most patients present because of cardiac muscle infiltra-tion and subsequent pump failure. Some patients pre-sent because of occlusive deposition of amyloid in cor-onary arteries. These patients present with ischemic symptoms of exertional angina and myocardial infarc-tion (Mueller et al. 2000). The epicardial coronary ar-teries are spared, and angiographic findings are normal. Exercise testing confirms ischemia. The diagnosis is usually not made before death. Vascular deposits in small vessels are demonstrable on biopsy of the right ventricular myocardium. We have seen 11 patients pre-senting with angina or unstable coronary syndromes. Low voltage on the electrocardiogram was seen in only 2. The mean time to death after the development of symptoms was 18 months. However, most patients were diagnosed at autopsy, demonstrating the failure to rec-ognize this clinical syndrome.

Digoxin has routinely been considered contraindi-cated in the management of amyloid heart disease be-cause of a high reported association with sudden cardi-ac death. Sudden death is a well-recognized complica-tion of cardiac amyloidosis, whether or not the patient receives digoxin. It is not possible to know with cer-tainty whether digoxin increases the risk of sudden death. Digoxin can decrease ventricular rate in the pres-ence of atrial fibrillation. Digoxin is unlikely to improve myocardial performance because systolic function is well preserved in amyloidosis until late in the disease.

The clinician needs to be aware that all patients with cardiac amyloid do not have the AL variety. There are familial forms of amyloid cardiomyopathy that are par-ticularly common in elderly men of African American descent (Jacobson et al. 1997). These patients present with clinical characteristics identical to those seen in AL (Jacobson et al. 1994). The patients lack a monoclo-nal protein in the serum and urine and have a mutant TTR with an isoleucine at position 123. There is also a syndrome of cardiac amyloid associated with the de-position of native TTR, so-called senile cardiac amyloi-dosis (Kyle et al. 1996). The echocardiographic features are indistinguishable, and the amyloid deposits, when viewed with Congo red, show no characteristic features. Once again, these patients have no monoclonal protein in the serum or urine and have TTR detected immuno-histochemically on the deposits (Gertz et al. 1989a). Gene studies show no mutations in the *TTR* gene, and the mechanism of deposition is not understood. One-fourth of patients older than age 90 years demonstrate such deposits in the myocardium. One needs to remem-ber that all forms of cardiac amyloidosis are not immu-noglobulin light chain derived (Smith et al. 1984).

7.6.2 Kidney

Proteinuria does not always equate with albuminuria, and when free monoclonal light chains are detected in the urine, the differential diagnosis of the proteinuria can be limited to cryoglobulinemia, amyloidosis, Ran-dall-type light chain deposition disease, and myeloma cast nephropathy. Immunofixation of the urine in pa-tients with proteinuria is important in the diagnostic evaluation. In AL, the second most frequently affected organ is the kidney, seen in 28% of Mayo Clinic patients, but the figures run as high as half of all amyloid patients seen by Bellotti and Merlini. Amyloid is found in 2.5%

to 2.8% of all kidney biopsy specimens. In nondiabetic adults with nephrotic syndrome, amyloidosis is seen in 12% of renal biopsies.

Survival in patients with renal amyloid correlates with the serum creatinine value at diagnosis. Patients presenting with a creatinine value less than 1.3 mg/dL have a median survival of 25.6 months (Gertz et al. 1992 a). Those with an increased creatinine value have a median survival of 14.9 months. The amount of 24-hour urine protein excretion has no impact on survival. However, patients with higher amounts of protein excretion have a shorter time from diagnosis to the development of end-stage renal disease (Gertz and Kyle 1990). Fourteen percent of our patients present with a serum creatinine value greater than or equal to 2 mg/dL. For all amyloid patients, the median urinary protein excretion is 0.8 g/24 h. Thirty percent of all our patients have greater than 3 g of protein excretion/24 h. Fewer than 5% of AL patients have a urinary protein loss less than 150 mg/d. Many of the patients with no proteinuria have isolated cardiac amyloid or isolated amyloid neuropathy. Two-thirds of the patients have a detectable light chain in the urine, and two-thirds have a detectable light chain in the serum. The higher the urinary protein loss, the more likely it is to find the monoclonal light chain. In amyloidosis patients excreting more than 1 g/d of urinary protein, a monoclonal light chain is found in the urine in 86%.

Interestingly, as greater degrees of urinary protein loss develop, the ratio of patients with κ to λ light chain amyloid changes. In patients with nephrotic-range proteinuria, 5 times as many have monoclonal λ as κ. The median urinary protein loss in patients who have κ amyloid is 1.1 g/d. Patients with a λ protein in the urine have a median urinary protein loss of 4.6 g/d. Although poorly understood, this suggests that the presence of a λ light chain predisposes to a higher frequency of kidney involvement. The median survival in patients who have a urinary λ light chain is 1 year compared with 2½ years in those patients with either no monoclonal protein in the urine or free κ light chain in the urine. There was no difference in the frequency of renal insufficiency in κ or λ light chain amyloid.

The major clinical consequence of nephrotic-range proteinuria is severe serum hypoalbuminemia. The loss of albumin results in a decrease in intravascular oncotic pressure. This leads to plasma transudation into the extracellular space, with the resultant edema. The edema generally requires diuretics for control, but this further

increases intravascular volume contraction and hypotension and decreases renal blood flow. Anasarca may develop. Bilateral catheter embolization of the renal arteries has been reported to decrease the loss of urinary protein and increase the serum total protein in a patient with advanced anasarca.

The principal long-term complication of continuous urinary protein loss in amyloidosis is tubular damage that results in end-stage renal disease. The presenting 24-hour urine protein and serum creatinine values predict which patients ultimately go on to end-stage renal disease. The median time from diagnosis of AL nephrotic syndrome to dialysis is 14 months. Median survival at Mayo from the start of dialysis is 8 months. Most deaths are due to the development of cardiac amyloid. There is no survival difference for patients receiving hemodialysis or peritoneal dialysis. Among 16 patients with AL who received chronic dialysis, the 1-year survival from diagnosis was 68%, with no difference between hemodialysis and peritoneal dialysis.

Patients younger than age 45 years had a better survival. There was a trend to improved survival with chemotherapy, which slowed progression to end-stage renal disease. Predictors of survival were age (younger than 70 years) and serum calcium and creatinine concentrations at presentation. The most important extrarenal complications of AL were heart failure, cardiac arrhythmias, and refractory hypotension. Gastrointestinal tract involvement was manifested by malabsorption. Dialysis was regularly complicated by intradialitic hypotension.

There is a poor correlation between the extent of amyloid deposits seen on kidney biopsy and the extent of the proteinuria. Even small amyloid deposits are associated with severe nephrotic syndrome. Although older literature suggested that the kidneys are enlarged in amyloidosis, today virtually all patients with nephrotic syndrome undergo ultrasonography, and the kidneys are virtually always normal sized. The urinary sediment in amyloid is bland, showing fat or fatty acid crystals but no casts or red cells. In a study of 118 patients with monoclonal gammopathies undergoing renal biopsy, 30% had AL. The median time from diagnosis to dialysis was 15 months; the median survival, 24 months; and the main cause of death, cardiac amyloid.

If amyloid does not involve the kidney at presentation, it is rare for it to occur during follow-up. In our population, only 2% of patients with amyloid subsequently develop proteinuria after presentation. With the advent of cardiac transplantation in AL patients, we have seen 2 patients who subsequently developed renal nephrotic syndrome. In the past, these patients would not have survived to develop this renal complication.

The proteinuria in amyloidosis results from amyloid penetrating the glomerular basement membrane. Adult Fanconi syndrome, renal vein thrombosis, and retroperitoneal fibrosis have all been reported to be associated with renal amyloid. Immunotactoid (fibrillary) glomerulopathy is a fibrillar deposition in the kidney that can be confused with AL. On electron microscopy, the fibrils of fibrillary glomerulopathy are twice the width of amyloid fibrils. These patients do not develop extrarenal disease, and the deposits are not positive on Congo red staining. A monoclonal protein is not associated with this. Randall-type light chain deposition disease represents the deposition of nonamyloid immunoglobulin light chains in a granular fashion along the tubular basement membrane. It can produce nephrotic syndrome and renal insufficiency. Both amyloid and light chain deposition have been reported in the same patient. Light chain deposition disease does not show fibrillar deposits on electron microscopy.

Abnormal uptake of amyloid P component reflecting graft amyloid was seen in 4 of 10 patients whose fibril precursor protein supply had not diminished. In patients with renal amyloidosis, there is a high prevalence of adrenal dysfunction. Of 22 patients with renal amyloid, 7 demonstrated poor cortisol reserve and 4 died of hypoadrenalism. Histologically, amyloid deposits were found in the adrenal glands in 7 patients.

7.6.3 Liver

Hepatomegaly is found by physical examination in one-fourth of patients with amyloidosis (Gertz and Kyle 1988). The hepatomegaly may be due to right-sided heart failure and high filling pressures. In our experience, symptomatic hepatic amyloid syndrome is present in 16% of patients. The most common clinical and laboratory presentations are unexplained hepatomegaly in conjunction with an increased serum alkaline phosphatase or γ-glutamyltransferase value. The most frequent clinical diagnosis before amyloidosis is recognized is malignancy with hepatic metastasis. There is a high concordance between hepatic and renal involvement, and when 2 organs are involved with amyloid, it is usually the liver and the kidney.

Half of patients with hepatic amyloidosis present with greater than 1 g of proteinuria in 24 hours. The presence of proteinuria in the patient who has hepatomegaly and an increased alkaline phosphatase value is an important clue to a systemic extrahepatic disorder. The 4 clinical clues that permit recognition of hepatic amyloidosis are: 1) presence of significant proteinuria; 2) presence of a monoclonal protein in the serum or urine; 3) presence of Howell-Jolly bodies in the peripheral blood film, reflecting splenic infiltration with amyloid and functional hyposplenism; and 4) hepatomegaly out of proportion to the degree of abnormality on liver function tests. Most patients present with increased alkaline phosphatase concentration. The aspartate aminotransferase and alanine transaminase concentrations are typically less than twice normal at the time of diagnosis, and the bilirubin value is virtually always normal. However, hyperbilirubinemia in a patient with hepatic amyloidosis is virtually always a preterminal finding.

An occasional patient with hepatic amyloidosis presents due to splenic rupture and intra-abdominal hemorrhage, rarely hepatic rupture, which is usually fatal. We have diagnosed hepatic rupture in AL using computed tomography that demonstrates a subcapsular hematoma (Gastineau et al. 1991b). The median liver size at the time of diagnosis of hepatic amyloidosis is 7 cm below the right costal margin, with more than half the patients having a liver span of 5 to 9 cm below the right costal margin. Ten percent of patients with biopsy-proven hepatic amyloid have no hepatomegaly and are diagnosed by virtue of the increased alkaline phosphatase concentration. In this subset of patients with hepatic amyloidosis, splenomegaly is seen in 11%. Frank nephrotic syndrome is associated in 36% of patients with hepatic amyloidosis. The median increase in the alkaline phosphatase value is 2.3 times the upper limit of normal. The alkaline phosphatase concentration represents the most important laboratory feature distinguishing between patients with and without involvement of the liver. The concentration of C-reactive protein is also significantly higher in patients whose livers are involved (Gertz and Kyle 1997). Although it has been suggested that patients with hepatic amyloidosis have a predilection for κ light chains, this is not in accord with our data, which continue to demonstrate λ preponderance, even with exclusively liver involvement. In our experience, liver biopsy is not a high-risk procedure, even though reports of major morbidities exist after percutaneous needle biopsy of amyloid.

The use of serum amyloid P component scanning demonstrates hepatic deposits of amyloid in virtually all patients, but clinically important deposits are far less common. Cholestatic jaundice, when seen, is a preterminal finding. Portal hypertension has been reported with varices and bleeding but is seen rarely in hepatic amyloidosis. The reason for this is unknown, but a reasonable supposition is that death ensues from extrahepatic amyloidosis before the development of portal hypertension. Ascites is common in amyloidosis, but this is usually a consequence of nephrotic syndrome and hypoalbuminemia with associated congestive heart failure and is generally not associated with hepatic involvement and portal hypertension. Liver biopsy shows perisinusoidal and portal deposition in most instances. Vascular involvement of the portal triads is seen frequently but is not a clinically important feature of hepatic amyloidosis. The median survival after diagnosis would be approximately 1 year.

The scintigraphic findings in amyloidosis of the liver are nonspecific and demonstrate irregular distribution of radionuclide and the occasional absence of splenic uptake. Standard imaging is not considered useful. Angiography demonstrates luminal irregularity and abrupt changes in the caliber of the branches of the hepatic artery, which are presumed related to compression by sinusoidal amyloid deposition. Estimates of the risk of complications from biopsy of the liver range from 0.31% to 3%. The presence of amyloidosis is not a contraindication to biopsy if it is clinically indicated. Spontaneous rupture after biopsy has not been reported in AL. In our hands, however, biopsy of the subcutaneous fat or the bone marrow yields a diagnosis in 90%, and only the remaining 10% require direct biopsy of the liver.

Patients with amyloidosis have been treated with transjugular intrahepatic portal systemic shunting. This decrease in portal pressures was reported to resolve ascites and hydrothorax. In 1 patient, bilateral nephrectomy performed for uncontrolled nephrotic syndrome improved liver function and normalized a markedly increased bilirubin value. The presence of hepatic involvement does not adversely affect the prognosis in amyloidosis. In a multivariate analysis, the presence of hepatomegaly had a significant impact on survival in the first year after diagnosis. This apparent contradiction is explained by the recognition that hepatomegaly may be due to congestive heart failure rather than anatomic involvement of the liver. In one study, hepatomegaly was reported due to passive congestion of the liver without hepatic amyloid in 3 of 9 patients at autopsy. Levy et al. found that 20% of patients with amyloidosis and palpable hepatomegaly did not have parenchymal amyloid at autopsy.

The presence of hyposplenism on the blood smear is specific for splenic amyloidosis. Conversely, the absence of hyposplenism is not a reliable indicator that the spleen is not involved. In one report, 12 patients with known diffuse splenic involvement did not show peripheral blood film evidence of hyposplenism. Technetium scanning, as noted, can demonstrate a marked reduction in splenic blood flow due to amyloid infiltration, but this correlates poorly with the presence of Howell-Jolly bodies. In summary, the cardinal features of hepatic amyloidosis are: 1) hepatomegaly with increased alkaline phosphatase value and minimal change in the transaminases, 2) proteinuria, 3) the presence of a monoclonal protein in the serum or the urine, and 4) the presence of hyposplenism.

7.6.4 Gastrointestinal Tract

Most patients with amyloidosis have amyloid deposits in the gastrointestinal tract on screening biopsy (Kyle et al. 1966). Most intestinal deposits are exclusively vascular, are present in the submucosa, and do not produce symptoms. Few patients with AL present with symptoms referable to the gastrointestinal tract. The presence of anorexia and weight loss correlates poorly with the presence of gastrointestinal tract amyloid deposits. Malabsorption, as defined by a low serum carotene value, is seen in less than 5% of patients with amyloid. Likewise, steatorrhea is seen in less than 5% of patients.

Symptoms of intestinal amyloid include intestinal pseudo-obstruction in many instances, and many patients have been reported for whom surgical intervention was undertaken for obstruction, only to have amyloid demonstrated at laparotomy. The symptoms of pseudo-obstruction are nausea and vomiting. Emesis usually results in the detection of undigested food. Abdominal distension and pain are common. Nausea is present even when fasting. The dysfunction of the gastrointestinal tract can result from direct mucosal infiltration or from dysmotility, a consequence of autonomic failure. The steatorrhea associated with amyloid clinically resembles malabsorption due to celiac disease, Whipple disease, or bacterial overgrowth.

We (Hayman et al. 2001b) reported on 19 patients with small bowel biopsy proof of amyloidosis of the AL type. This represented 1% of our total patient population, although we have seen many patients with clinical evidence of malabsorption for whom small bowel biopsy was not undertaken. The most common presenting symptoms were diarrhea, anorexia, dizziness, and abdominal pain. All patients had weight loss, with a median loss of 30 pounds. More than half had orthostatic hypotension. Intestinal malabsorption of vitamin K, leading to prolongation of the prothrombin time, was seen in one-fourth of the patients. A reduction in the value of factor X was seen in one-fourth of the patients. Only 1 patient had factor X activity of less than 30%. There was a poor concordance between intestinal amyloid and the presence of hepatic amyloid. Fewer than one-third of the patients had any increase of the serum alkaline phosphatase value, and only 15% had hepatomegaly. Therefore, intestinal involvement often occurs without involvement of the liver.

Imaging studies are generally not helpful in the diagnosis. Barium studies of the upper gastrointestinal tract occasionally demonstrate esophageal dysmotility or gastroesophageal reflux. Dilatation of the small bowel consistent with pseudo-obstruction is seen only rarely. The small bowel barium study reveals thickening or nodularity, dilatation with delayed transit, and increased fluid accumulation. Abdominal computed tomography is not helpful and shows mild splenomegaly or lymphadenopathy occasionally. Endoscopic procedures can demonstrate esophagitis, duodenitis, and gastritis but results are frequently normal.

In our experience, the median delay from symptomatic onset to histologic diagnosis of amyloidosis was 7 months, but in 1 patient the diagnosis required 4 years. Laparotomy was performed in 4 of the 19 patients, and in 3 of these 4, the diagnosis was not immediately made because Congo red stains were not performed on tissue taken at laparotomy. The hemoglobin value at diagnosis and weight loss had a significant influence on survival. Patients with a greater than 20-pound weight loss had a median survival of 10 months. Nutritional failure was the cause of death in 55% of our patients. One-fourth died of heart failure due to cardiac amyloid.

Occasionally, amyloidosis can present as ischemic colitis. In these patients, the amyloid deposits are obstructing the vessels of the laminae propria and muscularis mucosae. This leads to chronic mucosal ischemia with sloughing of the lining and hemorrhage. In these patients, radiographic studies demonstrate luminal narrowing, thickening of mucosal folds, and ulcerations. These are most often seen in the descending and rectosigmoid colon. Duodenal perforation caused by vascular obstruction as a result of amyloid has been reported. Once intestinal pseudo-obstruction develops, treatment of the underlying amyloid does not result in recovery of intestinal propulsion. Histologically, extensive replacement of the muscularis propria by amyloid is particularly prominent in the small intestine.

7.6.5 Nervous System

Amyloid involvement of the peripheral nervous system was first described in 1938. The frequency of neuropathy in AL ranges from 15% to 20%. Typically, patients with peripheral neuropathy are minimally symptomatic, and their clinical picture is overshadowed by concomitant cardiac or renal involvement. It is important in those patients whose presentation is predominantly neuropathy that consideration be given to the possibility of a familial amyloidosis syndrome. The finding of a monoclonal protein in the serum or urine is key, because this would not be expected in patients with a nonimmunoglobulin form of amyloidosis.

The standard for diagnosing amyloid neuropathy is the sural nerve biopsy, but the majority of patients with clinical and electromyographic evidence of peripheral neuropathy can be diagnosed by less invasive methods. The most frequent symptoms of amyloid neuropathy are paresthesias, muscle weakness, numbness, pain, orthostatic symptoms, urinary retention, and impotence. Syncope is seen in only 12% of patients. In one-fourth of patients, the peripheral neuropathy has a dysesthetic component manifested by a distal burning sensation. The lower extremities are involved first in nearly 90% of the patients, and symptoms of autonomic neuropathy are seen in two-thirds. Although rare, cranial nerve involvement has been reported in amyloidosis. Carpal tunnel syndrome is recognized in more than half of patients who have amyloid peripheral neuropathy, although it is occasionally difficult to recognize carpal tunnel syndrome when the neuropathic symptoms involve the upper extremities. One-third of patients have significant weight loss.

In patients presenting with amyloid peripheral neuropathy, the echocardiogram is abnormal in 44%. Renal involvement at the time of diagnosis of amyloid peripheral neuropathy is uncommon, occurring in approximately 5% of patients. The neuropathy of amyloid is demyelinating and results in increased cerebrospinal fluid protein in one-third of patients. Typical electromyographic changes consist of decreased amplitude of compound muscle action potentials, decreased or absent sensory responses, normal or mild slowing of nerve conduction velocity, and presence of fibrillation potentials on needle examination. Axonal degeneration is detected on the electromyogram in 96% of patients.

On sural nerve biopsy, all patients with amyloid neuropathy have deposits surrounding endoneurial capillaries or in the epineurium. There is usually a marked decrease in myelin fiber density and axonal degeneration on examination of teased fibers. The overall median survival of patients who present with dominant neuropathy is 25 months (Rajkumar et al. 1998 b). Chemotherapy rarely results in clinical improvement in the neuropathic symptoms. The neuropathy progresses over time. Marked restriction of mobility ultimately develops in three-fourths of patients, and one-third are ultimately bedridden. In multivariate analysis, the only factor that predicts survival in patients with dominant neuropathy is the serum albumin value. Those with a serum albumin concentration less than 3 g/dL have a median survival of 18 months compared with 31 months in those whose serum albumin value was greater than 3 g/dL (Fig. 7.10).

The presence of autonomic neuropathy associated with peripheral neuropathy is an important diagnostic clue in amyloidosis. Usually only diabetes produces significant autonomic features in association with peripheral neuropathy. The diagnosis is frequently delayed. The median duration of symptoms before diagnosis is 29 months. Sadly, this is longer than the median survival after diagnosis. It is critical that all patients with a peripheral neuropathy have screening immunofixation performed for the serum and urine. The finding of a monoclonal light chain restricts the differential diagnosis to monoclonal gammopathy of undetermined significance (MGUS)-associated neuropathy; polyneuropathy, organomegaly, endocrinopathy, M protein, and skin changes (POEMS) syndrome; and cryoglobulinemia.

We have seen patients with amyloid neuropathy who presented with a normal electromyogram, because amyloid preferentially causes loss of small myelinated fibers and unmyelinated fibers, and electromyography is better at detecting changes in large myelinated fibers. Patients can have symptoms and paresthesias with a normal electromyogram. In the hands of others, the sural nerve biopsy is not 100% sensitive for the diagnosis of amyloidosis; 9 patients have been reported, in 6 of whom a sural nerve biopsy showed no amyloid. Occasionally, amyloid may deposit at the level of the nerve root, which leads to distal demyelination without amyloid deposits distally in the sural nerve. Multiple sections of the sural nerve need to be examined because the deposits can be focal.

7.6.6 Respiratory Tract

Involvement of the respiratory tract usually is asymptomatic and does not typically cause clinical problems. In most patients who have histologic evidence of lung involvement, the symptoms are overshadowed by the usual concomitant presence of cardiac involvement. Histopathologic demonstration of the alveolar or interstitial deposits of amyloid is uncommon, and gas exchange generally is preserved until late in the disease. We reported our experience on histologically proven pulmonary amyloid (Utz et al. 1996). Of 55 patients seen, 20 had localized forms of pulmonary amyloid (Gertz et al. 1993), primarily nodular pulmonary amyloidosis not associated with systemic disease and associated with a benign prognosis. Patients with tracheobronchial amyloidosis were treated with neodymium:yttrium-aluminum-garnet (YAG) laser therapy or low-dose radiation for obstructive symptoms. Thirty-five patients had pul-

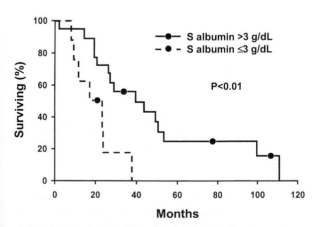

Fig. 7.10. The impact of serum (*S*) albumin on the survival of patients with isolated amyloid peripheral neuropathy. (From Rajkumar et al. [1998 b]. By permission of Excerpta Medica.)

monary involvement as part of a systemic immunoglobulin light chain amyloidosis. These patients presented radiographically as having an interstitial or reticulonodular pattern with or without pleural effusion. The median survival after diagnosis was 16 months. Bronchoscopic lung biopsy was a safe and effective diagnostic technique and was not associated with excessive bleeding.

The chest radiograph in pulmonary amyloidosis is not specific and simply reflects an interstitial process that can be misinterpreted as lower lobe fibrosis. Involvement of the minor salivary glands with amyloid is common. Histologic evidence of salivary gland involvement in amyloidosis is present in a high proportion, and a high proportion of patients report xerostomia. These patients have been misdiagnosed as having Sjögren syndrome. There appears to be a higher prevalence of pulmonary amyloidosis in patients whose amyloid is associated with an IgM monoclonal gammopathy or Waldenström macroglobulinemia (Gertz et al. 1993). Only diffuse interstitial pulmonary amyloid is associated with a monoclonal gammopathy. Monoclonal proteins are not associated with either tracheobronchial or nodular pulmonary amyloidosis. Dyspnea is a common symptom, usually cardiac in origin, but may also be due to disrupted gas exchange from interstitial amyloid. We found that low doses of prednisone produced symptomatic although not objective radiographic benefit.

In an autopsy study, pulmonary involvement was found in 11 of 12 patients with AL. Pathologically, the deposition of amyloid occurs in blood vessel walls and the alveolar septum. In these 12, clinical dyspnea was present in only 4 and was responsible for death in 1. Hemoptysis was reported in diffuse alveolar septal amyloid. Rarely, ventilatory failure was reported as a result of generalized muscular weakness and diaphragmatic involvement. Diffuse amyloid infiltration of the skeletal muscles and diaphragm was reported. Pleural infiltration with amyloid can produce pleural effusions. We have seen pulmonary hypertension with right-sided cardiac failure as a rare complication (Dingli et al. 2001). These patients had occlusive amyloid deposits in the pulmonary arteriolar circulation. None had echocardiographic evidence of left ventricular dysfunction. The median survival time in patients with pulmonary hypertension was 2.8 years. The mainstay of therapy is the administration of vasodilators with calcium channel blockers. However, patients with amyloidosis frequently are intolerant of these medications because of concomitant orthostatic hypotension. The diagnosis of pulmonary hypertension should be considered in patients with AL and unexplained dyspnea or fluid overload who have normal left ventricular diastolic and systolic function.

7.6.7 Coagulation System

Bleeding can be a serious complication of amyloidosis. Deficiency of factor X is well recognized (Greipp et al. 1981) but the most common manifestation of hemorrhage is purpura related to fragility of blood vessels resulting from the infiltration of the vessel wall by amyloid. Factor X deficiency is seen in less than 5% of patients. In a review, 8.7% of amyloid patients had factor X values less than 50%. Serious bleeding was seen only in patients whose factor X value was less than 25% of normal. Factor X deficiency is virtually always limited to those patients who have advanced hepatosplenic amyloidosis. Improvement in factor X values has been reported with splenectomy, the use of oral melphalan-prednisone, and stem cell transplantation. The most common abnormality of hemostasis in vitro is a prolonged thrombin time (Gastineau et al. 1991a). This appears to be related to an inhibitor of fibrin polymerization circulating in the plasma. Platelet defects including abnormal platelet aggregation have been reported, as have decreased levels of a_2-plasmin inhibitor and increased levels of plasminogen. Life-threatening bleeding is uncommon, with the exception of those patients who have a severe deficiency of factor X or those with ischemic colitis due to vascular obstruction in the bowel.

Thirty-six consecutive patients with biopsy-proven amyloidosis and monoclonal immunoglobulin light chains had coagulation studies. Hemorrhagic manifestations were mild to moderate in 9 and severe in only 1. Again, the most frequent laboratory abnormalities were prolongation of the thrombin time and the reptilase time. Severe depression of factor X was observed in only 1. The prothrombin times were prolonged in 8, and the activated partial thromboplastin time, in 25. No lupus anticoagulant was found.

The medical records of 2,132 patients with biopsy-proven AL were reviewed to identify patients with documented thromboembolism. Patients who had stroke, peripheral vascular disease, and myocardial infarction were excluded. Twenty-one males and 19 females were identified who had experienced an objectively documented thromboembolism. The median age was 65 years. In 11 of the 40, thromboembolism preceded the diagnosis of amyloid. In 9 of the 11, the event occurred 1 month or more before the diagnosis of amyloid. In 20 of 40 patients, thromboembolism occurred 1 month or more after the diagnosis of AL. Twenty-nine of the 40 had venous thrombosis: 15 calf, 5 subclavian, 3 popliteal, 3 inferior vena cava, 1 common femoral, and 1 arteriovenous fistula. Eleven of 40 had arterial thrombosis: 4 femoral, 1 popliteal, multiple arteries of the lower extremities in 2, and the atria in 2. Thirty-seven of the 40 patients had at least 1 additional risk factor for thrombosis, including nephrotic syndrome in 20, immobilization in 13, tobacco use in 6, heart failure in 8, estrogen use in 1, obesity in 4, aortic aneurysm in 1, prosthetic material in 4, and disseminated intravascular coagulation in 2. Five of the patients had detectable activated protein C resistance.

Eight patients died within 1 month after the thrombotic event. Eighteen of the 40 died within 1 year after the thrombotic event. The development of thrombosis in patients with AL appears to predict a significant mortality within the first month and year after the event. There were no characteristics of the distribution of the amyloid or of the type of light and heavy chain that predicted other than the development of thromboembolic events. The use of recombinant human factor VIIa in the management of amyloid-associated factor X deficiency was reported in a 63-year-old woman whose factor X value ranged between 4% and 10%. Recombinant human factor VIIa was administered preoperatively and every 3 hours postoperatively for 48 hours after a splenectomy. Recombinant human factor VIIa appears to be a safe and effective means of controlling bleeding in amyloid-associated factor X deficiency to allow for more definitive interventions.

7.7 Prognosis

When a patient presents with a syndrome compatible with amyloidosis and is found to have a monoclonal protein and the diagnosis is confirmed histologically (usually with fat aspiration or bone marrow biopsy), the next step is to assess the patient's prognosis. We (Gertz et al. 1991b) reviewed 153 patients with AL; the median survival of the group was 20 months, with a 5-year survival of 20%. Patients with overt congestive

heart failure had a median survival of 8 months, with a 5-year survival of 2.4%. Patients with the best outcome had amyloid neuropathy as the sole manifestation of their disease (median survival of 40 months and 5-year survival of 32%). The clinical classification of patients in the 4 groups (heart failure, nephrotic syndrome, peripheral neuropathy, and other) is useful for assessing long-term prognosis. There is a trend for superior survival in female patients. Heart failure, Howell-Jolly bodies on the peripheral blood film, bone marrow plasma cells >30%, free urine light chains, and circulating plasma cells are all adverse predictors of survival.

Kyle and Greipp (1983) reviewed 229 patients with AL and identified heart failure and orthostatic hypotension as being associated with a median survival of less than 1 year. Peripheral neuropathy, excluding patients with heart failure and nephrotic syndrome, was associated with a survival of 56 months. The coexistence of multiple myeloma had an adverse impact on survival. Jaw claudication (Gertz et al. 1986), which results from narrowing or obstruction of the facial branches of the external carotid artery with amyloid, can be seen in as many as 9% of patients with AL. The median survival for these patients is 42 months compared with 12 months for other patients. Patients who present with jaw claudication tend to have predominantly vascular deposits of amyloid and soft tissue nonvisceral deposits, including amyloid arthropathy and tongue enlargement (Salvarani et al. 1994).

Patients who are functionally hyposplenic, defined by the presence of Howell-Jolly bodies on the peripheral blood smear, had a median survival of 4.4 months (Gertz et al. 1983). The presence of hyposplenism is a marker for advanced hepatic and splenic involvement. The survival of 80 patients diagnosed by liver biopsy was 9 months, with a 5-year survival of 13%. Duston et al. reported on 51 patients with AL and peripheral neuropathy. Survival after diagnosis was 35 months, which was better than for patients presenting with other features of amyloidosis.

The cause of death in most patients with amyloidosis is cardiac related, either congestive heart failure caused by progressive cardiomyopathy or sudden death caused by ventricular fibrillation or asystole. The clinical outcome is driven by the extent of cardiac involvement, and echocardiography is an important part of the assessment of all patients with AL. Although only 17% of patients have overt heart failure at diagnosis, nearly 40% have echocardiographic abnormalities demonstrable by 2-dimensional and Doppler studies. Klein and Tajik (1991) studied 64 patients with AL and found that in early amyloidosis relaxation was abnormal, but in advanced amyloidosis, there was restrictive filling with a shortened deceleration time. The typical restrictive filling pattern of amyloid heart disease is seen in advanced stages only. Diastolic dysfunction in cardiac amyloid can be monitored serially using Doppler echocardiography (Klein et al. 1991). Patients can be divided into 2 groups on the basis of their deceleration time: either 150 ms or less (including restriction) or more than 150 ms. The 1-year survival of patients with a shortened deceleration time was 49% compared with 92% in those with greater than 150-ms deceleration time. The Doppler-derived left ventricular diastolic filling variables are important independent prognostic indicators in AL.

Doppler studies of right ventricular diastolic function have been reported. Filling abnormalities correlate well with the degree of amyloid infiltration measured by right ventricular free wall thickness. Restrictive physiology is seen in the advanced stages of the disease, and abnormal relaxation is seen in the earlier stages of the disease.

Surian et al. reviewed the findings and renal biopsy specimens from patients with amyloidosis. A better prognosis was associated with a lower percentage of glomerular capillary wall thickening, a higher incidence of amyloid deposits in vessels but not in glomerular capillaries, and deposits of IgG and C3 in mesangial and glomerular capillary walls. As noted previously, the serum creatinine concentration has a strong influence on survival. Urinary light chain excretion and serum creatinine concentration are powerful prognostic indicators. Patients with any increase in serum creatinine value have a reduced survival of 15 months. Patients who have a free light chain in the urine have a shorter survival than those who do not: 12 versus 35 months.

The presence of exertional syncope is a powerful predictor of imminent sudden death and is usually an indication for the placement of an implantable defibrillator, because most patients die within 2 months.

The plasma cell labeling index is a test capable of measuring the proliferative potential of bone marrow plasma cells in patients with AL. More than 95% of patients with amyloidosis have a demonstrable clonal excess of plasma cells in the bone marrow. When bone marrow and labeling index measurements were performed in 125 patients with AL, the median survival of patients with a labeling index of 0 (none of 500 plasma cells in the S phase of the cell cycle) was 30 months. Patients who had any plasma cells actively synthesizing DNA (labeling index greater than 0) had a median survival of 15 months (Gertz et al. 1989b).

One hundred forty-seven patients with biopsy-proven AL had peripheral blood mononuclear cells analyzed for the presence of cytoplasmic immunoglobulin-positive plasma cells by a sensitive slide-based immunofluorescent technique. Circulating monoclonal plasma cells were quantified as a percentage of circulating cytoplasmic immunoglobulin positive cells. Sixteen percent of patients had detectable circulating peripheral blood plasma cells. The median survival of patients with circulating cells was 10 months compared with 29 months for patients without circulating cells (McElroy et al. 1998). In a multivariate analysis (McElroy et al. 1998), peripheral blood plasma cells and serum β_2-microglobulin were independent prognostic factors for survival. The survival impact of peripheral blood plasma cells remains when patients with coexisting myeloma and dominant cardiac amyloidosis are excluded from the analysis. The prognostic value of circulating peripheral blood plasma cells may be an important consideration in selecting treatment options for patients with AL.

The median survival of patients with an increased serum β_2-microglobulin value at presentation was 11 months compared with 33 months in patients with a normal β_2-microglobulin value. The predictive survival value of an increased β_2-microglobulin concentration is independent of the presence of heart failure and renal insufficiency. In patients who have completely normal renal function, the median survival of patients with an increased β_2-microglobulin value was 9 months compared with 39 months for those patients with a normal β_2-microglobulin level. A combination of the β_2-microglobulin value and the presence or absence of circulating plasma cells allows patients to be classified into 3 separate groups with median survivals of 42, 21, and 4 months, respectively ($P<0.0001$) (Gertz et al. 1990).

The time between histologic diagnosis and referral for evaluation is an important prognostic variable. In patients with amyloidosis evaluated at Mayo Clinic, the median survival is nearly 2 years. However, when patients evaluated within 30 days of diagnosis are considered, the median survival is approximately 13 months. This suggests that there is referral bias that favors those patients physically able to come to a large amyloidosis treatment center. This type of information is important when interpreting the results of a clinical trial from 1 center (Kyle and Gertz 1995).

In a multivariate analysis of prognostic factors, the median survival of the entire group was 12 months, ranging from 4 months for those with heart failure to 50 months for those with peripheral neuropathy. The presence of congestive heart failure, a urinary monoclonal light chain, hepatomegaly, or multiple myeloma was an adverse factor affecting survival during the first year after diagnosis. After the first year, an increased serum creatinine concentration and the presence of multiple myeloma, orthostatic hypotension, and a monoclonal serum protein became predictors of poor survival. Stratification for the impact of these variables on survival is important when studies of therapy are compared. In summary, all patients being assessed for amyloidosis need echocardiography, including measures of diastolic performance, ejection fraction, and mitral deceleration time. The serum β_2-microglobulin value and the presence of overt congestive heart failure remain important predictors of outcome (Fig. 7.11) (Kyle et al. 1986).

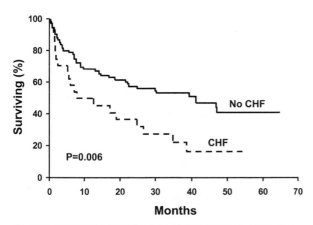

Fig. 7.11. Impact of congestive heart failure (*CHF*) on survival in patients with amyloidosis. (From Gertz M [2003] Multiple myeloma and amyloidosis. In Straus D [ed] The educational review manual in medical oncology – 2003. Castle Connolly Graduate Medical Publishing, New York. By permission of the publisher.)

7.8 Therapy

7.8.1 Adjunctive and Supportive Therapy for Systemic Amyloid

7.8.1.1 Cardiac Amyloid

The mainstay of the treatment of cardiac amyloidosis is a diuretic agent. Because many patients have associated orthostatic hypotension and intravascular volume contraction due to concomitant nephrotic syndrome, diuretic therapy is difficult. It is often associated with syncope and decreased renal blood flow, with an associated increase in serum creatinine concentration. Permanent pacemaker implantation may be required in patients with recurrent syncope (Mathew et al. 1997a, b). Afterload reduction using angiotensin-converting enzyme inhibitors is standard management of heart failure. Whether these agents have any role and provide similar improvements in survival in patients with amyloid remains unknown. The high frequency of hypotension is challenging for the use of therapeutic doses of angiotensin-converting enzyme inhibitors.

Doses of furosemide as high as 120 mg 3 times per day may be necessary for control of edema. When furosemide alone fails to control edema, the addition of metolazone can be beneficial. Digoxin is not generally helpful because systolic dysfunction is seen only late in the course of cardiac amyloidosis, and digoxin has no beneficial effect on the restrictive physiology and reduced diastolic filling seen in these patients. Calcium channel blockers such as nifedipine and diltiazem can aggravate the congestive heart failure in patients with AL. Studies have shown that nifedipine binds selectively to amyloid fibrils and results in higher intracellular concentrations of this agent (Gertz et al. 1985). Angiotensin-converting enzyme inhibitors (captopril, enalapril, and lisinopril) can reduce the afterload in patients with cardiac amyloid and have been shown to reduce mortality in patients with congestive cardiomyopathy on an ischemic basis. There have been reports of lisinopril resulting in reductions in proteinuria in patients with amyloid nephrotic syndrome.

The orthostatic hypotension associated with amyloidosis can be treated in part with fludrocortisone acetate in doses of 0.1 mg orally 2 to 3 times a day. Higher doses (0.4 to 2 mg daily) have also been used with success. This agent is poorly tolerated in elderly patients treated for hypotensive disorders and results in significant supine hypertension, fluid retention that can aggravate cardiac failure, edema, and severe degrees of hypokalemia. A second agent that has been used regularly to treat the hypotension in amyloidosis patients is midodrine. The recommended dose is 10 mg 3 times daily at approximately 4-hour intervals. Dosing should take place primarily during the daytime hours to avoid supine hypertension before sleep. The drug is rapidly absorbed from the gastrointestinal tract, with peak serum levels observed in 30 minutes. The dose is usually initiated at 2.5 mg and then increased as a function of therapeutic response in increments of 2.5 mg daily; the maximum recommended dose is 40 mg. The drug should be started at a lower dose in patients with renal insufficiency because active metabolites are excreted by the kidney. Side effects include tachycardia, supine hypertension, and restlessness.

Cardiac transplantation has been used for patients with isolated heart involvement with AL. Hosenpud et al. studied 7 patients with a mean age of 46 years who had transplantation for cardiac amyloid. Recurrent amyloid developed in the allograft in 2 patients at 3½ and 4 months; 1 of the 2 died 13 months after transplantation. There was 1 immediate postoperative death. Five patients were alive at a mean of 32 months after transplantation. One patient with AL who had transplantation was in functional class I 1 year later but had demonstrable amyloid deposits by electron microscopy 14 weeks after transplantation. A follow-up study of 10 patients with cardiac amyloid who had transplantation revealed recurrent amyloid in the allograft, and 4 of 9 patients survived for more than 1 month. One patient with AL survived 9 years after cardiac transplantation.

Ten patients with a mean age of 54 years received transplants during the 13-year period from 1984 to 1997. Two died perioperatively; the mean follow-up in the remaining 8 patients was 50 months. Recurrent amyloid deposits in the cardiac allografts were demonstrable in 5 patients at 5, 11, 12, 28, and 30 months posttransplantation. There was no echocardiographic evidence of infiltrative cardiomyopathy. Seven patients died between 3 and 116 months (median, 32 months) after transplantation. Four of the 7 deaths were related to extracardiac amyloid deposits. The 1-year actuarial survival was 60%; the 5-year actuarial survival, 30%. The high perioperative mortality of 20% is, in part, related to extracardiac amyloid. Heart transplantation is technically feasible but does require treatment of the underlying amyloidosis.

A 47-year-old woman was hospitalized with congestive heart failure. She had IgGλ cardiac amyloidosis. She received a heart transplant followed 6 months later by a stem cell transplant conditioned with melphalan (200 mg/m²). The latter was designed to prevent recurrent disease. Post stem cell transplantation, she had persistent thrombocytopenia of 25,000 cells/μL. The IgGλ monoclonal component decreased but was persistent. The patient died suddenly 2 years post stem cell transplantation, and her myocardium showed mild deposits of amyloid. At Mayo Clinic, 13 patients have received cardiac transplants. The long-term survival is statistically inferior to that of patients with nonamyloid heart disease, but the actuarial 5-year survival appears to be 50%, which is reasonable. We have done stem cell transplantations on 4 of these patients in an effort to prevent recurrent disease, and 2 of the 4 remain alive.

7.8.1.2 Renal Amyloid

In patients with renal amyloidosis, diuretics help control their edema. The outcome of hemodialysis in AL patients is inferior to the results seen in patients on dialysis as a result of primary renal disorders. The European experience has shown a 76% 2-year survival for all patients compared with only 53% in amyloidosis patients. In 1984, the first patient with amyloidosis and end-stage renal disease received continuous ambulatory peritoneal dialysis. In this early report, 3 of 3 patients were alive for 10 to 18 months. One patient subsequently received a renal transplant and survived 57 months. At autopsy, widespread deposits of amyloid were found.

The dialysis experience in 61 patients with amyloidosis revealed that 18 died within 1 month after the initiation of therapy; 43 patients had dialysis for more than 1 month (Gertz et al. 1992 a). There was no survival difference between hemodialysis and chronic ambulatory peritoneal dialysis. Younger patients had a better 5-year survival. Fifteen of the 43 patients were alive at a median of 61 months after dialysis began. The most important complications were the development of cardiac and gastrointestinal tract amyloid. We have not seen any survival difference between hemodialysis and peritoneal dialysis in our practice. Two-thirds of the deaths in our patients who were dialyzed were due to extrarenal progression of amyloid, the majority having cardiac amyloid.

The literature on renal transplantation in amyloidosis is scarce. Most reports originate from Europe and cover patients with AA. In a report of 12 patients, 2 of whom had AL, at 2 years after transplantation, 4 of the 12 were alive, and in 2 of the 4, the renal biopsy specimens showed amyloid deposits. Recurrence of amyloid in the transplanted kidney is well recognized. In a study of 11 amyloid patients who received transplants, 3 showed amyloid recurrence in the grafts at 11, 28, and 37 months. In 2 patients with AL who received a renal transplant, 1 patient developed deposition of amyloid in the transplanted kidney, resulting in renal failure and death. The second patient developed cardiac amyloidosis and died with good allograft function. In a study of 45 patients with amyloid who received a kidney transplant, the 3-year survival of the patients with amyloid was 51% and inferior to that of patients who received transplants for primary renal diseases. Age older than 40 years was the major factor determining poor survival. The median age of an AL patient is 62 years. Recurrence of amyloid in the transplanted kidney was established histologically in 4 patients. The estimate was that the recipient of a renal transplant had at a minimum a 20% chance of recurrence of amyloid at 1 year. Evidence of renal graft amyloid was sought by serum amyloid P scintigraphy in 15 patients with systemic amyloid who had undergone renal transplantation (Gillmore et al. 2000).

In a study from Scandinavia, 2 AL patients received transplants; renal biopsy specimens from the patients showed amyloid deposits. There were no factors that predicted recurrence of amyloid in the graft. Dorman et al. described 2 AL patients who received renal transplants. Glomerular amyloid developed in the first, resulting in failure of the transplanted kidney and ultimately the patient's death. The second patient died of progressive cardiac amyloidosis. Pasternack et al. published their results on 45 patients with amyloidosis who received a kidney transplant. The 3-year survival of the amyloidosis patients was 51%, inferior to that of patients with primary glomerular disease. Age older than 40 years was a major factor predicting poor survival. Recurrence of amyloid in a transplanted kidney was established histologically in 4 patients at 11 to 37 months posttransplantation. In patients surviving for 1 year, there was a minimum chance of 20% of acquiring amyloid in the transplanted kidney.

Angiotensin-converting enzyme inhibitors appear to reduce proteinuria in patients with nephrotic syndrome by producing a postglomerular vasodilatation. This can be complicated by severe hyperkalemia, and caution is required in monitoring. Enalapril decreased proteinuria in steroid-resistant nephrotic syndrome in focal and segmental glomerulosclerosis. The mechanism of action is thought to be renal hemodynamic and may be effective in amyloid nephropathy as well.

7.8.1.3 Gastrointestinal Tract Amyloid

The gastrointestinal tract is a common site for amyloid deposition. The most frequent symptom is alternating diarrhea and constipation. In most patients, this is due to autonomic failure, but in a small subset, massive deposits in the gastrointestinal tract result in a sprue-like syndrome. Loperamide, diphenoxylate, tincture of opium, and paregoric should be used but produce variable results. Octreotide (somatostatin analog) decreases diarrhea but requires multiple injections per day in the short-acting form, usually 200 to 300 μg divided in 2 to 3 doses. This agent also is provided in the long-acting depository form in 10-, 20-, and 30-mg doses in which an intergluteal dose can be administered every 4 weeks for 2 months and then every 4 weeks according to the response of the diarrhea. Three patients with amyloidosis were totally disabled as a result of diarrhea and fecal incontinence. In all 3 patients, ostomies were placed as a palliative intervention, with excellent patient satisfaction.

An occasional patient will have severe intestinal dysmotility that can only be managed with long-term total parenteral nutrition. Cisapride has been reported to be effective for treating chronic intestinal pseudo-obstruction, but we have not found cholinergic agents, metoclopramide, or cisapride to be effective.

7.8.2 Nonchemotherapy Treatment of AL

7.8.2.1 DMSO (Dimethyl Sulfoxide)

DMSO can solubilize amyloid deposits in vitro. In a mouse model of AA, DMSO produced partial resolution of amyloid deposits. When DMSO was added to the drinking water of mice with AA, existing deposits regressed. The best results with DMSO have been after its topical application in patients with cutaneous amyloidosis and after intravesical instillation in patients with localized urinary bladder amyloidosis. The results of DMSO therapy for patients with visceral disease remain inconclusive, and this agent is infrequently used in the management of amyloidosis.

7.8.2.2 Colchicine

Familial Mediterranean fever (FMF) is a unique form of autosomal dominant inherited amyloidosis characterized by recurrent peritonitis, pleuritis, synovitis, or migratory skin rash. The disorder commonly affects Sephardic Jews, Armenians, Arabs, and those of Turkish descent. There is no relationship between the appearance of attacks and the development of amyloidosis. Amyloidosis develops in a significant proportion of patients, although there is no relationship between the frequency of attacks and the development of amyloid. One-fourth of patients in whom amyloidosis develops have no history of polyserositis or arthritis. Twenty-five percent of renal amyloid diagnosed in the Middle East is related to FMF. Before the introduction of colchicine, the median survival of patients who had FMF amyloid was 25 months, with a 5-year survival of 20%. The clinical manifestations of amyloidosis seen in FMF are proteinuria-nephrotic syndrome and dialysis-dependent renal insufficiency.

Two double-blind placebo-controlled trials showed the efficacy of colchicine in preventing attacks of familial amyloidosis. In one study, the frequency of attacks was reduced by 82%, and in a second study serositis attacks decreased by 78%. Once colchicine was introduced for prevention of polyserositis, it was assessed for its value in preventing amyloidosis. Colchicine decreased the incidence of renal amyloid by nearly two-thirds, and the development of amyloidosis is infrequent in patients who are compliant with colchicine therapy. Colchicine is even capable of reversing the proteinuria in patients with established renal amyloid. Colchicine is capable of preventing deterioration of renal function. Of 350 children younger than age 16 years given prophylactic colchicine, amyloidosis did not develop. It has also been used after renal transplantation in FMF patients with end-stage renal disease to prevent recurrent disease. The agent is safe in children and pregnant women. In view of the success of colchicine in treating and preventing the amyloidosis associated with FMF, it was used in patients with AL. One patient with AL treated with colchicine had a decrease over 2 years in 24-hour urine protein loss from 6.7 to 1.4 g/d.

Fifty-three patients with AL seen at the Clinical Research Center of Boston University School of Medicine received colchicine and were compared with retrospective controls. Female sex and the time from diagnosis to the initiation of colchicine were associated with the

duration of survival. The median survival for colchicine-treated patients was 7 months compared with 6 months for non-colchicine-treated patients. This was not a prospective randomized study, and colchicine is infrequently used today in patients with AL.

7.8.3 Defining Responses in Amyloidosis

Defining responses in amyloidosis is challenging and is typically done using surrogate measurements. Responses to treatment in amyloidosis can be defined by improvement in organ function or by hematologic responses, as is done for patients with multiple myeloma. All patients who have a measurable serum or urine monoclonal protein need to be monitored after any therapeutic intervention for changes in the size of the M peak. For those patients who have only a free light chain that cannot be quantified readily, immunofixation must be performed serially to determine whether the monoclonal protein is present or absent. When M components are measurable, a response, just as in multiple myeloma, requires a 50% reduction in the size of the peak in the serum and in the urine. When M proteins are not measurable, a response requires complete eradication of the light chain by immunofixation in the serum or in the urine. Confirmation with the bone marrow showing less than 5% plasma cells supports the response criteria, although gene rearrangement and immunohistochemical studies frequently reflect the presence of a clonal population, even when the percentage of plasma cells is less than 2%.

Organ-based response criteria have been defined. For patients with amyloid nephrotic syndrome, a 50% reduction in the 24-hour albumin excretion with no increase in serum creatinine or decrease in serum albumin concentration is required. In patients with hepatic involvement, a response requires a 50% reduction in the increased serum alkaline phosphatase value with no increase in transaminase or bilirubin concentration. The liver size may not increase. To define echocardiographic regression of amyloidosis of the heart, a reduction in wall thickness needs to be documented. Because of interprocedural variability, at least a 2-mm decrease in the thickness of the septum or a 20% increase in the ejection fraction is required to define a response. Neuropathic responses can be documented by improved conduction velocities seen on electromyography.

7.8.4 Cytotoxic Chemotherapy in the Treatment of AL

Many case reports documenting the resolution or regression of amyloidosis after cytotoxic chemotherapy first began to appear in the mid 1970s. The rationale for the use of systemic chemotherapy, particularly alkylating agents, was to suppress the plasma cell clone in the bone marrow responsible for the production of the immunoglobulin light chain that deposits as amyloid fibrils. The time to a response with alkylating agent chemotherapy can be long, and one major problem is distinguishing between patients for whom therapy is destined to fail and those for whom an adequate trial has not been completed.

Buxbaum et al. performed in vitro studies on the synthesis of light chains from the plasma cells of a patient with amyloidosis. Light chain tetramers were found in the cytoplasm of the abnormal plasma cells. After alkylating agent-based chemotherapy, light chain synthesis was suppressed and was associated with a clinical response.

Fielder and Durie reported on 34 patients with AL; 7 patients responded to melphalan and prednisone chemotherapy and had a median survival of 28 months. The presence of cardiac amyloid was a powerful predictor of failure to respond to therapy. We also noted a correlation between the level of serum β_2-microglobulin and the likelihood of response. Benson described 7 patients with AL treated with melphalan and prednisone and colchicine. Two died of cardiomyopathy within 5 months of initiating chemotherapy, but 5 were alive 17 to 60 months after the initiation of therapy, and none of them showed progressive disease. Nephrotic syndrome resolved in 2, and liver function improved in 2. Six patients with biopsy-proven amyloid were treated with melphalan and prednisone. Four survived at least 4 years, and 2 died within 3 months after diagnosis. Four of the 6 patients had cardiac involvement, and 2 had renal involvement.

Melphalan-based therapy fails in most patients with amyloidosis. Even in subset analysis, no more than 30% of patients show evidence of a response, and this represents patients with isolated renal involvement and no increase in the serum creatinine concentration. One patient with chronic polyarthritis who was receiving melphalan therapy developed amyloidosis, demonstrating that melphalan could not prevent development of AL. Even in patients who show evidence of organ regression, a follow-up renal biopsy demonstrates persistent amyloid deposits. It is unknown whether clinical improvement is associated with histologic regression, because follow-up biopsies are done infrequently.

When we retrospectively reviewed our own experience with the treatment of amyloidosis, we found that the overall response rate in all patients with carefully defined response criteria was only 18%. When the serum creatinine value exceeded 3 mg/dL, a response rarely occurred, and increased serum creatinine concentration had an adverse impact on survival. In patients with nephrotic syndrome with normal serum creatinine values and a normal echocardiogram, the response rate was 39%. Responses were seen in patients with amyloid cardiomyopathy (15%) (Gertz et al. 1991b). It was rare for patients with symptomatic peripheral neuropathy to derive any clinical benefit from melphalan-based therapy. The median time to response in this study was 1 year; however, the median survival of responders is 89 months, with nearly 78% of the group surviving 5 years. Nonresponders had a median survival of 15 months, suggesting that alkylating agent-based chemotherapy for AL was beneficial and that chemotherapy is a reasonable consideration in all patients.

Over a 21-year period at Mayo Clinic, 841 patients with AL were seen. The actuarial survival for 810 patients was 51% at 1 year, 16% at 5 years, and 4.7% at 10 years. The 30 patients who survived for 10 years after the diagnosis of AL all received alkylating agent therapy. In 14, the monoclonal protein disappeared from the serum or urine. Of 10 patients with nephrotic syndrome, 4 had a 50% reduction in proteinuria. Congestive heart failure, older age, a creatinine value greater than 2 mg/dL, a bone marrow plasma cell percentage greater than 20%, and a platelet count greater than 500×10^9/L were unfavorable prognostic features.

Levy et al. reported on 10 patients with AL; 8 were treated with cyclophosphamide or melphalan, none of whom showed benefit. Four of these patients were subsequently treated with vincristine, doxorubicin, and dexamethasone as a 96-hour infusion. Two of the patients had a 50% reduction in the serum monoclonal protein. This regimen is an option for patients with AL. Its use may be limited as a result of the high proportion of patients with neuropathy or cardiomyopathy for whom VAD is contraindicated.

The first prospective randomized study of chemotherapy in amyloidosis was published in 1978; 55 patients with AL were randomized in a double-blind fashion to therapy with melphalan and prednisone or placebo. Although there was no difference in overall survival, patients given melphalan and prednisone continued on treatment for a longer time and received larger doses of therapy before the code was broken. Nephrotic syndrome disappeared in 2, urinary loss of albumin decreased by more than 50% in 8 others, and there were no responses in the placebo group. Of 13 patients who received 12 months of therapy with melphalan and prednisone, 6 improved, 3 were stable, and 4 had progression.

In a randomized crossover study of melphalan and prednisone versus colchicine, 101 patients were stratified according to their dominant clinical manifestation: congestive heart failure, peripheral neuropathy, nephrotic syndrome, and other. Patients were stratified by age older than or younger than 65 years. Forty-nine patients received melphalan and prednisone. Eight subsequently crossed over to colchicine. Fifty-two patients received colchicine, and 35 crossed over to melphalan and prednisone because of progressive disease. There was no difference in survival, and the 2 groups were analyzed in aggregate. When survival of patients receiving only 1 regimen was analyzed or when survival was analyzed from the time of the study entry to the time of death or progression, significant differences were evident that favored melphalan and prednisone.

A subsequent 3-arm study accrued 219 patients between 1982 and 1992 (Kyle et al. 1997). Patients were randomized to 1 of 3 regimens: 1) colchicine 0.6 mg twice daily with increasing doses to the point of gastrointestinal tract toxicity ($n=72$), 2) melphalan 0.15 mg/kg per day plus prednisone 0.8 mg/kg per day for 7 days every 6 weeks, with dose escalation to produce midcycle myelosuppression ($n=70$), and 3) melphalan plus prednisone plus colchicine, as in regimens 1 and 2 ($n=69$). Patients were stratified by age, sex, and major clinical manifestation. Half the patients had nephrotic-range proteinuria; 20% had congestive heart failure. The median survival for patients receiving melphalan- and prednisone-containing regimens was 17 months versus 8.5 months for colchicine alone. Melphalan-containing regimens were superior to colchicine in the treatment of AL.

A clinical trial randomizing patients to melphalan, prednisone, and colchicine or to colchicine alone stratified patients according to sex, time from diagnosis to study entry, and dominant organ system involvement (Skinner et al. 1996). Fifty patients received colchicine,

and 50 received the combination of all 3 agents. Melphalan and prednisone were given every 6 weeks for 1 year. The overall survival of all patients was 8.4 months, but survival was 6.7 months in the colchicine group and 12.2 months in the melphalan group. There was a survival advantage for those patients whose major system manifestations were either peripheral neuropathy or other. Multivariate analysis showed a significant impact of melphalan-based therapy and the absence of heart failure on survival.

Treatment with melphalan and prednisone is not innocuous. Of 153 melphalan-treated patients, cytogenetic abnormalities developed in the bone marrow in 10, consistent with melphalan damage to hematopoietic stem cells. Eight of the 10 died as a result of pancytopenia. One died of progressive renal amyloid, and 1 patient was alive. Four patients had acute leukemia, nonlymphocytic type, and 5 had myelodysplasia. Overall, significant bone marrow damage developed in 7% of all patients exposed to melphalan. The actuarial risk for myelodysplasia or acute leukemia in patients surviving 3½ years after the diagnosis of AL was 21%. The median survival after the diagnosis of myelodysplasia or leukemia was 8 months.

On the basis of a study in mice suggesting that vitamin E inhibited the development of amyloidosis, we treated 16 patients with vitamin E. None of the patients showed any objective regression of their disease, and the median survival of the group was 19 months. We also treated patients with interferon alfa-2b, and no responses were seen, suggesting this was not a valuable agent in the treatment of AL.

A 45-year-old man was diagnosed as having multiple myeloma, and a diagnosis of amyloidosis was proven in rectal and lip biopsies. Vincristine, doxorubicin, and dexamethasone therapy resulted in an objective response from the myeloma and the amyloidosis. In a patient with nephrotic syndrome, a renal biopsy revealed AL amyloid deposits of λ type. The patient received 4 cycles of vincristine, doxorubicin, and dexamethasone chemotherapy, and the proteinuria rapidly diminished during chemotherapy. Three of 4 patients with light chain amyloid nephrotic syndrome treated with the same chemotherapy obtained a partial response and were alive in remission at 4.1, 6.5, and 9.3 years.

Nine consecutive patients with biopsy-proven AL were treated with pulsed dexamethasone, 40 mg on days 1–4, 9–12, and 17–20, every 5 weeks for 3 to 6 cycles, followed by maintenance interferon, 3 to 6 million units 3 times a week. Three patients received maintenance dexamethasone, 40 mg per day for 4 days each month for 1 year. Improvement in AL organ involvement was seen in 8 of 9 patients. Of 7 with nephrotic-range proteinuria, 6 had a greater than 50% reduction in proteinuria with a median time to response of 4 months. Organ function improvement was seen in patients with gastrointestinal tract, hepatic, and neuropathic involvement. Neither of 2 patients with heart failure improved. This nonleukemogenic regimen leads to faster responses than melphalan and prednisone and may be just as effective (Dhodapkar et al. 1997). However, we treated 19 patients with high-dose dexamethasone in a similar fashion. In this cohort, only 3 of 19 patients showed an objective organ response. The median survival of the entire group was 11.2 months. High-dose dexamethasone is occasionally beneficial in patients without cardiac amyloid involvement. We attempted to use dexamethasone as a salvage regimen in patients who had previously failed to respond to melphalan and prednisone therapy. Twenty-five previously treated patients received high-dose dexamethasone. Three patients showed objective regression with organ-specific improvement of the disease. The median survival of the entire group was 13.8 months. Dexamethasone was occasionally beneficial as a salvage regimen in melphalan-treated patients.

We performed a prospective randomized study of 101 patients with AL to determine if intensified alkylating agent chemotherapy produced results superior to those with standard melphalan and prednisone. Patients were stratified by age, clinical manifestation, and the presence or absence of heart failure. Melphalan and prednisone were compared with vincristine, carmustine, melphalan, cyclophosphamide, and prednisone. At this point, 76 of the 101 patients have died, and the median overall survival for the entire group of 101 patients was 26.4 months. There was no difference between the 2 arms. The survival exceeds that of an unselected group of patients with amyloidosis and reflects the fact that patients who are enrolled in chemotherapy studies of amyloidosis have a better outcome, likely by virtue of their eligibility to participate in a clinical trial. In this group, 18 patients ultimately required dialysis, and all but 3 have since died. The most common cause of death while receiving dialysis was intractable hypotension related to cardiac involvement. A myelodysplastic syndrome was documented in 8 of the patients, and 7 have died. All deaths were related to myelodysplasia or to the development of acute leukemia. The 1 survivor

underwent a nonmyeloablative allogeneic transplantation 82 months after diagnosis of amyloidosis.

Gianni et al. reported on the use of 4'-iodo-4'-deoxy-doxorubicin in the treatment of amyloidosis. It appears to be most effective for patients with soft tissue deposits and less effective for those with visceral amyloidosis. We studied 45 patients receiving this agent and found a response rate of 15%. Further studies are under way with dose escalation to determine if higher doses can provide better response rates.

7.8.5 Stem Cell Transplantation for AL

Hematopoietic stem cell transplantation in patients with amyloidosis is unique. The majority of patients who receive transplants for the presence of a hematologic malignancy have significant dysfunction of their bone marrow, manifested by multiple cytopenias. These patients are generally selected with excellent cardiac, hepatic, and renal function and a performance status of 0 or 1. Unfortunately, most patients with amyloidosis present with precisely the opposite findings. These patients are hematologically normal, occasionally with a modest degree of anemia. Thrombocytosis is seen occasionally in those patients with hepatic involvement and hyposplenism. These patients, however, have significant visceral organ dysfunction, which puts them at higher risk for complications related to transplantation.

The first syngeneic transplant for amyloidosis was reported in 1995. The patient was conditioned with cyclophosphamide (120 mg/kg) and total body irradiation (12 Gy). This 32-year-old patient demonstrated resolution of nephrotic-range proteinuria and autonomic neuropathy, with disappearance of monoclonal light chains from serum and urine. A serum amyloid P-component scan showed a reduction in total body amyloid burden.

There have been 2 reports of allogeneic bone marrow transplantation for amyloidosis. One patient with purpura, macroglossia, and proteinuria of 1.4 g/d received 6 cycles of cyclophosphamide, vincristine, doxorubicin, and methylprednisolone and had a hematologic response. The patient received an allotransplant after being conditioned with melphalan (110 mg/m^2) and total body irradiation (12 Gy). The patient was alive at 29 months with a complete hematologic response. The second patient received a human leukocyte antigen identical allogeneic transplant after conditioning with melphalan (140 mg/m^2) and total body irradiation (8 Gy).

The urinary protein value decreased from 9.15 g to 1.3 g. The treatment was complicated by chronic skin and liver graft-versus-host disease, and the patient was alive 18 months posttransplantation. Given the current age restrictions associated with transplants and the need for good performance status and renal function, it is unlikely that allogeneic or nonmyeloablative allogeneic transplantation will be applicable to a significant proportion of AL patients.

7.8.5.1 Autologous Peripheral Blood Stem Cell Transplantation

Owing to the ease of collection, lower rate of tumor contamination, and faster engraftment observed with blood stem cells over autologous bone marrow, the majority of reported experiences used peripheral blood cells. Contamination of the apheresis product with clonotypic immunoglobulin-positive plasma cells has been demonstrated in AL patients after apheresis. CD34 cell selection can be performed in these patients, but whether this improves outcome is unknown (Comenzo et al. 1998a). In a prospective randomized study of purging in multiple myeloma patients, no benefit was seen, and it is thought unlikely that the results would be different for a population of patients with amyloidosis.

The largest experience with stem cell transplantation has been reported from Boston University. This group initially reported on 5 patients with AL treated with stem cell transplants, and all 5 showed a clinical response (Comenzo et al. 1996). Their experience was subsequently expanded to 25 patients, with a hematologic response rate of 62% and an organ response rate of 65% (Comenzo et al. 1998b). The last reported update reviewed 250 patients receiving high-dose melphalan (100–200 mg/m²). The median age of patients was 57 years; 53% had cardiac involvement on echocardiography. Three-month peritransplantation mortality was 14%; 11% of patients who began stem cell mobilization did not proceed to transplantation because of death or toxicities that prohibited safe transplantation. Major morbidities occurred in 23 patients during mobilization and collection, and 18 of the patients did not go on to transplantation. Four cardiac arrests occurred during stem cell infusion and 6 during the weeks after transplantation. Febrile neutropenia was seen in 62 patients, gastrointestinal tract hemorrhage in 17, and progressive renal failure requiring dialysis in 12. Sixty-six percent of the patients were alive with a mean follow-up of 23 months. The best responses were seen in patients with isolated renal amyloidosis. Subsequent patients have received transplants with lower doses of melphalan at 100 mg/m².

The first multicenter survey reporting the outcome of transplantation was published in 1998, and the results were sobering (Moreau et al. 1998). Twenty-one patients received transplants: 18 with melphalan alone and 3 with melphalan plus total body irradiation. The death rate from toxic reactions was 43%; 9 of 21 died within the first month after transplantation. Although 10 of the 12 survivors achieved a response, all 9 deaths were due to multiorgan failure, including 1 patient with severe bleeding. The median time from diagnosis of AL to transplantation was 11 months, suggesting some patient selection may have occurred, because half of patients with AL would succumb to the disease by the time they were ready for transplantation. The number of organs clinically involved at the time of transplantation was prognostic. For patients presenting with 2 or more clinical manifestations, the 4-year overall survival was 11.1%. The risk of death from toxic response when 2 or more organ dysfunctions were documented was greater than 75%, reflecting the need for careful patient selection before this procedure is used.

Twenty-seven patients who received high-dose melphalan were reported. There were 8 treatment-related deaths (30%). Deaths were due to multiorgan failure in 4, gastrointestinal tract hemorrhage in 2, and sepsis and cardiac complications in 1 each. A clonal response of bone marrow plasma cells was seen in 64% of patients and clinical organ regression in 57%; 17 of the 27 patients were alive when the report was published. Nine patients were reported who received transplants. Four of the 9 died within the 1st year after transplantation, for a treatment-related mortality of 44%. Five were alive with a median follow-up of 12.6 months. There were 4 responses and 1 progression. Three of the 4 patients who died had cardiac amyloid. The 4th had 3-organ involvement (renal, intestinal, and peripheral nerve). The development of multiorgan failure and gastrointestinal tract bleeding appears to be the result of toxic responses to transplantation occurring more frequently in patients with amyloidosis than in those who received transplants for other indications. Gastrointestinal tract bleeding is unusual after autologous transplantation, and it appears to be specific to patients with AL.

Of our first 45 patients who received transplants, 11 patients died at a median of 2 months posttransplantation. Gastrointestinal tract bleeding was seen in 9 patients (20%). The onset of bleeding occurred at a median of day +9. The median platelet count at the onset of bleeding was 22×10^9/L. Bleeding was seen in the lower gastrointestinal tract in 3, the upper gastrointestinal tract in 2, and in both in 4. Five patients underwent endoscopy, and all demonstrated an inflamed, friable esophageal and gastric mucosa. Four of the 9 patients in whom gastrointestinal tract bleeding developed died in the posttransplantation period, 3 of multiorgan failure. Factors that were associated with a higher risk of gastrointestinal tract bleeding were slow engraftment of platelets and female sex. The median number of red cell transfusions was 20 during the first 100 days posttransplantation in those with gastrointestinal tract bleeding. The mechanism of gastrointestinal tract bleeding in amyloidosis after stem cell transplantation is probably multifactorial. Vascular deposition of amyloid can make the vessels friable, and once conditioning chemotherapy causes significant mucosal damage, bleeding may occur. Abnormalities involving the coagulation system did not play a role in any of our patients.

Among the first 23 transplant recipients at Mayo Clinic, 3 did not go on to stem cell infusion because of poor performance status during mobilization (Gertz et al. 2000). Two died of progressive amyloid at 1 and 3 months. Of the 20 who went on to transplantation, renal amyloid, cardiac amyloid, peripheral neuropathy, and liver amyloid were seen in 14, 12, 3, and 1, respectively. Five of the 20 patients died posttransplantation. Two subsequently died of progressive amyloidosis, and 13 patients were alive, with 12 fulfilling the criteria of a hematologic or an organ response.

When we updated our results to 66 patients, renal, cardiac, peripheral nerve, hepatic, and autonomic amyloid were present in 68%, 48%, 17%, and 6%, respectively; 14% of the patients had an ejection fraction of less than 60% at transplantation. Two different mobilization schemes were used: 33 patients had mobilization with cyclophosphamide, 1.5 g/m² on 2 consecutive days, followed by sargramostim, 5 µg/kg per day; 33 patients received filgrastim, 10 µg/kg per day. Stem cells are collected when the peripheral blood CD34 count exceeds 10/µL. Our median CD34 collection was 6.4×10^6 cells/kg. In the patients mobilized with cyclophosphamide, the median number of aphereses required was 3, but in patients re-

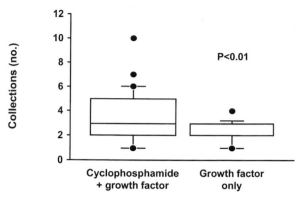

Fig. 7.12. Number of aphereses required to achieve the target stem cell numbers, using 2 mobilization schemes. (From Gertz MA, Lacy MQ, Dispenzieri A, Gastineau DA, Chen MG, Ansell SM, Inwards DJ, Micallef IN, Tefferi A, Litzow MR [2002] Stem cell transplantation for the management of primary systemic amyloidosis. Am J Med 113:549–555. By permission of Excerpta Medica.)

ceiving filgrastim alone, the median number of aphereses required was 2 – a significant difference (Fig. 7.12).

Graft function was assessed in all patients. One patient who died on day +6 was not evaluable for granulocyte engraftment. The remaining 65 patients achieved a granulocyte count of 0.5×10^9/L at a median of 12 days posttransplantation. Six patients died without achieving a platelet count of 20×10^9/L, and 1 patient is alive with a platelet count between 10×10^9/L and 20×10^9/L. Fifty-nine patients achieved a platelet count greater than 20×10^9/L at a median of day 14. Patients who had received oral melphalan chemotherapy before stem cell collection had slower engraftment of their platelet count. Nine of the 66 (14%) died as a direct result of transplant-related complications, including cardiac arrhythmia, gastrointestinal tract bleeding with multiorgan failure, pulmonary embolus, disseminated aspergillus, pneumonia, and aspiration pneumonia.

Nine of the patients required dialysis posttransplantation. Seven of these patients died. One had complete recovery, and 1 is alive on dialysis. Eight of the 9 patients had renal amyloid before transplantation. Patients who went on to dialysis had a median creatinine concentration of 1.7 mg/dL. In the patients who did not require dialysis, the median creatinine value was 1.1 mg/dL. A myelodysplastic syndrome developed in 1 patient 29 months posttransplantation. This patient had previously received melphalan chemotherapy orally. The median hospital stay was 14 days, with 15 of the patients hospitalized more than a month. The most common

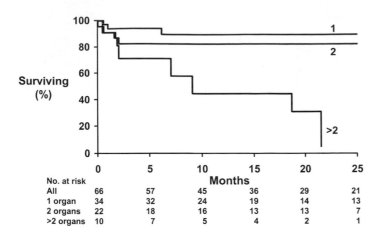

Fig. 7.13. Survival of 66 patients who received transplants for amyloidosis, stratified by number of organs involved pretransplantation. (From Gertz MA, Lacy MQ, Dispenzieri A, Gastineau DA, Chen MG, Ansell SM, Inwards DJ, Micallef IN, Tefferi A, Litzow MR [2002] Stem cell transplantation for the management of primary systemic amyloidosis. Am J Med 113:549–555. By permission of Excerpta Medica.)

No. at risk	0	5	10	15	20	25
All	66	57	45	36	29	21
1 organ	34	32	24	19	14	13
2 organs	22	18	16	13	13	7
>2 organs	10	7	5	4	2	1

Table 7.4. Toxic responses (SWOG ≥grade 2)

Toxic response	Frequency, % (no.)	
	200 mg/m^2 (n=23)	100 mg/m^2 (n=27)
Nausea/vomiting	83 (19)	52 (14)
Diarrhea	65 (15)	48 (13)
Mucositis	91 (21)	37 (10)
Pulmonary edema	35 (8)	26 (7)
Peripheral edema	48 (11)	15 (4)
Non-GI bleeding	17 (4)	0 (0)
GI bleeding	22 (5)	7 (2)
Hepatic	13 (3)	22 (6)
Renal	35 (8)	19 (5)
Metabolic	35 (8)	7 (2)
Sepsis	26 (6)	11 (3)

GI, gastrointestinal; SWOG, Southwest Oncology Group.

loss pretransplantation was 7.1 g/d and posttransplantation was 1.44 g/d. Twelve of the patients had a reduction in their urinary protein loss to less than 1 g/d. The median time to recognize a response was 3.6 months, but in 6 patients it took more than a year before a response was demonstrable. A multivariate analysis showed that only the serum creatinine value and the number of organs involved pretransplantation were significant predictors of adverse survival outcome (Fig. 7.13). Table 7.4 gives a compilation of reported toxicity associated with high-dose chemotherapy.

In spite of the high mortality associated with transplantation, the response rate we observed exceeds our previous experience with conventional-dose chemotherapy. These patients were highly selected to begin with, and it is difficult to be certain what the response rate and survival would be in an age- and organ-matched population. The most common type of response was resolution of the nephrotic syndrome. Table 7.5 summarizes reported data on stem cell transplantation in 294 patients.

Comenzo and Gertz developed a risk-adapted strategy for transplantation in patients with amyloidosis. In their review of 4 single-center studies, the mortality on day 100 was 21%. They proposed risk-adapted stratification using lower doses of melphalan supported with growth factor-mobilized stem cell components. Our guidelines for the selection of candidates for stem cell transplantation are given in Table 7.6, and the risk-adapted approach of Comenzo and Gertz is given in Table 7.7.

Patients receiving transplants for amyloidosis are a highly selected group by virtue of age, performance sta-

cause of bacteremia in 35 patients was staphylococcus. The percentage of patients surviving at 2 years was 91% with 1 organ involved, 82% with 2 organs involved, 33% with 3 organs involved, and 0% with 4 organs involved.

A total of 42 of the 66 patients had either a hematologic or an organ response. The responses were renal in 19; hepatic in 5; cardiac in 3; renal and cardiac in 2; renal and hepatic in 1; cardiac, renal, and neuropathic in 1; and autonomic in 1. Of 26 patients with renal amyloid who achieved a response, the median urinary protein

Table 7.5. Published series of autologous transplants for amyloidosis

Reference	Patients, no.	100-day treatment-related mortality	Overall survival (intention-to-treat)	Evaluable	Follow-up	Hematologic response	Amyloid organ disease involvement
Majolino et al.	1	1/1 (100%) CMV pneumonitis	0 at 74 days	1	74 days	PR at 2 weeks	Not reported
van Buren et al.	3 (1 syngeneic)	0/3 (0%)	2/2 (100%) at 24 mo	2	12 mo	2/2 (100%) CR	2/2 (100%) PR
Amoura et al.	9	3/9 (33%) ARF, sepsis, arrhythmia	5/9 (55%) at median 12.6 mo	5	Mean 8.9 mo	Not reported	4/5 (80%), 1/5 CR, 3/5 PR
Moreau et al. (1998)	21	9/21 (43%) Multiorgan failure, bleeding, arrhythmia	12/21 (57%) at median 14 mo	12	Median 14 mo	3/12 (25%) CR	10/12 (83%) PR+CR
Schulenburg et al.	1	1/1 (100%) GI perforation	0 at 4 days	0	NA	NA	NA
Patriarca et al.	1	0	1/1 (100%) at 22 mo	1	22 mo	1/1 (100%) CR	1/1 (100%) PR
Saba et al.	9	7/9 (78%) (3 during mobilization) Arrhythmia, CHF, hypotension	2/9 (22%) at >6 mo after referral	2	Not reported	Not reported	2/2 (100%) PR
Sezer et al.	1	0	1/1 (100%) at 3 mo	1	3 mo	1/1 (100%) CR	1/1 (100%) renal and cardiac PR
Gertz et al. (2000)	23 (3 never received transplants)	4/20 (20%) Pneumonia, multi-organ system failure, sudden death	13/23 (57%) at median 16 mo	20	Median >13 mo	8/20 (40%) CR	12/20 (60%) PR
Reich et al.	4	2/4 (50%) Acute MI, diffuse alveolar hemorrhage	2/4 (50%) at 7 and 19 mo	2	7 and 19 mo	1/2 (50%) PR	2/2 (100%) PR
Dember et al. (2001) and Sanchorawala et al. (2001)	205 (20 never received transplants)	28/205 (14%)	115/152 (76%) at >12 mo	115 at >12 mo	>12 mo	54/115 (47%) CR	18/50 (36%) renal CR at 12 mo (Dember)

ARF, acute renal failure; CHF, congestive heart failure; CMV, cytomegalovirus; CR, complete response; GI, gastrointestinal; MI, myocardial infarction; NA, not applicable; PR, partial response.

Table 7.6. Guidelines for selection of stem cell transplant recipients

Absolute contraindication
  Clinical congestive heart failure
  Total bilirubin >3.0 mg/dL
  Echocardiographic ejection fraction <45%

Relative contraindication
  Serum creatinine >2.0 mg/dL
  Interventricular septal thickness >15 mm
  Age >65 years
  More than 2 visceral organs involved

Table 7.7 Risk-adapted approach

Good risk (all of the following)
  1 or 2 Organs involved
  No cardiac involvement
  Creatinine clearance ≥51 mL/min
  Any age

Intermediate risk (all of the following)
  Younger than 61 years old
  1 or 2 Organs involved
  Asymptomatic cardiac or compensated cardiac
  Creatinine clearance <51 mL/min

Poor risk (one of the following)
  3 Organs* involved
  Advanced cardiac involvement

Melphalan dosing (mg/m²): based on risk group and age (years)

Good risk	Intermediate risk	Poor risk
200 if ≤60	140 if ≤50	Standard therapy
140 if 61–70	100 if 51–60	Clinical trials
100 if ≥71		

* Organ involvement includes heart, kidney, nerve, liver, vascular involvement of soft tissue.
Modified from Comenzo RL, Gertz MA (2002) Autologous stem cell transplantation for primary systemic amyloidosis. Blood 99:4276–4282. By permission of the American Society of Hematology.

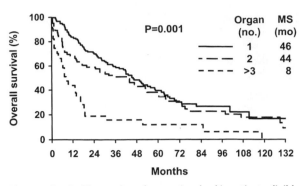

Fig. 7.14. Survival by number of organs involved in patients eligible for stem cell transplantation but treated with melphalan and prednisone. *MS*, median survival. (Modified from Dispenzieri A, Lacy MQ, Kyle RA, Therneau TM, Larson DR, Rajkumar SV, Fonseca R, Greipp PR, Witzig TE, Lust JA, Gertz MA [2001] Eligibility for hematopoietic stem-cell transplantation for primary systemic amyloidosis is a favorable prognostic factor for survival. J Clin Oncol 19:3350–3356. By permission of the American Society of Clinical Oncology.)

tus, number of organs involved, and the absence of class IV congestive heart failure. The survival of a true control group is uncertain. Dispenzieri et al. reviewed the amyloid database of Mayo Clinic from 1983 through 1997 to identify those patients who would have been eligible for peripheral blood stem cell transplantation. Inclusion criteria included biopsy-proven amyloid, symptomatic disease, absence of multiple myeloma, age younger than 70 years, septal thickness less than or equal to 15 mm, an ejection fraction greater than 55%, a serum creatinine value less than 2 mg/dL, and a direct bilirubin value less than 2 mg/dL. Two hundred twenty-nine patients were identified as eligible for transplantation among 1,288 patients, indicating the high proportion of patients not eligible for transplants. The median survival of the entire group was 42 months, with 5- and 10-year survival rates of 36% and 15%, respectively. Predictors of survival were the size of the M component in the 24-hour urine measurement, the number of involved organs (Fig. 7.14), the alkaline phosphatase value, the performance score, and the presence of weight loss. We found that the same patients who were eligible for stem cell transplantation were an inherently good-risk population who do relatively well with traditional-dose chemotherapy, substantially better than the expected median survival of 18 months for all patients. To accurately assess the effect of hematopoietic stem cell transplantation, a randomized trial would be required.

Table 7.8. Diagnostic pathway for primary amyloidosis

1. Consider primary amyloidosis in patients with
   Nephrotic-range proteinuria (nondiabetic)
   Cardiomyopathy (no ischemic history)
   Hepatomegaly (no filling defects on imaging)
   Peripheral neuropathy (nondiabetic)

2. Heighten suspicion
   Immunofixation of serum and urine

3. Confirm diagnosis histologically
   Fat aspirate and marrow biopsy stain with Congo red (90% sensitive)

4. Assess prognosis
   Echocardiography required (Doppler important)

5. Treat
   Melphalan and prednisone
   High-dose steroids
   Stem cell transplantation
   Organ transplantation

From Gertz MA, Lacy MQ, Dispenzieri A (2002) Amyloidosis. In Mehta J, Singhal S (eds) Myeloma. Martin Dunitz, London, pp 445–463. By permission of the publisher.

7.9 Conclusion

Amyloidosis should be suspected when a patient presents with unexplained nephrotic-range proteinuria, heart failure, neuropathy, or hepatomegaly (Table 7.8). The first screen should be immunofixation of serum or urine to detect a monoclonal protein. If a monoclonal protein is found, Congo red staining of bone marrow and subcutaneous fat aspiration should be performed. Prognosis should be assessed on 2-dimensional echocardiography. Systemic therapy is appropriate for most patients. High-dose myeloablative therapy with stem cell rescue is appropriate for selected patients, but firm evidence-based data do not exist to prove the survival benefit of stem cell transplantation.

References

Cohen AS (1992) History of amyloidosis. J Intern Med 232:509–510

Cohen AS, Calkins E. Cited by Sipe JD, Cohen AS (2000) Review: history of the amyloid fibril. J Struct Biol 130:88–98

Comenzo RL, Vosburgh E, Simms RW, Bergethon P, Sarnacki D, Finn K, Dubrey S, Faller DV, Wright DG, Falk RH, Skinner M (1996) Dose-intensive melphalan with blood stem cell support for the treatment of AL amyloidosis: one-year follow-up in five patients. Blood 88:2801–2806

Comenzo RL, Michelle D, LeBlanc M, Wally J, Zhang Y, Kica G, Karandish S, Arkin CF, Wright DG, Skinner M, McMannis J (1998a) Mobilized CD34+ cells selected as autografts in patients with primary light-chain amyloidosis: rationale and application. Transfusion 38:60–69

Comenzo RL, Vosburgh E, Falk RH, Sanchorawala V, Reisinger J, Dubrey S, Dember LM, Berk JL, Akpek G, LaValley M, O'Hara C, Arkin CF, Wright DG, Skinner M (1998b) Dose-intensive melphalan with blood stem-cell support for the treatment of AL (amyloid light-chain) amyloidosis: survival and responses in 25 patients. Blood 91:3662–3670

Connors LH, Richardson AM, Theberge R, Costello CE (2000) Tabulation of transthyretin (TTR) variants as of 1/1/2000. Amyloid 7:54–69

Cueto-Garcia L, Tajik AJ, Kyle RA, Edwards WD, Greipp PR, Callahan JA, Shub C, Seward JB (1984) Serial echocardiographic observations in patients with primary systemic amyloidosis: an introduction to the concept of early (asymptomatic) amyloid infiltration of the heart. Mayo Clin Proc 59:589–597

Cueto-Garcia L, Reeder GS, Kyle RA, Wood DL, Seward JB, Naessens J, Offord KP, Greipp PR, Edwards WD, Tajik AJ (1985) Echocardiographic findings in systemic amyloidosis: spectrum of cardiac involvement and relation to survival. J Am Coll Cardiol 6:737–743

Dember LM, Sanchorawala V, Seldin DC, Wright DG, LaValley M, Berk JL, Falk RH, Skinner M (2001) Effect of dose-intensive intravenous melphalan and autologous blood stem-cell transplantation on AL amyloidosis-associated renal disease. Ann Intern Med 134:746–753

Dhodapkar MV, Jagannath S, Vesole D, Munshi N, Naucke S, Tricot G, Barlogie B (1997) Treatment of AL-amyloidosis with dexamethasone plus alpha interferon. Leuk Lymphoma 27:351–356

Dingli D, Utz JP, Gertz MA (2001) Pulmonary hypertension in patients with amyloidosis. Chest 120:1735–1738

Dubrey SW, Davidoff R, Skinner M, Bergethon P, Lewis D, Falk RH (1997) Progression of ventricular wall thickening after liver transplantation for familial amyloidosis. Transplantation 64:74–80

Fonseca R, Ahmann GJ, Jalal SM, Dewald GW, Larson DR, Therneau TM, Gertz MA, Kyle RA, Greipp PR (1998) Chromosomal abnormalities in systemic amyloidosis. Br J Haematol 103:704–710

Fonseca R, Rajkumar SV, Ahmann GJ, Jalal SM, Hoyer JD, Gertz MA, Kyle RA, Greipp PR, Dewald GW (2000) FISH demonstrates treatment-related chromosome damage in myeloid but not plasma cells in primary systemic amyloidosis. Leuk Lymphoma 39:391–395

Gastineau DA, Gertz MA, Daniels TM, Kyle RA, Bowie EJ (1991a) Inhibitor of the thrombin time in systemic amyloidosis: a common coagulation abnormality. Blood 77:2637–2640

Gastineau DA, Gertz MA, Rosen CB, Kyle RA (1991b) Computed tomography for diagnosis of hepatic rupture in primary systemic amyloidosis. Am J Hematol 37:194–196

Gertz MA (1992) Secondary amyloidosis (AA). J Intern Med 232:517–518

Gertz MA, Kyle RA (1988) Hepatic amyloidosis (primary [AL], immunoglobulin light chain): the natural history in 80 patients. Am J Med 85:73–80

Gertz MA, Kyle RA (1990) Prognostic value of urinary protein in primary systemic amyloidosis (AL). Am J Clin Pathol 94:313–317

Gertz MA, Kyle RA (1991) Secondary systemic amyloidosis: response and survival in 64 patients. Medicine (Baltimore) 70:246–256

Gertz MA, Kyle RA (1997) Hepatic amyloidosis: clinical appraisal in 77 patients. Hepatology 25:118–121

Gertz MA, Kyle RA, Greipp PR (1983) Hyposplenism in primary systemic amyloidosis. Ann Intern Med 98:475–477

Gertz MA, Falk RH, Skinner M, Cohen AS, Kyle RA (1985) Worsening of congestive heart failure in amyloid heart disease treated by calcium channel-blocking agents. Am J Cardiol 55:1645

Gertz MA, Kyle RA, Griffing WL, Hunder GG (1986) Jaw claudication in primary systemic amyloidosis. Medicine (Baltimore) 65:173–179

Gertz MA, Kyle RA, Edwards WD (1989a) Recognition of congestive heart failure due to senile cardiac amyloidosis. Biomed Pharmacother 43:101–106

Gertz MA, Kyle RA, Greipp PR (1989b) The plasma cell labeling index: a valuable tool in primary systemic amyloidosis. Blood 74:1108–1111

Gertz MA, Kyle RA, Greipp PR, Katzmann JA, O'Fallon WM (1990) Beta 2-microglobulin predicts survival in primary systemic amyloidosis. Am J Med 89:609–614

Gertz MA, Greipp PR, Kyle RA (1991a) Classification of amyloidosis by the detection of clonal excess of plasma cells in the bone marrow. J Lab Clin Med 118:33–39

Gertz MA, Kyle RA, Greipp PR (1991b) Response rates and survival in primary systemic amyloidosis. Blood 77:257–262

Gertz MA, Kyle RA, O'Fallon WM (1992a) Dialysis support of patients with primary systemic amyloidosis. A study of 211 patients. Arch Intern Med 152:2245–2250

Gertz MA, Kyle RA, Thibodeau SN (1992b) Familial amyloidosis: a study of 52 North American-born patients examined during a 30-year period. Mayo Clin Proc 67:428–440

Gertz MA, Kyle RA, Noel P (1993) Primary systemic amyloidosis: a rare complication of immunoglobulin M monoclonal gammopathies and Waldenström's macroglobulinemia. J Clin Oncol 11:914–920

Gertz MA, Grogan M, Kyle RA, Tajik AJ (1997) Endomyocardial biopsy-proven light chain amyloidosis (AL) without echocardiographic features of infiltrative cardiomyopathy. Am J Cardiol 80:93–95

Gertz MA, Lacy MQ, Dispenzieri A (1999) Amyloidosis: recognition, confirmation, prognosis, and therapy. Mayo Clin Proc 74:490–494

Gertz MA, Lacy MQ, Gastineau DA, Inwards DJ, Chen MG, Tefferi A, Kyle RA, Litzow MR (2000) Blood stem cell transplantation as therapy for primary systemic amyloidosis (AL). Bone Marrow Transplant 26:963–969

Gillmore JD, Madhoo S, Pepys MB, Hawkins PN (2000) Renal transplantation for amyloid end-stage renal failure – insights from serial serum amyloid P component scintigraphy. Nucl Med Commun 21:735–740

Gillmore JD, Lovat LB, Persey MR, Pepys MB, Hawkins PN (2001) Amyloid load and clinical outcome in AA amyloidosis in relation to circulating concentration of serum amyloid A protein. Lancet 358:24–29

Greipp PR, Kyle RA, Bowie EJ (1981) Factor-X deficiency in amyloidosis: a critical review. Am J Hematol 11:443–450

Hawkins PN, Lavender JP, Pepys MB (1990) Evaluation of systemic amyloidosis by scintigraphy with ^{123}I-labeled serum amyloid P component. N Engl J Med 323:508–513

Hawkins PN, Aprile C, Capri G, Vigano L, Munzone E, Gianni L, Pepys MB, Merlini G (1998) Scintigraphic imaging and turnover studies with iodine-131 labelled serum amyloid P component in systemic amyloidosis. Eur J Nucl Med 25:701–708

Hayman SR, Bailey RJ, Jalal SM, Ahmann GJ, Dispenzieri A, Gertz MA, Greipp PR, Kyle RA, Lacy MQ, Rajkumar SV, Witzig TE, Lust JA, Fonseca R (2001a) Translocations involving the immunoglobulin heavy-chain locus are possible early genetic events in patients with primary systemic amyloidosis. Blood 98:2266–2268

Hayman SR, Lacy MQ, Kyle RA, Gertz MA (2001b) Primary systemic amyloidosis: a cause of malabsorption syndrome. Am J Med 111:535–540

Isobe T, Osserman EF (1974) Patterns of amyloidosis and their association with plasma-cell dyscrasia, monoclonal immunoglobulins and Bence-Jones proteins. N Engl J Med 290:473–477

Jacobson DR, Gertz MA, Buxbaum JN (1994) Transthyretin VAL107, a new variant associated with familial cardiac and neuropathic amyloidosis. Hum Mutat 3:399–401

Jacobson DR, Pastore RD, Yaghoubian R, Kane I, Gallo G, Buck FS, Buxbaum JN (1997) Variant-sequence transthyretin (isoleucine 122) in late-onset cardiac amyloidosis in black Americans. N Engl J Med 336:466–473

Klein AL, Tajik AJ (1991) Doppler assessment of diastolic function in cardiac amyloidosis. Echocardiography 8:233–251

Klein AL, Hatle LK, Burstow DJ, Seward JB, Kyle RA, Bailey KR, Luscher TF, Gertz MA, Tajik AJ (1989) Doppler characterization of left ventricular diastolic function in cardiac amyloidosis. J Am Coll Cardiol 13:1017–1026

Klein AL, Hatle LK, Taliercio CP, Taylor CL, Kyle RA, Bailey KR, Seward JB, Tajik AJ (1990) Serial Doppler echocardiographic follow-up of left ventricular diastolic function in cardiac amyloidosis. J Am Coll Cardiol 16:1135–1141

Klein AL, Hatle LK, Taliercio CP, Oh JK, Kyle RA, Gertz MA, Bailey KR, Seward JB, Tajik AJ (1991) Prognostic significance of Doppler measures of diastolic function in cardiac amyloidosis. A Doppler echocardiography study. Circulation 83:808–816

Klein AL, Canale MP, Rajagopalan N, White RD, Murray RD, Wahi S, Arheart KL, Thomas JD (1999) Role of transesophageal echocardiography in assessing diastolic dysfunction in a large clinical practice: a 9-year experience. Am Heart J 138:880–889

Kyle RA, Bayrd ED (1975) Amyloidosis: review of 236 cases. Medicine (Baltimore) 54:271–299

Kyle RA, Gertz MA (1995) Primary systemic amyloidosis: clinical and laboratory features in 474 cases. Semin Hematol 32:45–59

Kyle RA, Greipp PR (1983) Amyloidosis (AL): clinical and laboratory features in 229 cases. Mayo Clin Proc 58:665–683

Kyle RA, Rajkumar SV (1999) Monoclonal gammopathies of undetermined significance. Hematol Oncol Clin North Am 13:1181–1202

Kyle RA, Spencer RJ, Dahlin DC (1966) Value of rectal biopsy in the diagnosis of primary systemic amyloidosis. Am J Med Sci 251:501–506

Kyle RA, Greipp PR, O'Fallon WM (1986) Primary systemic amyloidosis: multivariate analysis for prognostic factors in 168 cases. Blood 68:220–224

Kyle RA, Gertz MA, Linke RP (1992a) Amyloid localized to tenosynovium at carpal tunnel release: immunohistochemical identification of amyloid type. Am J Clin Pathol 97:250–253

Kyle RA, Linos A, Beard CM, Linke RP, Gertz MA, O'Fallon WM, Kurland LT (1992b) Incidence and natural history of primary systemic amyloidosis in Olmsted County, Minnesota, 1950 through 1989. Blood 79:1817–1822

Kyle RA, Beard CM, O'Fallon WM, Kurland LT (1994) Incidence of multiple myeloma in Olmsted County, Minnesota: 1978 through 1990, with a review of the trend since 1945. J Clin Oncol 12:1577–1583

Kyle RA, Spittell PC, Gertz MA, Li CY, Edwards WD, Olson LJ, Thibodeau SN (1996) The premortem recognition of systemic senile amyloidosis with cardiac involvement. Am J Med 101:395–400

Kyle RA, Gertz MA, Greipp PR, Witzig TE, Lust JA, Lacy MQ, Therneau TM (1997) A trial of three regimens for primary amyloidosis: colchicine alone, melphalan and prednisone, and melphalan, prednisone, and colchicine. N Engl J Med 336:1202–1207

Levin M, Franklin EC, Frangione B, Pras M (1972) The amino acid sequence of a major nonimmunoglobulin component of some amyloid fibrils. J Clin Invest 51:2773–2776

Mathew V, Chaliki H, Nishimura RA (1997a) Atrioventricular sequential pacing in cardiac amyloidosis: an acute Doppler echocardiographic and catheterization hemodynamic study. Clin Cardiol 20:723–725

Mathew V, Olson LJ, Gertz MA, Hayes DL (1997b) Symptomatic conduction system disease in cardiac amyloidosis. Am J Cardiol 80:1491–1492

McElroy EA Jr, Witzig TE, Gertz MA, Greipp PR, Kyle RA (1998) Detection of monoclonal plasma cells in the peripheral blood of patients with primary amyloidosis. Br J Haematol 100:326–327

Moreau P, Leblond V, Bourquelot P, Facon T, Huynh A, Caillot D, Hermine O, Attal M, Hamidou M, Nedellec G, Ferrant A, Audhuy B, Bataille R, Milpied N, Harousseau JL (1998) Prognostic factors for survival and response after high-dose therapy and autologous stem cell transplantation in systemic AL amyloidosis: a report on 21 patients. Br J Haematol 101:766–769

Mueller PS, Edwards WD, Gertz MA (2000) Symptomatic ischemic heart disease resulting from obstructive intramural coronary amyloidosis. Am J Med 109:181–188

Olson LJ, Gertz MA, Edwards WD, Li CY, Pellikka PA, Homes DR Jr, Tajik AJ, Kyle RA (1987) Senile cardiac amyloidosis with myocardial dysfunction: diagnosis by endomyocardial biopsy and immunohistochemistry. N Engl J Med 317:738–742

Pellikka PA, Holmes DR Jr, Edwards WD, Nishimura RA, Tajik AJ, Kyle RA (1988) Endomyocardial biopsy in 30 patients with primary amyloidosis and suspected cardiac involvement. Arch Intern Med 148:662–666

Pepys MB, Hawkins PN, Booth DR, Vigushin DM, Tennent GA, Soutar AK, Totty N, Nguyen O, Blake CC, Terry CJ (1993) Human lysozyme gene mutations cause hereditary systemic amyloidosis. Nature 362:553–557

Rajkumar SV, Gertz MA, Kyle RA (1998a) Primary systemic amyloidosis with delayed progression to multiple myeloma. Cancer 82:1501–1505

Rajkumar SV, Gertz MA, Kyle RA (1998b) Prognosis of patients with primary systemic amyloidosis who present with dominant neuropathy. Am J Med 104:232–237

Ranlov I, Alves IL, Ranlov PJ, Husby G, Costa PP, Saraiva MJ (1992) A Danish kindred with familial amyloid cardiomyopathy revisited: identification of a mutant transthyretin-methionine 111 variant in serum from patients and carriers. Am J Med 93:3–8

Salvarani C, Gabriel SE, Gertz MA, Bjornsson J, Li CY, Hunder GG (1994) Primary systemic amyloidosis presenting as giant cell arteritis and polymyalgia rheumatica. Arthritis Rheum 37:1621–1626

Sanchorawala V, Wright DG, Seldin DC, Dember LM, Finn K, Falk RH, Berk J, Quillen K, Skinner M (2001) An overview of the use of high-dose melphalan with autologous stem cell transplantation for the treatment of AL amyloidosis. Bone Marrow Transplant 28:637–642

Skinner M, Anderson J, Simms R, Falk R, Wang M, Libbey C, Jones LA, Cohen AS (1996) Treatment of 100 patients with primary amyloidosis: a randomized trial of melphalan, prednisone, and colchicine versus colchicine only. Am J Med 100:290–298

Smith TJ, Kyle RA, Lie JT (1984) Clinical significance of histopathologic patterns of cardiac amyloidosis. Mayo Clin Proc 59:547–555

Solomon A, Weiss DT, Pepys MB (1992) Induction in mice of human light-chain-associated amyloidosis. Am J Pathol 140:629–637

Stangou AJ, Hawkins PN, Heaton ND, Rela M, Monaghan M, Nihoyannopoulos P, O'Grady J, Pepys MB, Williams R (1998) Progressive cardiac amyloidosis following liver transplantation for familial amyloid polyneuropathy: implications for amyloid fibrillogenesis. Transplantation 66:229–233

Utz JP, Swensen SJ, Gertz MA (1996) Pulmonary amyloidosis. The Mayo Clinic experience from 1980 to 1993. Ann Intern Med 124:407–413

Light Chain Deposition Disease

Steven R. Zeldenrust, M.D., Ph.D., Donna J. Lager, M.D., Nelson Leung, M.D.

Contents

8.1   Epidemiology   197

8.2   Etiology   197

8.3   Clinical Presentation   198

8.4   Diagnosis   198

8.5   Differential Diagnosis   200

8.6   Therapy   201

References   202

Light chain deposition disease (LCDD) results from the deposition of monoclonal immunoglobulin light chains in various organs. The nonfibrillary nature of the deposits differentiates LCDD from primary amyloidosis, in which the characteristic congophilic fibrils occur. First described in the kidney in 1973 (Antonovych et al. 1974), LCDD was recognized as a systemic disease by Randall et al. in 1976. Many cases are associated with multiple myeloma or lymphoproliferative disease, but up to 50% of patients have no evidence of a neoplastic plasma cell proliferative disorder at diagnosis (Buxbaum et al. 1990; Confalonieri et al. 1988; Ganeval et al. 1984; Gipstein et al. 1982; Tubbs et al. 1981).

8.1 Epidemiology

The frequency of LCDD is not known. Renal biopsy revealed LCDD in 5 of 260 patients with idiopathic proteinuria (Mallick et al. 1978). In a study of 47 patients with plasma cell dyscrasia, 10 had LCDD on renal biopsy (Pirani et al. 1987). In a group of 57 patients with multiple myeloma, 3% had evidence of LCDD at necropsy (Ivanyi 1990). There appears to be a higher incidence of the disease in males than females, with approximately a 2:1 ratio in some series (Buxbaum et al. 1990; Heilman et al. 1992; Pozzi et al. 1995). Age at presentation varies widely, with most series reporting a range from the 4th to 8th decades and a median age of about 50 years.

Survival also tends to vary widely, with patients who have overt multiple myeloma having the worst outcomes and those with no identifiable underlying plasma cell proliferative process occasionally exhibiting long-term survival. In a series of 19 patients, 11 of whom had multiple myeloma, Pozzi et al. (1995) reported a median survival of 18.1 ± 20.7 months. Heilman et al. (1992) reported somewhat better results in 19 patients, 12 of whom did not have multiple myeloma, with 5-year actuarial survival of 70%. The better outcome in this series likely reflects the lower percentage of patients with multiple myeloma.

8.2 Etiology

In contrast to primary amyloidosis, in which the fibrils are most often associated with λ light chain, the majority of cases (80% to 85%) of LCDD result from κ light chain deposits (Preud'homme et al. 1994). In particular, the VκIV subgroup appears to be overrepresented in patients with LCDD (Denoroy et al. 1994). Analysis of mutations in the primary sequence of the pathologic κ light chains from patients with LCDD suggests that alterations in the structure of the variable (V) region impart a predisposition to deposition (Bellotti et al. 1991; Cogne et al. 1991; Khamlichi et al. 1992). Detailed analysis of the κ light chain structure from some patients reveals an increased number of hydrophobic residues, suggesting that direct interactions between the V regions may enhance deposition (Deret et al. 1997). The hypothesis of a direct role of structural aberrations of the V region has been further strengthened by the finding that in vivo synthesis in the mouse of a κ light chain from a patient with LCDD is sufficient to result in deposition, whereas a control κ light chain did not result in similar deposits (Khamlichi et al. 1995). Further work has shown that a single point mutation in the V region of the κ light chain significantly destabilizes the structure of the protein and confers an increased susceptibility to in vitro aggregate formation (Helms and Wetzel 1996).

Posttranslational modification has also been implicated in promoting deposition. Isolation and characterization of the κ light chain from a patient with LCDD revealed aberrant glycosylation (Cogne et al. 1991). The authors postulated that the carbohydrate moieties act to promote aggregation, although the mechanism behind this process is not known. Analysis of the light chains extracted from tissue deposits in other patients with LCDD has revealed the presence of intact light chains and light chain fragments, suggesting proteolysis is involved in promoting deposition (Cogne et al. 1991; Picken et al. 1989). Additional studies have shown that plasma cells from patients with LCDD produce light chains of various discrete masses, suggesting that aberrant expression or posttranslational modification occurs at the level of the plasma cell (Buxbaum 2001).

8.3 Clinical Presentation

The vast majority of patients with LCDD present with renal disease manifested as renal insufficiency, proteinuria, microscopic hematuria, or nephrotic syndrome. Most often, the diagnosis is made at the time of renal biopsy. The characteristic renal lesion is nodular glomerulosclerosis. Progressive renal failure typically results in most cases and usually leads to dialysis.

Occasionally, patients present with symptomatic deposition in other organs, with the heart and liver being the most common sites of extrarenal involvement. Patients with hepatic involvement typically present with asymptomatic hepatomegaly or liver function test ab-

normalities; increased alkaline phosphatase concentration is the most common finding. Rare reports of fulminant hepatic failure resulting from LCDD have been published (Pelletier et al. 1988).

Cardiac involvement is most often recognized in patients with evidence of congestive heart failure. The most frequent cardiac manifestation is restrictive cardiomyopathy. Arrhythmias and conduction defects are also seen, including atrial and ventricular fibrillation, atrioventricular block, and tachyarrhythmias. It has been suggested that cardiac involvement is present in the majority of cases and likely underappreciated as a result of the overwhelming renal effects in many cases (Buxbaum et al. 2000).

Case reports of isolated involvement of the lung have also been published. Pulmonary involvement appears to be rare and most often asymptomatic. Deposits can be diffuse, with interstitial or pleural-based deposits, or discrete nodular aggregates (Kijner and Yousem 1988; Linder et al. 1983).

Ocular involvement has been reported, with uveal deposits and retinal vasculopathy resulting from vascular deposition (Daicker et al. 1995; Enzenauer et al. 1990). Rare reports of cutaneous lesions, musculoskeletal involvement, and neurologic abnormalities have also been published (Randall et al. 1976; Rivest et al. 1993).

8.4 Diagnosis

The diagnosis of LCDD requires the identification of amorphous, nonfibrillar monoclonal light chain deposits in biopsy specimens of affected organs. Immunohistochemistry is required to confirm the diagnosis in most cases. Staining for complement components is negative, which differentiates LCDD from immune complex disease. Staining with Congo red fails to produce the characteristic apple-green birefringence seen in amyloidosis. Electron microscopy has been used in some instances to discern the granular, nonfibrillar structure of deposits.

Serum protein electrophoresis is positive in only 25% of patients, but 60% to 85% have an identifiable monoclonal protein on immunofixation of the serum or urine (Buxbaum et al. 1990; Heilman et al. 1992; Pozzi et al. 1995). A substantial minority of patients (15% to 20%) have no demonstrable monoclonal protein on careful examination of the serum and urine at the time of diagnosis. However, serial studies may eventually

Fig. 8.1. Glomerulus with several periodic acid-Schiff-positive mesangial nodules and mild mesangial hypercellularity. (×200.)

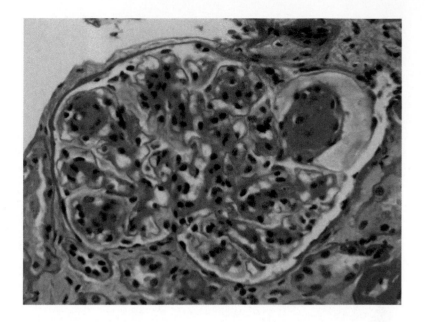

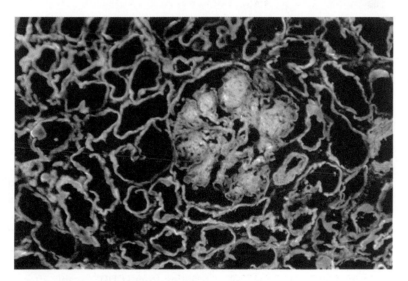

Fig. 8.2. Immunofluorescent staining for κ light chain demonstrates linear staining of tubular basement membranes and mesangial nodule

reveal a monoclonal protein after significant time has elapsed.

Approximately 50% of patients with LCDD have bone marrow plasmacytosis at diagnosis. Depending on the definition being used, 30% to 60% fulfill the criteria for multiple myeloma at diagnosis.

The most common finding on light microscopy of kidney biopsy specimens is nodular mesangial expansion with periodic acid-Schiff–positive material (Fig. 8.1). Nodular glomerulosclerosis and thickening of the tubular basement membrane have been the most

frequently reported lesions, but in an analysis of 23 patients with LCDD the incidence was only 43% and 56%, respectively (Strom et al. 1994). Other common features seen on renal biopsy specimens include a membranoproliferative glomerulonephritis pattern of injury, tubulointerstitial nephritis, tubular atrophy, and vascular sclerosis. Occasionally, cellular crescents can also be present (Heilman et al. 1992; Strom et al. 1994).

Immunohistochemical or immunofluorescent staining with antisera specific for κ and λ light chains can be helpful in confirming the diagnosis in many cases of

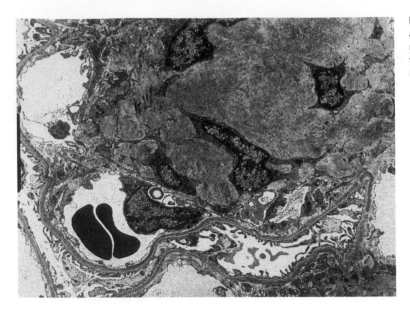

Fig. 8.3. Electron microscopy demonstrates amorphous osmiophilic deposits in a mesangial nodule. Osmiophilic deposits are also present in the lamina rara interna of the glomerular basement membrane

suspected LCDD. Linear staining of both the glomerular and tubular basement membrane is seen in the overwhelming majority of cases (Fig. 8.2). Rare patients have staining of only the glomerular basement membrane or the tubular basement membrane.

Electron microscopy is needed to confirm the nonfibrillar nature of the deposits in some cases (Fig. 8.3). The characteristic lesion seen on electron microscopy is granular deposits in the lamina rara interna of the glomerular basement membrane and along the outer side of the tubular basement membrane (Confalonieri et al. 1988).

Plain radiographs of the skeleton can be useful to exclude coexistent multiple myeloma, which produces the characteristic lytic lesions. A report from Germany revealed that magnetic resonance imaging may be helpful in distinguishing bony lesions resulting from LCDD from those of multiple myeloma (Baur et al. 1998). Focal areas of low signal intensity were found on T1- and T2-weighted spin echo images in a patient with LCDD, and they corresponded to areas of nonfibrillar light chain deposition seen on bone marrow biopsy. These areas failed to enhance significantly after administration of gadopentetate, in contrast to the lesions of multiple myeloma, which typically show diffuse enhancement.

8.5 Differential Diagnosis

The clinical differential diagnosis of LCDD includes myeloma cast nephropathy, primary amyloidosis, light and heavy chain deposition disease (LHCDD), and heavy chain deposition disease (HCDD). The characteristic feature of myeloma cast nephropathy is atypical, fractured polychromatic tubular casts on light microscopy that show intense staining with monoclonal κ or λ antisera on immunohistochemical analysis. In a recent series of 34 patients with renal immunoglobulin deposition disease, 11 showed features of both LCDD and myeloma cast nephropathy (Lin et al. 2001). As mentioned previously, the renal deposits of primary amyloidosis are fibrillar and show the characteristic apple-green birefringence on polarized light microscopy after staining with Congo red. Some patients exhibit deposits that are characteristic of both amyloid and LCDD (Faa et al. 1991; Gallo et al. 1988; Hofmann-Guilaine et al. 1985; Jacquot et al. 1985; Kirkpatrick et al. 1986; Smith and Malcolm 1986; Strom et al. 1994). The deposits seen in LHCDD and HCDD appear identical to those in LCDD but show staining with antisera specific for one of the immunoglobulin heavy chains.

8.6 Therapy

The low incidence of LCDD precludes testing of therapeutic strategies in a randomized fashion. The few series of clinical outcomes in the literature are retrospective analyses. As mentioned previously, patients with multiple myeloma and LCDD have a significantly worse prognosis than those with LCDD alone. There is no currently accepted standard treatment for LCDD.

The role of cytotoxic chemotherapy remains unclear. In a series of 19 patients with LCDD treated with systemic chemotherapy (mainly intermittent melphalan and prednisone), 12 of whom did not have multiple myeloma, Heilman et al. (1992) reported a 70% estimated survival at 5 years. The predominant benefit of chemotherapy appeared to be in patients with a serum creatinine concentration less than 4.0 mg/dL at diagnosis, with 5 of 8 patients in this group showing stabilization or improvement in renal function.

An Italian group reported little benefit from cytotoxic chemotherapy in 19 patients, 11 of whom had multiple myeloma (Pozzi et al. 1995). They reported transient improvement in renal function after 1 month of therapy in 5 patients, with an additional 8 patients showing stable renal function. Improvement was more frequent, but not statistically significant, in patients also receiving plasma exchange. Ultimately, 12 patients died within the 1st year of follow-up, with most survivors showing progressive renal impairment and ultimately requiring dialysis. The authors concluded that chemotherapy was beneficial in a minority of patients.

In another series of 13 patients, 8 of whom received chemotherapy, there was no clear association between treatment response and survival (Buxbaum et al. 1990). Renal transplantation was reported in 3 patients, only 2 of whom showed significant responses to chemotherapy before transplantation. All 3 patients survived for more than 5 years.

High-dose chemotherapy with stem-cell rescue has become the treatment of choice for young multiple myeloma patients; response and survival are superior to those of standard chemotherapy (Attal et al. 1996). It seems reasonable to conclude that similar effects would be seen in patients with coexisting multiple myeloma and LCDD; however, patients with LCDD are frequently too ill at presentation to be considered for aggressive chemotherapy. One patient with LCDD involving the heart, liver, and kidney was treated with intensive chemotherapy and stem-cell rescue by a French group (Mariette et al. 1995). The patient achieved a complete response to treatment and showed normalization of both cardiac and liver function; repeat biopsies showed resolution of the cardiac deposits and scant liver involvement. Renal function improved significantly but did not return to normal, suggesting that the heart and liver are able to recover more effectively from the damage induced by the light chain deposits. A similar effect was reported in a Japanese patient with multiple myeloma and LCDD affecting the heart (Nakamura et al. 2002). Cardiac function returned to normal after successful treatment of his myeloma with conventional chemotherapy.

The role of renal transplantation remains controversial in the management of LCDD. Although reports of prolonged renal allograft survival have been published, recurrence of LCDD in renal allograft is also well documented (Gerlag et al. 1986). As yet, no consensus has been reached regarding the appropriate indication for renal transplantation in these patients (Buxbaum et al. 1990; David-Neto et al. 1989). The largest single-center experience published to date described recurrence of LCDD in 6 of 8 transplant recipients. Recurrence was detected 3 to 48 months posttransplantation (mean, 25.4 months). Three of these patients required dialysis and 1 patient received a second kidney transplant. The 2 patients without recurrence were doing well at 9 and 19 years posttransplantation (Kanakiriya et al. 2000). A similar recurrence rate was seen in a review of LCDD patients who underwent kidney transplantation. Recurrent disease developed in 4 of 5 patients. Three of them went on dialysis and the other had evidence of advanced renal allograft dysfunction. The patient with no recurrence was alive with good renal function at 44 months posttransplantation. Average allograft survival in this review was 30.5 months (range, 5 to 50 months) (Short et al. 2001). No patient from either study had evidence of multiple myeloma at the time of kidney transplantation.

The limited data from these studies suggest that although prolonged benefits can be seen in a few patients after renal transplantation, the risk of recurrence is high and most patients experience graft loss. The decision to perform renal transplantation should be made on an individual basis. Patients should be well educated on the risk of recurrence to allow an informed decision and to avoid false expectations. Light chain production should be controlled before attempting renal transplantation. Patients with persistent circulating light chain are at high risk for recurrence and should be considered poor candidates for renal transplantation.

A better understanding of the disease process responsible for the development of LCDD is needed to develop more effective treatments for this disease. In the interim, the use of chemotherapy may be of some benefit in selected patients. More experience with renal transplantation in LCDD is needed to allocate appropriately the already scarce donor resources available.

References

Antonovych TT, Lin RC, Parrish E, Mostofi K (1974) Light chain deposits in multiple myeloma (abstract). Lab Invest 30:370A

Attal M, Harousseau JL, Stoppa AM, Sotto JJ, Fuzibet JG, Rossi JF, Casassus P, Maisonneuve H, Facon T, Ifrah N, Payen C, Bataille R (1996) A prospective, randomized trial of autologous bone marrow transplantation and chemotherapy in multiple myeloma. Intergroupe Français du Myelome. N Engl J Med 335:91–97

Baur A, Stabler A, Lamerz R, Bartl R, Reiser M (1998) Light chain deposition disease in multiple myeloma: MR imaging features correlated with histopathological findings. Skeletal Radiol 27:173–176

Bellotti V, Stoppini M, Merlini G, Zapponi MC, Meloni ML, Banfi G, Ferri G (1991) Amino acid sequence of k Sci, the Bence Jones protein isolated from a patient with light chain deposition disease. Biochim Biophys Acta 1097:177–182

Buxbaum JN (2001) Abnormal immunoglobulin synthesis in monoclonal immunoglobulin light chain and light and heavy chain deposition disease. Amyloid 8:84–93

Buxbaum JN, Chuba JV, Hellman GC, Solomon A, Gallo GR (1990) Monoclonal immunoglobulin deposition disease: light chain and light and heavy chain deposition diseases and their relation to light chain amyloidosis. Clinical features, immunopathology, and molecular analysis. Ann Intern Med 112:455–464

Buxbaum JN, Genega EM, Lazowski P, Kumar A, Tunick PA, Kronzon I, Gallo GR (2000) Infiltrative nonamyloidotic monoclonal immunoglobulin light chain cardiomyopathy: an underappreciated manifestation of plasma cell dyscrasias. Cardiology 93:220–228

Cogne M, Preud'homme JL, Bauwens M, Touchard G, Aucouturier P (1991) Structure of a monoclonal kappa chain of the V kappa IV subgroup in the kidney and plasma cells in light chain deposition disease. J Clin Invest 87:2186–2190

Confalonieri R, Barbiano di Belgiojoso G, Banfi G, Ferrario F, Bertani T, Pozzi C, Casanova S, Lupo A, De Ferrari G, Minetti L (1988) Light chain nephropathy: histological and clinical aspects in 15 cases. Nephrol Dial Transplant 3:150–156

Daicker BC, Mihatsch MJ, Strom EH, Fogazzi GB (1995) Ocular pathology in light chain deposition disease. Eur J Ophthalmol 5:75–81

David-Neto E, Ianhez LE, Chocair PR, Saldanha LB, Sabbaga E, Arap S (1989) Renal transplantation in systemic light-chain deposition (SLCD): a 44 month follow-up without recurrence. Transplant Proc 21:2128–2129

Denoroy L, Deret S, Aucouturier P (1994) Overrepresentation of the V kappa IV subgroup in light chain deposition disease. Immunol Lett 42:63–66

Deret S, Chomilier J, Huang DB, Preud'homme JL, Stevens FJ, Aucouturier P (1997) Molecular modeling of immunoglobulin light chains implicates hydrophobic residues in non-amyloid light chain deposition disease. Protein Eng 10:1191–1197

Enzenauer RJ, Stock JG, Enzenauer RW, Pope J Jr, West SG (1990) Retinal vasculopathy associated with systemic light chain deposition disease. Retina 10:115–118

Faa G, Van Eyken P, De Vos R, Fevery J, Van Damme B, De Groote J, Desmet VJ (1991) Light chain deposition disease of the liver associated with AL-type amyloidosis and severe cholestasis. J Hepatol 12:75–82

Gallo G, Picken M, Frangione B, Buxbaum J (1988) Nonamyloidotic monoclonal immunoglobulin deposits lack amyloid P component. Mod Pathol 1:453–456

Ganeval D, Noel LH, Preud'homme JL, Droz D, Grunfeld JP (1984) Light-chain deposition disease: its relation with AL-type amyloidosis. Kidney Int 26:1–9

Gerlag PG, Koene RA, Berden JH (1986) Renal transplantation in light chain nephropathy: case report and review of the literature. Clin Nephrol 25:101–104

Gipstein RM, Cohen AH, Adams DA, Adams T, Grabie MT (1982) Kappa light chain nephropathy without evidence of myeloma cells: response to chemotherapy with cessation of maintenance hemodialysis. Am J Nephrol 2:276–281

Heilman RL, Velosa JA, Holley KE, Offord KP, Kyle RA (1992) Long-term follow-up and response to chemotherapy in patients with light-chain deposition disease. Am J Kidney Dis 20:34–41

Helms LR, Wetzel R (1996) Specificity of abnormal assembly in immunoglobulin light chain deposition disease and amyloidosis. J Mol Biol 257:77–86

Hofmann-Guilaine C, Nochy D, Jacquot C, Tricottet V, Bariety J, Camilleri JP (1985) Association light chain deposition disease (LCDD) and amyloidosis: one case. Pathol Res Pract 180:214–219

Ivanyi B (1990) Frequency of light chain deposition nephropathy relative to renal amyloidosis and Bence Jones cast nephropathy in a necropsy study of patients with myeloma. Arch Pathol Lab Med 114:986–987

Jacquot C, Saint-Andre JP, Touchard G, Nochy D, D'Auzac de Lamartinie C, Oriol R, Druet P, Bariety J (1985) Association of systemic light-chain deposition disease and amyloidosis: a report of three patients with renal involvement. Clin Nephrol 24:93–98

Kanakiriya S, Lager D, Fervenza F (2000) Long term outcome of renal transplantation in light chain deposition disease (LCDD) (abstract). J Am Soc Nephrol 11:693A

Khamlichi AA, Aucouturier P, Silvain C, Bauwens M, Touchard G, Preud'homme JL, Nau F, Cogne M (1992) Primary structure of a monoclonal kappa chain in myeloma with light chain deposition disease. Clin Exp Immunol 87:122–126

Khamlichi AA, Rocca A, Touchard G, Aucouturier P, Preud'homme JL, Cogne M (1995) Role of light chain variable region in myeloma with light chain deposition disease: evidence from an experimental model. Blood 86:3655–3659

Kijner CH, Yousem SA (1988) Systemic light chain deposition disease presenting as multiple pulmonary nodules: a case report and review of the literature. Am J Surg Pathol 12:405–413

Kirkpatrick CJ, Curry A, Galle J, Melzner I (1986) Systemic kappa light chain deposition and amyloidosis in multiple myeloma: novel morphological observations. Histopathology 10:1065–1076

Lin J, Markowitz GS, Valeri AM, Kambham N, Sherman WH, Appel GB, D'Agati VD (2001) Renal monoclonal immunoglobulin deposition disease: the disease spectrum. J Am Soc Nephrol 12:1482–1492

Linder J, Croker BP, Vollmer RT, Shelburne J (1983) Systemic kappa light-chain deposition: an ultrastructural and immunohistochemical study. Am J Surg Pathol 7:85–93

Mallick NP, Dosa S, Acheson EJ, Delamore IW, McFarlane H, Seneviratne CJ, Williams G (1978) Detection, significance and treatment of paraprotein in patients presenting with 'idiopathic' proteinuria without myeloma. Q J Med 47:145–175

Mariette X, Clauvel JP, Brouet JC (1995) Intensive therapy in AL amyloidosis and light-chain deposition disease (letter). Ann Intern Med 123:553

Nakamura M, Satoh M, Kowada S, Satoh H, Tashiro A, Sato F, Masuda T, Hiramori K (2002) Reversible restrictive cardiomyopathy due to light-chain deposition disease. Mayo Clin Proc 77:193–196

Pelletier G, Fabre M, Attali P, Ladouch-Badre A, Ink O, Martin E, Etienne JP (1988) Light chain deposition disease presenting with hepatomegaly: an association with amyloid-like fibrils. Postgrad Med J 64:804–808

Picken MM, Frangione B, Barlogie B, Luna M, Gallo G (1989) Light chain deposition disease derived from the kappa I light chain subgroup: biochemical characterization. Am J Pathol 134:749–754

Pirani CL, Silva F, D'Agati V, Chander P, Striker LM (1987) Renal lesions in plasma cell dyscrasias: ultrastructural observations. Am J Kidney Dis 10:208–221

Pozzi C, Fogazzi GB, Banfi G, Strom EH, Ponticelli C, Locatelli F (1995) Renal disease and patient survival in light chain deposition disease. Clin Nephrol 43:281–287

Preud'homme JL, Aucouturier P, Touchard G, Striker L, Khamlichi AA, Rocca A, Denoroy L, Cogne M (1994) Monoclonal immunoglobulin deposition disease (Randall type): relationship with structural abnormalities of immunoglobulin chains (editorial). Kidney Int 46:965–972

Randall RE, Williamson WC Jr, Mullinax F, Tung MY, Still WJS (1976) Manifestations of systemic light chain deposition. Am J Med 60:293–299

Rivest C, Turgeon PP, Senecal JL (1993) Lambda light chain deposition disease presenting as an amyloid-like arthropathy. J Rheumatol 20:880–884

Short AK, O'Donoghue DJ, Riad HN, Short CD, Roberts IS (2001) Recurrence of light chain nephropathy in a renal allograft: a case report and review of the literature. Am J Nephrol 21:237–240

Smith NM, Malcolm AJ (1986) Simultaneous AL-type amyloid and light chain deposit disease in a liver biopsy: a case report. Histopathology 10:1057–1064

Strom EH, Fogazzi GB, Banfi G, Pozzi C, Mihatsch MJ (1994) Light chain deposition disease of the kidney: morphological aspects in 24 patients. Virchows Arch 425:271–280

Tubbs RR, Gephardt GN, McMahon JT, Hall PM, Valenzuela R, Vidt DG. (1981) Light chain nephropathy. Am J Med 71:263–269

Waldenström Macroglobulinemia

Jerry M. Winkler, M.D., Rafael Fonseca, M.D.

Contents

9.1 Introduction 206

9.2 Epidemiology 206
9.2.1 Incidence 206
9.2.2 Mortality 206
9.2.3 Sex Ratio 206
9.2.4 Race Ratio 206
9.2.5 Age Ratio 206
9.2.6 Survivorship 206

9.3 Etiology 206
9.3.1 IgM Monoclonal Gammopathy
       of Undetermined Significance ... 206
9.3.2 Chemical and Physical Factors ... 206
9.3.3 Genetics 207

9.4 Screening/Prevention 207

9.5 Molecular Biology and Genetics 207
9.5.1 Normal Counterpart to the
       Clonal Cells 207
9.5.2 Cytogenetics 207
9.5.3 Molecular Genetics 207

9.6 Clinical Presentation 207
9.6.1 Hyperviscosity Syndrome 208
9.6.2 Signs and Symptoms Due
       to the Clonal Expansion 210
9.6.3 Paraneoplastic
       and Other Manifestations 210

9.7 Classification and Staging 210

9.8 Diagnosis 211
9.8.1 Laboratory Tests 211

9.8.1.1 Hematologic Laboratory
         Abnormalities 211
9.8.1.2 Paraproteinemia 211
9.8.1.3 Bone Marrow Aspiration
         and Biopsy 212
9.8.2 Radiologic Studies 213

9.9 Differential Diagnosis 213

9.10 Secondary Malignancies 213

9.11 Therapy 215
9.11.1 Observation 215
9.11.2 Chemotherapy 215
9.11.2.1 Alkylating Agents 215
9.11.2.2 Combination Alkylator
          Chemotherapy 215
9.11.2.3 Fludarabine 215
9.11.2.4 Cladribine 218
9.11.2.5 Combination Therapy
          With Purine Nucleoside
          Analogs 219
9.11.2.6 Rituximab 219
9.11.2.7 Thalidomide 220
9.11.2.8 Corticosteroids 220
9.11.3 Autologous Stem Cell
       Transplantation 220
9.11.4 Surgery: Splenectomy 221
9.11.5 Supportive Care:
       Plasma Exchange 221

9.12 Prognosis 221
9.12.1 Prognostic Models 221
9.12.2 Disease Transformation 222

9.13 Conclusion 222

References 222

9.1 Introduction

Waldenström macroglobulinemia (WM) is a B-cell lymphoproliferative disorder characterized by a monoclonal lymphoplasmacytosis, which produces a monoclonal IgM paraproteinemia (Dimopoulos et al. 2000; Gertz et al. 2000; Owen et al. 2000). Its characteristic signs and symptoms include a hypoproliferative anemia, organomegaly (lymph nodes, liver, and spleen), and hyperviscosity due to high IgM concentrations (Dimopoulos et al. 2000; Gertz et al. 2000; Owen et al. 2000). We review the published literature on this disorder, with special emphasis on emerging therapeutic options.

The Swedish physician Jan Waldenström first described the disease. His classic 1944 report described 2 patients with oronasal bleeding, lymphadenopathy, low fibrinogen values, anemia, and an abnormal serum protein of high molecular weight. This description remains apt today, because there are no molecular features to define this disorder independent of the clinical syndrome.

9.2   Epidemiology

9.2.1 Incidence

The lack of standardized diagnostic criteria and the frequency of asymptomatic cases make prevalence estimates difficult, although WM is indeed rare. Only about 1,500 cases per year are reported in the United States, which is about one-sixth the number of myeloma cases reported in the same span (Dimopoulos et al. 2000; Groves et al. 1998; Herrinton and Weiss 1993).

9.2.2 Mortality

Because most WM patients are age 60 years or older and have comorbid conditions, it is estimated that one-fifth of the deaths attributed to WM may in fact be due to unrelated causes (Dimopoulos et al. 2000). Taking this into account, it can be estimated conservatively that 500 to 1,000 deaths from WM occur per year in the United States. This calculation likely underestimates the true mortality rate because of the significant number of cases that go undiagnosed.

9.2.3 Sex Ratio

WM appears to have a slight male predominance. Age-adjusted incidence rates for WM (per 1 million person-years) have been reported as 3.4 to 6.1 for males and 1.7 to 2.5 for females, with the rates increasing sharply with age (Groves et al. 1998; Herrinton and Weiss 1993).

9.2.4 Race Ratio

WM is more common among those of white than African or Mexican-mestizo descent (Dimopoulos et al. 2000; Groves et al. 1998; Herrinton and Weiss 1993).

9.2.5 Age Ratio

The disease predominantly affects the elderly (median age at presentation, 63 years), although we have seen patients as early as in their 2nd and 3rd decades of life (Gertz MA, Fonseca R, unpublished data).

9.2.6 Survivorship

The median survival is approximately 5 years, but about 10% of patients remain alive at 15 years (Kyle et al. 2000) (Table 9.1, see p. 208, 209).

9.3   Etiology

9.3.1 IgM Monoclonal Gammopathy of Undetermined Significance

The only clear risk factor for WM is monoclonal gammopathy of undetermined significance (MGUS) of the IgM type. IgM MGUS is more likely to evolve to WM and not to myeloma or amyloidosis (Kyle et al. 2002), and patients have a 46-fold higher relative risk of WM developing than in the general population. It is hypothesized that a proportion of patients with IgM MGUS actually represent early stages of WM. Overall, the prevalence of IgM MGUS is 4-fold that of WM.

9.3.2 Chemical and Physical Factors

The etiology of WM remains unknown. The rarity of this disorder has precluded inferences regarding infectious or environmental exposures. No specific genetic syndromes predisposing to this disease have been identified. Although occupational exposure has been postulated as a risk factor for some cases, there is little evidence to support this hypothesis (Tepper and Moss 1994).

9.3.3 Genetics

The majority of WM cases appear to be sporadic. However, some reports in the literature suggest familial clustering in a minority of cases. Families with several affected members have been described, and there appears to be some concordance among monozygotic twins (Blattner et al. 1980; Brown et al. 1967; Linet et al. 1993; Ogmundsdottir et al. 1999; Renier et al. 1989; Taleb et al. 1991). The disease may be due to genetic aberrations in developing B cells, but no recurrent abnormality is seen in all cases.

9.4 Screening/Prevention

Currently, no screening or preventive recommendations are available for this disease. In patients with a known IgM MGUS, expectant observation is warranted, with careful monitoring of symptoms, monoclonal protein, and hemoglobin value (Kyle and Garton 1987; Kyle et al. 2002).

9.5 Molecular Biology and Genetics

9.5.1 Normal Counterpart to the Clonal Cells

Although a precise definition of the normal counterpart of the malignant cell in WM has not been established, the cells most resemble postgerminal center B cells that have not undergone isotype class switching or memory B cells. Somatic hypermutation is evident in the clonal cells of WM, with little intraclonal heterogeneity at these loci (Aoki et al. 1995; Wagner et al. 1994). Consistent with their nonswitched phenotype, WM cells lack rearrangements at the switch μ regions (Schop et al. 2002).

9.5.2 Cytogenetics

Multiple reports describe cytogenetic findings in patients with WM, but none are universal or specific for the disease (Bottura 1966; Contrafatto 1977; Louviaux et al. 1998; Mansoor et al. 2001; Wong and So 2001). In the majority of cases, the karyotype analyses are normal (or uninformative), but inherent technical difficulties cause variable results. More recently, deletion of the long arm of chromosome 6 has been identified as a recurrent abnormality (Mansoor et al. 2001; Wong and So 2001). In a large cohort of WM patients studied by interphase fluorescent in situ hybridization, this deletion was the most common abnormality, present in 40% to 60% of cases (Schop et al. 2002).

Lymphoplasmacytic lymphoma has a t(9;14)(p13;q32) in at least 50% of cases (Offit et al. 1992). However, such cases have lacked monoclonal IgM paraprotein, so its relevance to WM is unclear (Iida et al. 1999). We have tested more than 40 patients with WM for the t(9;14)(p13;q32) by a specific interphase fluorescent in situ hybridization technique, and none of the samples had the abnormality (Schop et al. 2002). Sporadic reports of WM cases mention IgH (Chong et al. 1998; Nishida et al. 1989) or t(11;18)(q21;q21) (Hirase et al. 1996, 2000), translocations more typical of other B-cell neoplasms. Our group has been unable to find either abnormality in a large cohort of patients by interphase fluorescent in situ hybridization, indicating they are not common in WM (Schop et al. 2002).

9.5.3 Molecular Genetics

Little is known about the molecular genetic nature of WM. We have found that methylation of the tumor suppressor gene *p16* and *TP53* mutations are rare (Fonseca R, unpublished data). Ongoing studies address the role of gene expression profiles in patients with WM.

9.6 Clinical Presentation

With advancing disease, organomegaly, anemia, and hyperviscosity may develop (Gertz et al. 2000). The clinical features associated with WM can be divided into those that are related to clonal infiltration and compromise of the bone marrow and other organs, the effects of paraproteinemia on the peripheral blood (typically, but

Table 9.1. Clinical features of patients who have Waldenström macroglobulinemia

Series	N	Criteria for diagnosis		Study dates	Median age (range), y
		Monoclonal protein, g/dL	Marrow		
Newly diagnosed or untreated					
Facon et al. (1993)	167	>0.5	>25% or LPs	1969–89	–
Morel et al. (2000)	232	>0.5	>25% or LPs	1964–89	67 (30–100)
Gobbi et al. (1994)	144	>1.0	>30%	1976–91	61 (35–92)
Garcia-Sanz et al. (2001)	217	>3.0	>20% or LPs	1989–99	69
Kyrtsonis et al. (2001)	60	>0.5	+	1976–99	65 (43–91)
Dhodapkar et al. (2001)	118	+	+	1992–98	–
Kyle et al. (2000)	46	+	+	1971–93	63
Relapsed and refractory disease					
Leblond et al. (2001)	92	>0.5	Infiltrate	1993–97	64 (34.6–75)
Dhodapkar et al. (2001)	64	+	+	1992–98	–
Dimopoulos et al. (1993 b)	28	+	+	–	60 (43–79)
Leblond et al. (1998)	71	>0.5	+	1991–95	68 (42–81)
Leblond et al. (2001)	92	>0.5	+	1993–97	64.3 (34.6–75)
Dimopoulos et al. (1995)	46	–	–	1990–94	60 (34–81)
Hellmann et al. (1999)	13	>1.5	>30%	–	61.3 (46–73)

BJ, Bence Jones; cryo, cryoglobulin; LAD, lymphadenopathy; LPs, plasmacytoid lymphocytes; OS, overall survival; PC, plasma cells; Visc, viscosity.

[a] Measured in only 120 patients.

[b] Measured in only 70 patients.

[c] Defined as <12 g/dL (women) and <13.5 g/dL (men).

[d] Less than 100 in this series.

[e] More than 4 cps.

[f] Defined as <10 g/dL.

not limited to, hyperviscosity), and various other paraneoplastic phenomena.

9.6.1 Hyperviscosity Syndrome

One of the most characteristic features of WM is the presence of the hyperviscosity syndrome (Gertz and Kyle 1995). The dominant features are oronasal bleeding, retinal hemorrhage, and neurologic abnormalities (Fig. 9.1, see p. 210). At the retinal level, venous engorge-ment, retinal hemorrhage, and retinal vein occlusion occur (Robinson and Halpern 1992). The syndrome is seen in only 10% to 20% of patients at diagnosis (Dimopoulos et al. 2000) and does not necessarily correlate with the serum concentration of M protein or viscosity levels (Table 9.2, see p. 211). Increased viscosity in and of itself is not an indication for plasmapheresis or other treatment, and symptoms develop in different patients at different viscosity levels. Viscosity values of less than 4 cps are rarely associated with symptoms, whereas many patients with viscosity values of 5 to 8 cps, and

OS median, mo	M/F ratio	LAD, %	Spleen, %	Liver, %	↑Visc, %	Anemia (Hb <12 g/dL), %	% Patients PC <50%	κ/λ ratio	BJ, %	Cryo, %
60	1.27	23	26	13	8	58	22	3.0	41[a]	21[b]
–	2.46	–	22	21	10	67	20	5.7	36	6
–	1.09	–	–	–	–	–	–	4.7	41	–
–	2.00	25	19	24	31	38	–	–	31	5
108 (86–136)	1.40	22	18	13	12	85[c]	12[d]	3.5	54	5
~60	1.38	30	26	12	23	81	26	2.1	–	7
64.8	2.33	15	20	24	39[e]	89	–	6.5	–	10
43	2.06	36	17	11	–	51[f]	22[d]	–	–	–
~60	1.27	14	14	6	15	81	17	2.1	–	6
32	1.56	32	18	–	–	50[f]	46	–	–	–
23	–	(53 for all 3)			19	56[f]	–	–	–	–
45	2.06	36	17	11	–	51[f]	–	–	–	–
28	0.85	46	28	–	24	52[f]	–	–	–	4
–	1.25	33	22	–	–	33	–	–	–	–

the vast majority of patients with viscosity values greater than 8 cps, are symptomatic (Gertz and Kyle 1995). Therefore, repeated viscosity screening in patients with an IgM value less than 4,000 mg/dL is probably not needed (Gertz and Kyle 1995). Once the protein concentration is determined above which an individual patient crosses the "viscosity threshold," it can be used for future reference (Gertz and Kyle 1995). Minor reductions in the concentration of the serum M protein can have dramatic effects on serum viscosity and symptoms.

Viscosity is defined as the intrinsic resistance of a fluid to flow, described as a comparative ratio. The viscosity of normal plasma compared with water is 1.8. When IgM is abundant, the molecule's relatively large size alters the colligative properties of the plasma. The rheology of the hyperviscosity syndrome was described by Gertz and Kyle (1995). The viscosity of the blood can increase greatly with overzealous correction of anemia by transfusion of packed red blood cells; thus, transfusions must be used with caution in patients with high hyperviscosity. In these situations, the use of prophylactic plasmapheresis needs to be considered.

WM patients may have a constellation of neurologic symptoms attributable to hyperviscosity, many of which are ill-defined. Patients can complain of an array of symptoms, including headache or head "lightness" or "fullness." Focal neurologic deficits, including facial nerve paralysis, deafness, and other cranial neuropathies in this setting, were described originally by Waldenström (1948). Hyperviscosity can also lead to reversible clinical stroke or dementia.

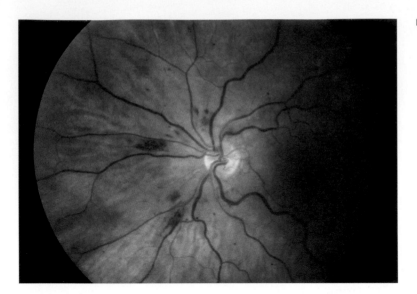

Fig. 9.1. Retinal bleeding

9.6.2 Signs and Symptoms Due to the Clonal Expansion

Anemia in WM is associated with the degree of clonal infiltration of the bone marrow. The anemia can vary from mild to severe and results in fatigue proportional to the level of anemia. Anemia (hemoglobin less than 10 g/dL) has been reported in 27% to 38% of patients (Facon et al. 1993; Garcia-Sanz et al. 2001). The anemia tends to be more pronounced because of the hemodilution caused by the paraprotein. The anemia is the most common reason for initiation of therapy (median hemoglobin, 10 g/dL) (Facon et al. 1993; Garcia-Sanz et al. 2001; Kyle and Garton 1987). Anemia can be responsive to erythropoietin administration. Increased viscosity reduces erythropoietin production and contributes to the anemia of WM (Singh et al. 1993). In heavily pretreated patients, one should always consider the possibility of myelodysplasia. Likewise, thrombocytopenia can be observed at the time of diagnosis but is rare then or later in the disease course as a result of progression or drug toxicity (Table 9.1).

Organomegaly is seen in about one-third of patients, most commonly hepatomegaly (20%) and splenomegaly (15%) (Facon et al. 1993; Garcia-Sanz et al. 2001) (Table 9.1). Up to 15% of patients may have associated lymphadenopathy, ranging from mild to bulky. Pulmonary involvement, characterized by a lymphoplasmacytic infiltrate staining positive for IgM, is also possible in WM.

9.6.3 Paraneoplastic and Other Manifestations

In up to 5% of WM patients, IgM-associated peripheral neuropathies and other syndromes can develop. There are several mechanisms by which WM could cause peripheral neuropathy, including IgM antimyelin-associated glycoprotein activity, IgM activity against other antigens in the nerve sheath, amyloidosis, and cryoglobulinemia (Dimopoulos et al. 2000; Gertz et al. 1999; Kyle and Garton 1987).

9.7 Classification and Staging

Currently, there is no widely accepted or useful clinical staging system for WM. The aforementioned disease continuum ranges from IgM MGUS to WM (Kyle et al. 2002). Identification of the IgM MGUS patients whose disease will eventually transform to WM is not currently possible. Within this continuum, WM is usually diagnosed when end organ damage develops, either due to viscosity or clonal expansion (e.g., anemia, organomegaly) (Kyle and Garton 1987). Some cases fulfilling the diagnostic criteria may remain indolent (Kyle and Garton 1987). Such cases do not require immediate therapy and should be considered analogous to smoldering multiple myeloma.

Recently, Garand and colleagues (2000) described an entity with similarities to WM in which patients have

Table 9.2. Hyperviscosity symptoms in Waldenström macroglobulinemia

Bleeding manifestations

  Oronasal

  Gastrointestinal tract bleeding

  Postoperative

Visual manifestations

  Visual loss

  Retinal vein thrombosis or hemorrhage

  Diplopia

  Exudates and papilledema

Inner ear and balance

  Ataxia

  Vertigo

  Deafness

Neurologic

  Headache

  Syncope

  Stupor or coma

  Cerebral hemorrhage

  Seizure

Cardiac

  High-output failure

Modified from Gertz et al. (2000). By permission of AlphaMed Press.

a B-cell lymphoproliferative disorder that produces an excess amount of monoclonal IgG. Although patients may have hyperviscosity associated with monoclonal IgG or IgA, these patients are not normally considered as having WM.

9.8 Diagnosis

The diagnosis of WM can be challenging, because there is no standardized set of minimum criteria. Currently, the diagnosis is made on the basis of the clinical features and the characteristic lymphoplasmacytic proliferation and serum IgM M protein (Dimopoulos et al. 2000; Gertz et al. 2000).

9.8.1 Laboratory Tests

Patients thought to have WM should have baseline laboratory tests consisting of complete blood cell count and serum chemistry profile, including creatinine, bilirubin, aspartate aminotransferase, alkaline phosphatase, and calcium. Serum β_2-microglobulin is also measured, because it is useful as a prognostic factor (Dhodapkar et al. 2001; Garcia-Sanz et al. 2001).

9.8.1.1 Hematologic Laboratory Abnormalities

Although there are several factors contributing to the anemia seen in WM patients, erythroid hypoproliferation due to the intramedullary lymphoplasmacytic clonal expansion is thought to be the main cause. However, hemoglobin dilution by the increased plasma volume (Dimopoulos et al. 2000; Gertz et al. 2000) and decreased renal tubular erythropoietin production (Singh et al. 1993) is also important. Peripheral destruction in the form of hypersplenism and hemolytic anemia is possible but less common as a cause for anemia in these patients (Facon et al. 1993; Garcia-Sanz et al. 2001; Kyle et al. 2000). Because of the expanded plasma volume, patients may be asymptomatic at low hemoglobin values.

Red cell rouleaux (French for "rolls") formation is characteristically seen in the peripheral smear. Likewise, the sedimentation rate is usually increased in WM patients, rendering this test useless for the evaluation of infection or systemic inflammation. The sedimentation rate alterations seem to be independent of the protein concentration, and great elevations may be seen even with relatively low M protein values. For this reason, WM has been confused occasionally with polymyalgia rheumatica or temporal arteritis.

9.8.1.2 Paraproteinemia

There is no minimal concentration of monoclonal IgM required for the diagnosis of WM (Kyle and Garton 1987). Some investigators have established a lower limit of 3 g/dL (Gobbi et al. 1994; Kyle et al. 2000); others have used lower values. Many consider a serum monoclonal IgM exceeding a concentration of 1.5 g/dL to be characteristic of WM, because this limit appears useful in differentiating it from other neoplasms with plasmacytoid differentiation. A recent consensus conference at the National Institutes of Health recommended a concentration of at least 1.5 g/dL be used as a minimal diagnostic criterion (Fonseca R, unpublished data). Another consensus meeting suggested that monoclonal lymphoplasmacytes in association with any monoclonal IgM protein (irrespective of its concentration) establish the diagnosis of WM (Fonseca R, unpublished data).

To properly characterize an M protein newly detected on protein electrophoresis, immunofixation is typically done. Nephelometry is also recommended to quantify levels of IgG, IgA, and IgM. Because a high concentration of a monoclonal IgM (narrow bands) can saturate the densitometry reading, it may underestimate the true concentration of the monoclonal IgM. In such cases, nephelometry is a more accurate test. However, because discrepancies between the quantitative values obtained from serum protein electrophoresis and nephelometry are possible, only one of these tests should be used for subsequent disease monitoring. Viscosity determination is helpful at baseline and should be repeated if symptoms consistent with hyperviscosity are present.

It is a common misconception that patients with WM do not shed light chains in the urine. In fact, between 40% and 80% of patients have Bence Jones proteinuria. Therefore, a 24-hour urine collection should be analyzed by protein electrophoresis and immunofixation to detect possible Bence Jones proteins (Facon et al. 1993; Garcia-Sanz et al. 2001) (Table 9.1).

9.8.1.3 Bone Marrow Aspiration and Biopsy

A bone marrow trephine aspiration and biopsy is performed routinely at the time of diagnosis and whenever there are changes in clinical status, to estimate the degree of clonal involvement. The primary pathologic abnormality in WM is a clonal proliferation of B cells that secrete monoclonal IgM (Dimopoulos et al. 2000; Gertz et al. 2000; Owen et al. 2000). The morphology is typically lymphoplasmacytic, although the spectrum goes from lymphocytic to mature plasmacytic (Dimopoulos et al. 2000; Gertz et al. 2000; Owen et al. 2000) (Fig. 9.2).

It has been suggested that 30% marrow infiltration by clonal lymphocytes (in addition to the monoclonal IgM paraproteinemia) be required to make the diagnosis (Gobbi et al. 1994), although others consider any degree of lymphoplasmacytic bone marrow infiltration with an associated monoclonal IgM spike as sufficient (Facon et al. 1993). The existence of many B-cell neoplasms with plasmacytic differentiation that do not otherwise resemble macroglobulinemia complicates this issue further.

In the aspirate samples, flow cytometric studies can characterize the neoplastic cells and differentiate them from other B-cell neoplasms. Typically, clonal cells in WM express pan B-cell surface markers (CD19, CD20, CD22) in association with monoclonal light chains on the cell surface and in the cytoplasm. Cell surface expression of CD10 (common in follicular lymphoma), CD23 (common in chronic lymphocytic leukemia), and CD5 (common in chronic lymphocytic leukemia and mantle cell lymphoma) is usually absent. CD138 (syndecan-1) can be detected in the plasma cell compartment (Feiner et al. 1990; Owen et al. 2000, 2001; Pangalis et al. 1999). Although CD5 is not seen in the majority of cases, it has been detected occasionally in cases fulfilling the diagnostic criteria, has been reported, and has been observed by us as well (Remstein E, personal communication) (Feiner et al. 1990; Owen et al. 2000, 2001; Pangalis et al. 1999) (Table 9.3).

Although the plasma cell labeling index is a useful prognostic factor in myeloma, its role in WM remains undefined (Greipp et al. 1993). In our institutional experience, most WM patients have low labeling index values consistent with a nonproliferating clone (0% in greater than 80% of patients) (Fonseca R, unpublished data). Karyotype analysis has diagnostic utility, and it should be done in previously treated patients thought to have therapy-associated myelodysplasia or acute leukemia.

Fig. 9.2. Lymphoplasmacytosis.

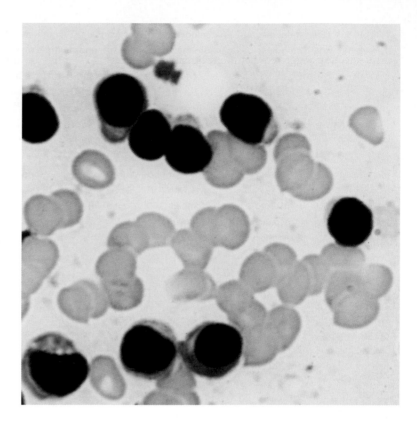

9.8.2 Radiologic Studies

In contrast to myeloma, lytic bone disease is unusual in WM; therefore, routine skeletal radiographs or bone scans are not needed unless the patient reports bone pain.

9.9 Differential Diagnosis

The Revised European-American Lymphoma classification system (Harris et al. 1994) formally designates WM as lymphoplasmacytic lymphoma because of its morphologic and immunophenotypic features. The diagnosis of WM is straightforward in cases with high-concentration paraproteinemia and the classic lymphoplasmacytic infiltrate. It may be difficult to differentiate WM from marginal zone lymphomas on a purely pathologic basis, because the immunophenotype may be identical. Differentiation of WM from mantle cell lymphoma and B-cell chronic lymphocytic leukemia is usually straightforward, because the latter 2 always express CD5 and

lack the strong immunoglobulin expression of WM. Mantle cell lymphoma should also have strong nuclear positivity for *cyclin D* by immunohistochemistry and a t(11;14)(q13;q32). Follicular B-cell lymphoma can be differentiated readily from WM; the former has characteristic nodal architecture on light microscopy, cell surface expression of CD10, and positive nuclear staining for *bcl-2* expression as a consequence of the t(14;18)(q32;q21) (Table 9.3).

9.10 Secondary Malignancies

There are no associations between WM and other malignancies except those arising as a complication of treatment. Alkylating agents, the main chemotherapeutic tools against WM, are well known to cause chromosomal breaks. A dreaded long-term complication of the use of chlorambucil is the development of myelodysplasia and acute myeloid leukemia. In a study of 46 patients, 9% developed this complication: acute leukemia in 3 and refractory anemia in 1 (Kyle et al. 2000). Other

Table 9.3. Differential diagnosis: pathologic features of mantle cell lymphoma, B-cell chronic lymphocytic leukemia, marginal zone lymphoma, Waldenström macroglobulinemia, and multiple myeloma

Feature	Mantle cell lymphoma	B-cell CLL	Follicular B-cell lymphoma	Marginal zone B-cell lymphoma	WM	Multiple myeloma
Paraprotein	None	Small IgG or IgM	Usually none	+/– Small IgM	IgM (large)	IgA, IgG[a]
Morphology	Centrocyte-like; small- to medium-sized lymphocytes	Small lympho-cyte with clumped chromatin	Follicle center cells (follicular pattern)	Monocytoid B cell; hetero-geneous	Plasmacytoid lymphocytes and plasma cells	Plasma cells
Surface Ig	+	+	+	+	+	+
Cytoplasmic Ig	–	–	–	–	++	+++
CD19	+	+	+	+	+	–
CD20	++	+	++	+	+	(15% CD20⁺)
CD23	–	+	–/+	–	–	–
CD22	+	–	–	+	+	–
CD38	–	–/+	–	–	+	++
CD138	–	–	–	–	+	++
CD5	+	+	–	–	Usually –	–
CD10	–/+	–	+	–	–	–
Cytogenetic aberrations	t (11;14) (q13;q32), cyclin D1+	13q–, 6q–, +12, 11q23–	t(14;18) (q32;q21), Bcl 2+	t(11;18) (q21;q21), +3	6q–	t(4;14) (p16.3;q32), t(11;14) (q13;q32), t(14;16) (q32;q23), other+14q32, 13q–, aneuploidy
SHM	–	+ (50%) –(50%)	++	++	+++	+++
Bone marrow involvement	25%	~ 100%	85%	50%	>90%	100%
Bone lytic lesions	No	No	No	No	5%	70%

CLL, chronic lymphocytic leukemia; SHM, somatic hypermutation; WM, Waldenström macroglobulinemia.
[a] Unusual, but can have IgD, IgE, or IgM.

reports have confirmed this association between alkylator therapy and subsequent acute myelogenous leukemia (Horsman et al. 1983). Acute myelogenous leukemia arising from myelodysplasia is clearly the greatest risk of alkylating agent therapy, but fortunately it occurs in a small minority of patients. However, as better treatments become available and prolong survival, the risk appears to increase with time.

9.11 Therapy

9.11.1 Observation

There are some patients in whom expectant observation is all that is warranted because of the absence of symptoms. With currently available therapies, the treatment is considered palliative and should be used only for the symptomatic patient and to prevent hyperviscosity. As is also seen in myeloma, some patients with WM should be considered as having the smoldering variant of the disease (Gertz et al. 2000; Kyle and Greipp 1980). However, expectant observation requires regular office visits and laboratory determinations of disease markers (e.g., hemoglobin and serum IgM levels) to continuously ascertain the need for treatment.

9.11.2 Chemotherapy

9.11.2.1 Alkylating Agents

Oral alkylating agents remain the most widely used therapy for WM (Table 9.4). The effectiveness of oral chlorambucil has been confirmed in 2 studies involving 174 patients (Facon et al. 1993; Kyle et al. 2000). Overall median survival was comparable in these studies (60 and 65 months). Kyle and colleagues (2000) showed that chlorambucil significantly improved hemoglobin concentration (61% of patients) and reduced splenomegaly (67%) and lymphadenopathy (71%); patients receiving chlorambucil daily ultimately fared no better than patients receiving it "pulsed" every 6 weeks.

9.11.2.2 Combination Alkylator Chemotherapy

The combination of vincristine, carmustine, melphalan, cyclophosphamide, and prednisone (VBMCP) has been used extensively in myeloma and was tested for WM in 2 studies. The first demonstrated an 82% overall response

rate (22% complete responses) in 33 patients given VBMCP every 5 weeks for 2 years, followed by maintenance dosing every 10 weeks (Case et al. 1991). The projected 10-year survival rate was 58%. The second study used monthly melphalan, cyclophosphamide, and prednisone for 1 year in 34 WM patients, followed by continuous chlorambucil maintenance (Petrucci et al. 1989). The overall response rate was 74% (26% complete responses), with a median event-free survival of 66 months. Combination chemotherapy appears less effective as salvage therapy, however. Leblond and colleagues (2001) randomized 45 patients in whom single-agent alkylator therapy failed to now receive cyclophosphamide, doxorubicin (Adriamycin), and prednisone (CAP) for 6 cycles versus fludarabine. Only 11% of patients receiving CAP attained partial responses that were of short duration (median, 3 months).

9.11.2.3 Fludarabine

Purine nucleoside analogs (fludarabine, cladribine, and pentostatin) are highly effective in low-grade lymphomas and B-cell chronic lymphocytic leukemia. In 1990, the use of fludarabine for WM was explored. In one report, 5 of 11 patients showed a 50% M-spike reduction, sustained for more than 12 months (Kantarjian et al. 1990) (Table 9.5). In a separate report, Dimopoulos et al. (1993b) described a 36% response rate (median duration, 38 months) in 28 patients. Subsequent larger studies ($n = 71$ and 182) (Dhodapkar et al. 2001; Leblond et al. 1998) reported a response rate with fludarabine of 30% to 35%. Most studies required a median of 5 months of treatment before response to fludarabine became evident (Dhodapkar et al. 2001; Kantarjian et al. 1990; Leblond et al. 2001; Thalhammer-Scherrer et al. 2000), and all studies had low complete response rates (defined as the complete resolution of the M spike and lymphocytic infiltrates) (Dhodapkar et al. 2001; Dimopoulos et al. 1993b; Foran et al. 1999; Kantarjian et al. 1990; Leblond et al. 1998, 2001; Thalhammer-Scherrer et al. 2000; Zinzani et al. 1995). Among the studies of fludarabine with at least 12 months median follow-up, the median duration of remission ranged from 19 to 44.5 months, with median overall survival ranging from 23 to 60 months (Foran et al. 1999; Leblond et al. 1998, 2001; Thalhammer-Scherrer et al. 2000).

Subgroup analysis of an earlier study suggested that relapsed patients refractory to alkylator therapy were less likely to respond to fludarabine (Dimopoulos et

Table 9.4. Treatment with alkylators in patients who have Waldenström macroglobulinemia

Series	Regimen	N	Overall response rate, %	Median response duration, mo	Median overall survival, mo	Median event-free survival, mo	Remarks
Facon et al. (1993)	Chlorambucil 0.1 mg/kg per d, continuous	110	75	NR	60	NR	–
Kyle et al. (2000)	Chlorambucil 0.1 mg/kg per d, continuous	24	79	26[a]	65	NR	–
	OR						
	Chlorambucil 0.3 mg/kg per d×7d, repeat q6wk	22	68	46[a]	65	NR	
Case et al. (1991)	BCNU/CTX/Vinc then Melph/Pred repeated q5wk×2y	33	82	39 (5±114)/ 43 (15–60)[b]	NR	NR	Projected 10-y overall survival, 58%
Petrucci et al. (1989)	Melph/CTX/Pred×7d, repeat q4wk×12, then daily chlorambucil/Pred	34	68	NR	NR	66	Median response duration and overall survival not reached at time of report
Leblond et al. (2001)	CTX+DOX on d1, then Pred (d1–5), q4wk	45	11	3	45	~5.5	MCP vs. fludarabine as salvage; no significant overall survival difference

BCNU, carmustine; CTX, cyclophosphamide; DOX, doxorubicin; MCP, melphalan/cyclophosphamide/prednisone; Melph, melphalan; NR, not reported; Pred, prednisone; Vinc, vincristine.

[a] Based on 50% IgM reduction.

[b] Partial responders/complete responders.

al. 1993b). Other small studies showed higher response rates among treatment-naive patients compared with previously treated patients (Foran et al. 1999). A recent large comparison study found the response rates in untreated and previously treated arms were comparable (38% vs. 33%, $P=0.62$), but patients older than age 70 years were less likely to respond to fludarabine (hazard ratio, 0.34; $P=0.02$) (Dhodapkar et al. 2001).

Because of low uninvolved immunoglobulin levels and disease-related granulocytopenia, WM patients are susceptible to infectious complications. Because purine nucleoside analogs markedly reduce the number of circulating $CD4^+$ T cells, fludarabine treatment may further impair immunity, leading to opportunistic infections such as *Pneumocystis carinii* pneumonia. Other opportunistic infections are possible.

Table 9.5. Treatment with fludarabine in patients who have Waldenström macroglobulinemia

Series	Fludarabine regimen	N	Overall response rate, %	Median response duration, mo	Median overall survival, mo	Median event-free survival, mo	Remarks
Kantarjian et al. (1990)	30 mg/m^2 IV bolus qd×5d, repeated q4wk	11	45	10[a]	NR	NR	–
Leblond et al. (2001)	25 mg/m^2 IV bolus×5d, q4wk	45	31	19	41	~6.5	CAP vs. fludarabine as salvage, no overall survival difference
Dhodapkar et al. (2001)	30 mg/m^2 qd×5d, repeat q28d	182	35	NR	60	NR	No difference between pre-Tx and Tx-naive
Dimopoulos et al. (1993b)	20–30 mg/m^2 IV×5d OR 30 mg/m^2 qd×3d	28	36	38	32	NR	–
Zinzani et al. (1995)	25 mg/m^2 per d×5d, q21–28d×6 courses	12	42	10.5	NR	NR	Median FU only 6 mo
Leblond et al. (1998)	25 mg/m^2 IV bolus×5d, repeated q4wk until max response	71	30	32	23	NR	Pretreatment Hb and platelets correlated with survival
Thalhammer-Scherrer et al. (2000)	25 mg/m^2 per d×5d, repeat q4wk	7	86	44.5	NR	NR	–
Foran et al. (1999)	25 mg/m^2 per d×5d, q4wk to max response+2 more cycles	19	79	>36	NR	NR	–

CAP, cyclophosphamide/doxorubicin/prednisone; FU, follow-up; Hb, hemoglobin; IV, intravenous; max, maximum; NR, not reported; Tx, treatment.

[a] Four of five responders still in remission at study termination.

9.11.2.4 Cladribine

Initially introduced for the treatment of hairy cell leukemia, cladribine is structurally similar to fludarabine. Its use for WM was reported in 29 patients, 9 of whom were treatment-naive and received continuous 7-day infusion for 2 cycles (Dimopoulos et al. 1993a) (Table 9.6). The overall response rate was 59% (100% among newly diagnosed patients versus 40% among the pretreated). Subsequent studies found response rates more typical of those seen with fludarabine (range, 29%–52%) and were unable to confirm the initial report of higher response rates among previously untreated patients (Betticher et al. 1997; Delannoy et al. 1994; Hellmann et al. 1999; Laurencet et al. 1999; Liu et al. 1998). Also, grade 3 or

greater marrow toxicity became an important dose-limiting toxicity (Delannoy et al. 1994; Hellmann et al. 1999; Laurencet et al. 1999; Liu et al. 1998).

Alternative cladribine dosing regimens were also evaluated. No difference in response rate was seen between patients receiving cladribine as a 2-hour infusion of 5.6 mg/m^2 per day for 5 days and those receiving continuous infusions of 4 mg/m^2 per day for 7 days (Delannoy et al. 1994). Cladribine administered as a 2-hour bolus infusion (obviating the need for a central venous catheter) was studied initially in 21 patients who received 0.12 mg/kg per day for 5 days over 3 consecutive months (Liu et al. 1998). The overall response rate was 55% (including 1 complete response), with responses sustained for a median of 28 months; however, grade 3

Table 9.6. Treatment with cladribine in patients who have Waldenström macroglobulinemia

Series	Cladribine regimen	N	Overall response rate, %	Median response duration, mo	Median overall survival, mo	Remarks
Liu et al. (1998)	0.12 mg/kg per d (2-h bolus)×5d, q mo×3–8 cycles	21	52	28	48	–
Betticher et al. (1997)	0.1 mg/kg SC bolus×5d q4wk, max 6 cycles	25	40	8	NR	–
Dimopoulos et al. (1993a)	0.1 mg/kg IV qd×7d, 2 cycles	29	59	NR	NR	–
Delannoy et al. (1994)	4 mg/m^2 per d IV×7d OR 5.6 mg/m^2 per d IV over 2 h×5d	18	39	2	NR	Continuous vs. bolus infusions; no difference in outcomes
Dimopoulos et al. (1994)	0.1 mg/kg per d IV×7d cont, 2 cycles	14	29	11	NR	Brief report of fludarabine failures/ relapses
Hellmann et al. (1999)	0.14 mg/kg per d (2-h bolus)×5d, repeated q28–35d for 3–5 cycles	22	41	12	NR	–
Laurencet et al. (1999)	0.1 mg/kg per d d1–3+CTX 500 mg/m^2 d1+Pred 40 mg/m^2 d1–5	3	100	NR	NR	–

Cont, continuous; CTX, cyclophosphamide; IV, intravenous; max, maximum; NR, not reported; Pred, prednisone; SC, subcutaneous.

or 4 neutropenia occurred in 60% of patients (Liu et al. 1998). A subsequent study of a similar bolus regimen found a 41% overall response rate (no complete response), with many patients experiencing severe thrombocytopenia (77%) and thrombocytopenia (32%, with one attributable fatality) (Hellmann et al. 1999). Long-term cladribine administration via subcutaneous (SC) injection (0.1 mg/kg daily for 5 days, maximum of 6 cycles) was evaluated in 25 previously treated patients. After a median of 3 cycles, 40% achieved a partial response, with a median remission duration of 8 months. Grade 2 or greater infections developed in 16% of patients (Betticher et al. 1997).

Cladribine combination regimens have been studied less extensively. Bolus administration of cladribine (0.12 mg/kg over 2 hours for 5 days, repeated monthly for 4 cycles) followed by interferon maintenance therapy resulted in a 90% response rate (1 complete) in a series of 10 previously untreated patients. Another study of 3 patients given cladribine (0.1 mg/kg SC for 3 days) in combination with cyclophosphamide (500 mg/m² for 1 day) and prednisone (40 mg/m² for 5 days) for up to 6 cycles achieved a 100% response rate (all partial) (Laurencet et al. 1999).

Patients who are resistant to fludarabine are unlikely to benefit from cladribine. In a cross-resistance study, 14 patients in whom fludarabine therapy failed received 2 courses of cladribine. Although 3 of 4 patients whose disease progressed after a previous response to fludarabine responded to cladribine, only 1 of 10 patients with fludarabine-resistant disease responded (Dimopoulos et al. 1994).

Cladribine is thus effective as frontline treatment for WM but is associated with myelosuppression, fever, and T-cell immunodeficiency (Bryson and Sorkin 1993). Cladribine treatment for WM should probably be limited to 2 cycles to avoid profound myelosuppression. Renal and neurologic effects and local skin reactions have also been reported. Interestingly, cladribine-induced T-lymphocyte suppression appears to be associated with autoimmune phenomena. Four WM patients were reported in whom immune-mediated hemolysis developed after cladribine therapy (median, 40 months after initial administration); 1 patient responded to oral corticosteroids and 2 died (Tetreault and Saven 2000).

9.11.2.5 Combination Therapy With Purine Nucleoside Analogs

Regimens have been studied that combine alkylating agents with purine nucleoside analogs. In a dose-escalation study, bolus administration of cladribine (5.6 mg/m² per day) was followed by a 1-hour infusion of cyclophosphamide for 3 days. Cyclophosphamide initially was given at 200 mg/m², and the dose escalated in 100-mg/m² increments. The overall response rate was 58% (Van Den Neste et al. 2000). However, after the administration of cladribine (5.6 mg/m²), the development of granulocytopenia limited the maximum tolerated cyclophosphamide dose to 300 mg/m². Repeated cycles could not be given in 31% of patients because of prolonged thrombocytopenia, and severe infections were seen in 4% of cycles. Studies are planned combining cyclophosphamide, cladribine, and rituximab.

9.11.2.6 Rituximab

Because the clonal cells of WM express surface CD20, the anti-CD20 monoclonal antibody rituximab has the potential to target malignant cells selectively while causing limited myelosuppression (Table 9.7). The first trial in 7 previously treated WM patients (who received either 4 or 8 weekly infusions of rituximab) showed that the medication was indeed well tolerated, with no infectious complications (Byrd et al. 1999). Partial responses were noted in 3 patients, with a median progression-free survival of 6.6 months.

In the first of 2 recent studies of rituximab for WM, 8 of 30 patients (27%) had a partial response (>50% IgM decline), and 10 of 30 (33%) had a minor response (>25% IgM decline) after a median of 4 rituximab infusions. Of note, 47% of these patients had previously received a nucleoside analog. Although no complete responses were seen, posttreatment marrow examination showed the lymphoplasmacytic infiltration decreased from 60% to 15%. In addition, hematocrit improved in 63% of patients (with 6 of 7 transfusion-dependent patients becoming independent) and platelet counts improved in 50%. However, the median time to treatment failure for responding patients was 8 months (5 months for stable patients) (Treon et al. 2001). The second trial reported a 44% response rate in 27 untreated patients and confirmed the improvements in hemoglobin, IgM, bone marrow involvement, and peripheral neuropathy seen in earlier studies. No significant myelosuppression

Table 9.7. Treatment with rituximab in patients who have Waldenström macroglobulinemia

Series	Rituximab regimen	N	Overall response rate, %	Median response duration, mo	Median overall survival, mo	Median event-free survival, mo
Dimopoulos et al. (2002)	375 mg/m² IV×4 wk, repeated×1 for responders	27	44	NR	NR	NR
Byrd et al. (1999)	375 mg/m² IV q wk×4 wk	7	57	11	NR	6.6
Treon et al. (1999)	375 mg/m² IV q wk×4 wk	30	27	8	NR	NR

IV, intravenous; NR, not reported.

occurred, and the median time to progression was longer in this study (16 months). Interestingly, patients with IgM values greater than 4 g/dL were significantly less likely to respond ($P = 0.03$) (Dimopoulos et al. 2002).

Because of its acceptable toxicity profile, the lack of therapy-associated myelosuppression and myelodysplasia, and patients' acceptance, rituximab use for WM has become widespread (Treon and Anderson 2000). Furthermore, it is being used increasingly in younger patients and in earlier stages of disease. The main toxicity of rituximab is the infusion syndrome, consisting of rigors, fever, and hypotension during the first treatment. It is usually well controlled with corticosteroids and antihistamines, and subsequent cycles are usually well tolerated. It is currently unknown whether rituximab should be used as frontline treatment of WM.

Patients with minimal marrow infiltration (< 25% of the cellularity) may be candidates for radioimmunoconjugate anti-CD20 (e.g., yttrium) as a potentially more effective, although myelosuppressive, alternative to the monoclonal antibody alone (White 1999). Studies to determine the safety of this approach will be needed.

9.11.2.7 Thalidomide

Thalidomide is an immunomodulatory and antiangiogenic agent that is effective in salvage therapy for multiple myeloma. A recent phase 2 trial of thalidomide (200–600 mg/d) in 20 WM patients (10 previously treated) showed an overall response rate of 25%; unfortunately, the time to progression was less than 3 months (Dimopoulos et al. 2001). Thalidomide appears to be minimally effective as a single agent in WM.

9.11.2.8 Corticosteroids

Although historically macroglobulinemia has not been considered a steroid-responsive malignancy, reports do exist suggesting situations in which steroids alone can be beneficial, particularly in patients with severe pancytopenia who would not be candidates for cytotoxic therapy. In one such study, vincristine (0.25 mg/m²) and bleomycin (5 units) were given for 4 consecutive days with alternate-day oral prednisone (1,000 mg/m²). Both WM patients in this study had a greater than 50% decrease in M protein and bone marrow infiltration, with remission durations ranging from 4 to greater than 35 weeks. In patients with severe pancytopenia who are not candidates for other therapy, a trial of corticosteroids may be beneficial in this disorder. Corticosteroids may also profoundly reduce the immune complex vasculitis seen in WM patients with associated cryoglobulinemia (O'Reilly and MacKenzie 1967).

9.11.3 Autologous Stem Cell Transplantation

After the success and proven survival benefit of stem cell transplantation in multiple myeloma, this treatment was tried in patients with WM, with encouraging results. Six patients (median age, 52 years) were reported (Desikan et al. 1999); 2 were pretreated minimally and 4 had relapsed after purine nucleoside analog therapy. Two patients (both previously treated with fludarabine) failed to mobilize initially and required 2 attempts. All 6 subsequently received transplants: 5 were conditioned with melphalan (200 mg/m²) including 1 tandem transplant, and 1 patient received melphalan (140 mg/m²) with total body irradiation. There was no treatment-related mortality. Five of the 6 engrafted promptly, and all 6 achieved a partial response. Five of the 6 were still alive at the time of the report, with 4 remaining event-free for a range of 2 to 52 months. This suggests that WM patients can safely be mobilized and receive transplants, although patients with prior exposure to purine nucleoside analogs and alkylating agents may be poor candidates.

In another study (Dreger et al. 1999), 7 patients received 2 to 3 cycles of Dexa-BEAM (dexamethasone, carmustine [BiCNU], etoposide, ARA-C, melphalan) chemotherapy with stem cell collection, followed by high-dose cyclophosphamide and total body irradiation. Engraftment was prompt, and there were no treatment-related deaths. A decreased serum IgM concentration occurred in all evaluable patients, but immunofixation demonstrated a persistent M protein in 5 patients. All patients were alive without progression at publication (range, 3 to 30 months).

9.11.4 Surgery: Splenectomy

Although splenectomy does not address the marrow infiltration associated with macroglobulinemia, it may benefit some patients with hypersplenic syndromes or spleen-dominant disease. Splenectomy normalized the clotting function of 1 WM patient with an associated factor VIII deficiency, and another patient with giant splenomegaly experienced a hematologic response post-splenectomy (Brody et al. 1979; Nagai et al. 1991). Two subsequent WM patients with massive splenomegaly refractory to chemotherapy underwent splenectomy. The monoclonal IgM disappeared, and these patients remained free of disease at 12 and 13 years (Humphrey and Conley 1995). This suggests that the spleen may facilitate IgM secretion and that splenectomy is a viable option for patients with massive splenomegaly, particularly those whose disease progresses during chemotherapy.

9.11.5 Supportive Care: Plasma Exchange

Total plasma exchange has no impact on the tumor burden or the immunoglobulin-producing cells in macroglobulinemia, but it has a significant role in the management of patients with prominent symptoms of hyperviscosity. Such patients may be newly diagnosed and in need of urgent therapy or may have exhausted all options for systemic chemotherapy. Among newly presenting WM patients, bleeding is the most common manifestation of hyperviscosity. Such situations require urgent plasma exchange because of the high incidence of blindness after retinal hemorrhage and macular detachment (Thomas et al. 1983). When acute hyperviscosity symptoms develop (usually at viscosity values >4 cps), IgM reductions of as little as 20% can reduce the viscosity by up to 50% because the serum viscosity does not correlate linearly with IgM values (Avnstorp et al. 1985). Plasma exchange thus remains a valuable adjunctive technique in the management of macroglobulinemia.

9.12 Prognosis

9.12.1 Prognostic Models

The prognosis of patients who have WM varies, with some patients having significantly shorter survival than others. Morel and colleagues (2000) developed a prognostic model for patients with WM. In their study of 232 patients treated with alkylating agents (no purine nucleoside analogs) before 1989, they found age older than 65 years, albumin concentration less than 40 g/L, and cytopenias (hemoglobin <12 g/dL, platelet counts <150×10³, and leukocyte counts <4×10³) were important independent prognostic factors. By assigning points for each cell lineage affected by a cytopenia (e.g., 1 point for anemia, 2 points for anemia and leukopenia), patients could be grouped into 3 prognostic categories: low (0–1 points, 27% of patients); intermediate (2 points, 27% of patients); or high risk (3 or 4 points, 46% of patients). The proportion of patients alive at 5 years was 87%, 62%, and 25% for the low-, intermediate-, and high-risk groups, respectively (Table 9.8). The median actuarial overall survival was 61 months, and there was no difference in overall survival between the patients who were monitored initially and those who received immediate treatment. Other prognostic factors in the univariate model were β_2-microglobulin (>3 mg/L), serum IgM, and plasma volume greater than 50 mL/kg. Factors not prognostic were the presence of Bence Jones protein, splenomegaly, "B" symptoms, light-chain type, cryoglobulinemia, pattern of marrow involvement, and other cytologic features. In patients younger than 65 years, only the presence of 2 or more cytopenias was important.

An alternative prognostic scoring system, developed by Gobbi and colleagues (1994), considers weight loss,

Table 9.8. Prognostic models for patients who have Waldenström macroglobulinemia

Prognostic system proposed by Dhodapkar et al. (2001)			
Stage	β_2-microglobulin, mg/dL	Other	5-year overall survival, %
A	<3	Hemoglobin>12 g/dL	87
B	<3	Hemoglobin<12 g/dL	64
C	≥3	Serum IgM≥4,000 mg/dL	53
D	≥3	Serum IgM<4,000 mg/dL	21
Prognostic system proposed by Morel et al. (2000)			
Category	Points		
Low risk	0–1		87
Intermediate risk	2		62
High risk	3–4		25

cryoglobulinemia, anemia (hemoglobin <10 g/dL), and age older than 60 years. Low-risk patients have 0 or 1 adverse feature; the others are considered high risk. Finally, Dhodapkar and colleagues (2001) evaluated prognostic factors in a group of 182 patients who were treated with fludarabine. They found an overall response rate of 36%, with 2% of patients attaining a complete response. Patients older than age 70 years had significantly lower overall response rates and shorter survivals. Serum β_2-microglobulin greater than or equal to 3 mg/L, hemoglobin less than 12 g/dL, and IgM greater than 4,000 mg/dL were also associated with a shorter survival. Using these 3 factors, they developed a system to predict 5-year overall survival (Table 9.8).

9.12.2 Disease Transformation

Evolution of WM to more aggressive lymphoproliferative disorders has been reported (Abe et al. 1982). In many of these instances, extramedullary features of disease ensue, such as pleural effusions. The prognosis in such cases is poor.

9.13 Conclusion

Clear-cut guidelines cannot be issued for all patients because of the lack of randomized phase 3 studies. The mainstays of therapy remain alkylating agents and purine nucleoside analogs, usually administered singly and in sequence. Data do not exist that permit selection of one modality rather than another. Whether combination therapies will be superior to single-agent therapy is unknown. The ultimate role of rituximab in the management of this disease remains to be defined.

References

Abe M, Takahashi K, Mori N, Kojima M (1982) "Waldenström's macroglobulinemia" terminating in immunoblastic sarcoma. A case report. Cancer 49:2580–2586

Aoki H, Takishita M, Kosaka M, Saito S (1995) Frequent somatic mutations in D and/or JH segments of Ig gene in Waldenström's macroglobulinemia and chronic lymphocytic leukemia (CLL) with Richter's syndrome but not in common CLL. Blood 85:1913–1919

Avnstorp C, Nielsen H, Drachmann O, Hippe E (1985) Plasmapheresis in hyperviscosity syndrome. Acta Med Scand 217:133–137

Betticher DC, Hsu Schmitz SF, Ratschiller D, von Rohr A, Egger T, Pugin P, Stalder M, Hess U, Fey MF, Cerny T, for the Swiss Group for Clinical Cancer Research (SAKK) (1997) Cladribine (2-CDA) given as subcutaneous bolus injections is active in pretreated Waldenström's macroglobulinaemia. Br J Haematol 99:358–363

Blattner WA, Garber JE, Mann DL, McKeen EA, Henson R, McGuire DB, Fisher WB, Bauman AW, Goldin LR, Fraumeni JF Jr (1980) Waldenström's macroglobulinemia and autoimmune disease in a family. Ann Intern Med 93:830–832

Bottura C (1966) The genetic nature of Waldenström's macroglobulinemia. [Spanish] Prensa Med Argent 53:223–224

Brody JI, Haidar ME, Rossman RE (1979) A hemorrhagic syndrome in Waldenström's macroglobulinemia secondary to immunoadsorption of factor VIII. Recovery after splenectomy. N Engl J Med 300:408–410

Brown AK, Elves MW, Gunson HH, Pell-Ilderton R (1967) Waldenström's macroglobulinaemia. A family study. Acta Haematol 38:184–192

Bryson HM, Sorkin EM (1993) Cladribine. A review of its pharmacodynamic and pharmacokinetic properties and therapeutic potential in haematological malignancies. Drugs 46:872–894

Byrd JC, White CA, Link B, Lucas MS, Valasquez WS, Rosenberg J, Grillo-Lopez AJ (1999) Rituximab therapy in Waldenström's macroglobulinemia: preliminary evidence of clinical activity. Ann Oncol 10:1525–1527

Case DC Jr, Ervin TJ, Boyd MA, Redfield DL (1991) Waldenström's macroglobulinemia: long-term results with the M-2 protocol. Cancer Invest 9:1–7

Chong YY, Lau LC, Lui WO, Lim P, Lim E, Tan PH, Tan P, Ong YY (1998) A case of t(8;14) with total and partial trisomy 3 in Waldenström macroglobulinemia. Cancer Genet Cytogenet 103:65–67

Contrafatto G (1977) Marker chromosome of macroglobulinemia identified by G-banding. Cytogenet Cell Genet 18:370–373

Delannoy A, Ferrant A, Martiat P, Bosly A, Zenebergh A, Michaux JL (1994) 2-Chlorodeoxyadenosine therapy in Waldenström's macroglobulinaemia. Nouv Rev Fr Hematol 36:317–320

Desikan R, Dhodapkar M, Siegel D, Fassas A, Singh J, Singhal S, Mehta J, Vesole D, Tricot G, Jagannath S, Anaissie E, Barlogie B, Munshi NC (1999) High-dose therapy with autologous haemopoietic stem cell support for Waldenström's macroglobulinaemia. Br J Haematol 105:993–996

Dhodapkar MV, Jacobson JL, Gertz MA, Rivkin SE, Roodman GD, Tuscano JM, Shurafa M, Kyle RA, Crowley JJ, Barlogie B (2001) Prognostic factors and response to fludarabine therapy in patients with Waldenström macroglobulinemia: results of United States intergroup trial (Southwest Oncology Group S9003). Blood 98:41–48

Dimopoulos MA, Kantarjian H, Estey E, O'Brien S, Delasalle K, Keating MJ, Freireich EJ, Alexanian R (1993a) Treatment of Waldenström macroglobulinemia with 2-chlorodeoxyadenosine. Ann Intern Med 118:195–198

Dimopoulos MA, O'Brien S, Kantarjian H, Pierce S, Delasalle K, Barlogie B, Alexanian R, Keating MJ (1993b) Fludarabine therapy in Waldenström's macroglobulinemia. Am J Med 95:49–52

Dimopoulos MA, Weber DM, Kantarjian H, Keating M, Alexanian R (1994) 2-Chlorodeoxyadenosine therapy of patients with Waldenström macroglobulinemia previously treated with fludarabine. Ann Oncol 5:288–289

Dimopoulos MA, Weber D, Delasalle KB, Keating M, Alexanian R (1995) Treatment of Waldenström's macroglobulinemia resistant to standard therapy with 2-chlorodeoxyadenosine: identification of prognostic factors. Ann Oncol 6:49–52

Dimopoulos MA, Panayiotidis P, Moulopoulos LA, Sfikakis P, Dalakas M (2000) Waldenström's macroglobulinemia: clinical features, complications, and management. J Clin Oncol 18:214–226

Dimopoulos MA, Zomas A, Viniou NA, Grigoraki V, Galani E, Matsouka C, Economou O, Anagnostopoulos N, Panayiotidis P (2001) Treatment of Waldenström's macroglobulinemia with thalidomide. J Clin Oncol 19:3596–3601

Dimopoulos MA, Zervas C, Zomas A, Kiamouris C, Viniou NA, Grigoraki V, Karkantaris C, Mitsouli C, Gika D, Christakis J, Anagnostopoulos N (2002) Treatment of Waldenström's macroglobulinemia with rituximab. J Clin Oncol 20:2327–2333

Dreger P, Glass B, Kuse R, Sonnen R, von Neuhoff N, Bolouri H, Kneba M, Schmitz N (1999) Myeloablative radiochemotherapy followed by reinfusion of purged autologous stem cells for Waldenström's macroglobulinaemia. Br J Haematol 106:115–118

Facon T, Brouillard M, Duhamel A, Morel P, Simon M, Jouet JP, Bauters F, Fenaux P (1993) Prognostic factors in Waldenström's macroglobulinemia: a report of 167 cases. J Clin Oncol 11:1553–1558

Feiner HD, Rizk CC, Finfer MD, Bannan M, Gottesman SR, Chuba JV, Amorosi E (1990) IgM monoclonal gammopathy/Waldenström's macroglobulinemia: a morphological and immunophenotypic study of the bone marrow. Mod Pathol 3:348–356

Foran JM, Rohatiner AZ, Coiffier B, Barbui T, Johnson SA, Hiddemann W, Radford JA, Norton AJ, Tollerfield SM, Wilson MP, Lister TA (1999) Multicenter phase II study of fludarabine phosphate for patients with newly diagnosed lymphoplasmacytoid lymphoma, Waldenström's macroglobulinemia, and mantle-cell lymphoma. J Clin Oncol 17:546–553

Garand R, Sahota SS, Avet-Loiseau H, Talmant P, Robillard N, Moreau A, Gaillard F, Stevenson FK, Bataille R (2000) IgG-secreting lymphoplasmacytoid leukaemia: a B-cell disorder with extensively mutated VH genes undergoing Ig isotype-switching frequently associated with trisomy 12. Br J Haematol 109:71–80

Garcia-Sanz R, Montoto S, Torrequebrada A, de Coca AG, Petit J, Sureda A, Rodriguez-Garcia JA, Masso P, Perez-Aliaga A, Monteagudo MD, Navarro I, Moreno G, Toledo C, Alonso A, Besses C, Besalduch J, Jarque I, Salama P, Rivas JA, Navarro B, Bladé J, Miguel JF (2001) Waldenström macroglobulinaemia: presenting features and outcome in a series with 217 cases. Br J Haematol 115:575–582

Gertz MA, Kyle RA (1995) Hyperviscosity syndrome. J Intensive Care Med 10:128–141

Gertz MA, Lacy MQ, Dispenzieri A (1999) Amyloidosis: recognition, confirmation, prognosis, and therapy. Mayo Clin Proc 74:490–494

Gertz MA, Fonseca R, Rajkumar SV (2000) Waldenström's macroglobulinemia. Oncologist 5:63–67

Gobbi PG, Bettini R, Montecucco C, Cavanna L, Morandi S, Pieresca C, Merlini G, Bertoloni D, Grignani G, Pozzetti U, Caporali R, Ascari E (1994) Study of prognosis in Waldenström's macroglobulinemia: a proposal for a simple binary classification with clinical and investigational utility. Blood 83:2939–2945

Greipp PR, Lust JA, O'Fallon WM, Katzmann JA, Witzig TE, Kyle RA (1993) Plasma cell labeling index and beta 2-microglobulin predict survival independent of thymidine kinase and C-reactive protein in multiple myeloma. Blood 81:3382–3387

Groves FD, Travis LB, Devesa SS, Ries LA, Fraumeni JF Jr (1998) Waldenström's macroglobulinemia: incidence patterns in the United States, 1988–1994. Cancer 82:1078–1081

Harris NL, Jaffe ES, Stein H, Banks PM, Chan JK, Cleary ML, Delsol G, DeWolf-Peeters C, Falini B, Gatter KC (1994) A revised European-American classification of lymphoid neoplasms: a proposal from the International Lymphoma Study Group. Blood 84:1361–1392

Hellmann A, Lewandowski K, Zaucha JM, Bieniaszewska M, Halaburda K, Robak T (1999) Effect of a 2-hour infusion of 2-chlorodeoxyadenosine in the treatment of refractory or previously untreated Waldenström's macroglobulinemia. Eur J Haematol 63:35–41

Herrinton LJ, Weiss NS (1993) Incidence of Waldenström's macroglobulinemia. Blood 82:3148–3150

Hirase N, Miyamura T, Ishikura H, Yufu Y, Nishimura J, Nawata H (1996) Primary macroglobulinemia with t(11;18)(q21;q21). [Japanese] Rinsho Ketsueki 37:340–345

Hirase N, Yufu Y, Abe Y, Muta K, Shiokawa S, Nawata H, Nishimura J (2000) Primary macroglobulinemia with t(11;18)(q21;q21). Cancer Genet Cytogenet 117:113–117

Horsman DE, Card RT, Skinnider LF (1983) Waldenström macroglobulinemia terminating in acute leukemia: a report of three cases. Am J Hematol 15:97–101

Humphrey JS, Conley CL (1995) Durable complete remission of macroglobulinemia after splenectomy: a report of two cases and review of the literature. Am J Hematol 48:262–266

Iida S, Rao PH, Ueda R, Chaganti RS, Dalla-Favera R (1999) Chromosomal rearrangement of the PAX-5 locus in lymphoplasmacytic lymphoma with t(9;14)(p13;q32). Leuk Lymphoma 34:25–33

Kantarjian HM, Alexanian R, Koller CA, Kurzrock R, Keating MJ (1990) Fludarabine therapy in macroglobulinemic lymphoma. Blood 75:1928–1931

Kyle RA, Garton JP (1987) The spectrum of IgM monoclonal gammopathy in 430 cases. Mayo Clin Proc 62:719–731

Kyle RA, Greipp PR (1980) Smoldering multiple myeloma. N Engl J Med 302:1347–1349

Kyle RA, Greipp PR, Gertz MA, Witzig TE, Lust JA, Lacy MQ, Therneau TM (2000) Waldenström's macroglobulinaemia: a prospective study comparing daily with intermittent oral chlorambucil. Br J Haematol 108:737–742

Kyle RA, Therneau TM, Rajkumar SV, Offord JR, Larson DR, Plevak MF, Melton LJ III (2002) A long-term study of prognosis in monoclonal gammopathy of undetermined significance. N Engl J Med 346:564–569

Kyrtsonis MC, Vassilakopoulos TP, Angelopoulou MK, Siakantaris P, Kontopidou FN, Dimopoulou MN, Boussiotis V, Gribabis A, Konstantopoulos K, Vaiopoulos GA, Fessas P, Kittas C, Pangalis GA (2001) Waldenström's macroglobulinemia: clinical course and prosnostic factors in 60 patients. Experience from a single hematology unit. Ann Hematol 80:722–727

Laurencet FM, Zulian GB, Guetty-Alberto M, Iten PA, Betticher DC, Alberto P (1999) Cladribine with cyclophosphamide and prednisone in the management of low-grade lymphoproliferative malignancies. Br J Cancer 79:1215–1219

Leblond V, Ben-Othman T, Deconinck E, Taksin AL, Harousseau JL, Delgado MA, Delmer A, Maloisel F, Mariette X, Morel P, Clauvel JP, Duboisset P, Entezam S, Hermine O, Merlet M, Yakoub-Agha I, Guibon O, Caspard H, Fort N, for the Groupe Coopératif Macroglobulinémie (1998) Activity of fludarabine in previously treated Waldenström's macroglobulinemia: a report of 71 cases. J Clin Oncol 16:2060–2064

Leblond V, Levy V, Maloisel F, Cazin B, Fermand JP, Harousseau JL, Remenieras L, Porcher R, Gardembas M, Marit G, Deconinck E, Desablens B, Guilhot F, Philippe G, Stamatoullas A, Guibon O (2001) Multicenter, randomized comparative trial of fludarabine and the combination of cyclophosphamide-doxorubicin-prednisone in 92 patients with Waldenström macroglobulinemia in first relapse or with primary refractory disease. Blood 98:2640–2644

Linet MS, Humphrey RL, Mehl ES, Brown LM, Pottern LM, Bias WB, McCaffrey L (1993) A case-control and family study of Waldenström's macroglobulinemia. Leukemia 7:1363–1369

Liu ES, Burian C, Miller WE, Saven A (1998) Bolus administration of cladribine in the treatment of Waldenström macroglobulinaemia. Br J Haematol 103:690–695

Louviaux I, Michaux L, Hagemeijer A, Criel A, Billiet J, Scheiff JM, Deneys V, Delannoy A, Ferrant A (1998) Cytogenetic abnormalities in Waldenström's disease (WD): a single centre study on 45 cases (abstract). Blood 92 Suppl:184b

Mansoor A, Medeiros LJ, Weber DM, Alexanian R, Hayes K, Jones D, Lai R, Glassman A, Bueso-Ramos CE (2001) Cytogenetic findings in lymphoplasmacytic lymphoma/Waldenström macroglobulinemia. Chromosomal abnormalities are associated with the polymorphous subtype and an aggressive clinical course. Am J Clin Pathol 116:543–549

Morel P, Monconduit M, Jacomy D, Lenain P, Grosbois B, Bateli C, Facon T, Dervite I, Bauters F, Najman A, deGramont A, Wattel E (2000) Patients with the description of a new scoring system and its validation on 253 other patients. Blood 96:852–858

Nagai M, Ikeda K, Nakamura H, Ohnishi H, Amino Y, Irino S, Sato A, Uda H (1991) Splenectomy for a case with Waldenström macroglobulinemia with giant splenomegaly (letter to the editor). Am J Hematol 37:140

Nishida K, Taniwaki M, Misawa S, Abe T (1989) Nonrandom rearrangement of chromosome 14 at band q32.33 in human lymphoid malignancies with mature B-cell phenotype. Cancer Res 49:1275–1281

Offit K, Parsa NZ, Filippa D, Jhanwar SC, Chaganti RS (1992) t(9;14)(p13;q32) denotes a subset of low-grade non-Hodgkin's lymphoma with plasmacytoid differentiation. Blood 80:2594–2599

Ogmundsdottir HM, Sveinsdottir S, Sigfusson A, Skaftadottir I, Jonasson JG, Agnarsson BA (1999) Enhanced B cell survival in familial macroglobulinaemia is associated with increased expression of Bcl-2. Clin Exp Immunol 117:252–260

O'Reilly RA, MacKenzie MR (1967) Primary macrocryogelglobulinemia. Remission with adrenal corticosteroid therapy. Arch Intern Med 120:234–238

Owen RG, Johnson SA, Morgan GJ (2000) Waldenström's macroglobulinaemia: laboratory diagnosis and treatment. Hematol Oncol 18:41–49

Owen RG, Barrans SL, Richards SJ, O'Connor SJ, Child JA, Parapia LA, Morgan GJ, Jack AS (2001) Waldenström macroglobulinemia. Development of diagnostic criteria and identification of prognostic factors. Am J Clin Pathol 116:420–428

Pangalis GA, Angelopoulou MK, Vassilakopoulos TP, Siakantaris MP, Kittas C (1999) B-chronic lymphocytic leukemia, small lymphocytic lymphoma, and lymphoplasmacytic lymphoma, including Waldenström's macroglobulinemia: a clinical, morphologic, and biologic spectrum of similar disorders. Semin Hematol 36:104–114

Petrucci MT, Avvisati G, Tribalto M, Giovangrossi P, Mandelli F (1989) Waldenström's macroglobulinaemia: results of a combined oral treatment in 34 newly diagnosed patients. J Intern Med 226:443–447

Renier G, Ifrah N, Chevailler A, Saint-Andre JP, Boasson M, Hurez D (1989) Four brothers with Waldenström's macroglobulinemia. Cancer 64:1554–1559

Robinson MK, Halpern JI (1992) Retinal vein occlusion. Am Fam Physician 45:2661–2666

Schop RF, Kuehl WM, Van Wier SA, Ahmann GJ, Price-Troska T, Bailey RJ, Jalal SM, Qi Y, Kyle RA, Greipp PR, Fonseca R (2002) Waldenström macroglobulinemia neoplastic cells lack immunoglobulin heavy chain locus translocations but have frequent 6q deletions. Blood 100:2996–3001

Singh A, Eckardt KU, Zimmermann A, Gotz KH, Hamann M, Ratcliffe PJ, Kurtz A, Reinhart WH (1993) Increased plasma viscosity as a reason for inappropriate erythropoietin formation. J Clin Invest 91:251–256

Taleb N, Tohme A, Abi Jirgiss D, Kattan J, Salloum E (1991) Familial macroglobulinemia in a Lebanese family with two sisters presenting Waldenström's disease. Acta Oncol 30:703–705

Tepper A, Moss CE (1994) Waldenström's macroglobulinemia: search for occupational exposure. J Occup Med 36:133–136

Tetreault SA, Saven A (2000) Delayed onset of autoimmune hemolytic anemia complicating cladribine therapy for Waldenström macroglobulinemia. Leuk Lymphoma 37:125–130

Thalhammer-Scherrer R, Geissler K, Schwarzinger I, Chott A, Gisslinger H, Knobl P, Lechner K, Jager U (2000) Fludarabine therapy in Waldenström's macroglobulinemia. Ann Hematol 79:556–559

Thomas EL, Olk RJ, Markman M, Braine H, Patz A (1983) Irreversible visual loss in Waldenström's macroglobulinaemia. Br J Ophthalmol 67:102–106

Treon SP, Anderson KC (2000) The use of rituximab in the treatment of malignant and nonmalignant plasma cell disorders. Semin Oncol 27 Suppl 12:79–85

Treon SP, Shima Y, Preffer FI, Doss DS, Ellman L, Schlossman RL, Grossbard ML, Belch AR, Pilarski LM, Anderson KC (1999) Treatment of plasma cell dyscrasias by antibody-mediated immunotherapy. Semin Oncol 26 Suppl 14:97–106

Treon SP, Agus DB, Link B, Rodrigues G, Molina A, Lacy MQ, Fisher DC, Emmanouilides C, Richards AI, Clark B, Lucas MS, Schlossman R, Schenkein D, Lin B, Kimby E, Anderson KC, Byrd JC (2001) CD20-Directed antibody-mediated immunotherapy induces responses and facilitates hematologic recovery in patients with Waldenström's macroglobulinemia. J Immunother 24:272–279

Van Den Neste E, Louviaux I, Michaux JL, Delannoy A, Michaux L, Sonet A, Bosly A, Doyen C, Mineur P, Andre M, Straetmans N, Coche E, Venet C, Duprez T, Ferrant A (2000) Phase I/II study of 2-chloro-2′-deoxyadenosine with cyclophosphamide in patients with pretreated B cell chronic lymphocytic leukemia and indolent non-Hodgkin's lymphoma. Leukemia 14:1136–1142

Wagner SD, Martinelli V, Luzzatto L (1994) Similar patterns of V kappa gene usage but different degrees of somatic mutation in hairy cell leukemia, prolymphocytic leukemia, Waldenström's macroglobulinemia, and myeloma. Blood 83:3647– 3653

Waldenström J (1944) Incipient myelomatosis or "essential" hyperglobulinemia with fibrinogenopenia – a new syndrome? Acta Med Scand 117:216–247

Waldenström J (1948) Zwei interessante Syndrome mit Hyperglobulinämie: Purpura hyperglobulinaemica und Makroglobulinämie. Schweiz Med Wochenschr 78:927–928

White CA (1999) Rituximab immunotherapy for non-Hodgkin's lymphoma. Cancer Biother Radiopharm 14:241–250

Wong KF, So CC (2001) Waldenström macroglobulinemia with karyotypic aberrations involving both homologous 6q. Cancer Genet Cytogenet 124:137–139

Zinzani PL, Gherlinzoni F, Bendandi M, Zaccaria A, Aitini E, Salvucci M, Tura S (1995) Fludarabine treatment in resistant Waldenström's macroglobulinemia. Eur J Haematol 54:120–123

Cryoglobulinemia

Angela Dispenzieri, M.D., Morie A. Gertz, M.D.

Contents

10.1 Introduction 228

10.2 Epidemiology 228

10.3 Etiology 230
    10.3.1 Physical and Chemical Factors (Physical Properties of Cryoglobulins) 231
    10.3.2 Cross-Reactive Idiotypes and Oligoclonal B Cells 231
    10.3.3 Relationships Among Predisposing Conditions and Cryoglobulinemia 232
    10.3.3.1 Laboratory Studies . . . 232
    10.3.3.2 Connective Tissue Disease 234
    10.3.4 Putting the Associations Together 234
    10.3.5 Genetics 236

10.4 Clinical Presentation 237
    10.4.1 Skin 237
    10.4.2 Arthralgias 239
    10.4.3 Nervous System 239
    10.4.4 Renal 240

10.4.5 Liver 242
10.4.6 Other 242

10.5 Classification and Staging: Clinical and Pathologic 243

10.6 Diagnosis 243
    10.6.1 Laboratory Tests 243
    10.6.2 Laboratory Detection 243

10.7 Differential Diagnosis 244

10.8 Second Malignancies 244

10.9 Treatment 245
    10.9.1 Treatment of Life-Threatening Disease 246
    10.9.2 Interferon-α 248
    10.9.3 Ribavirin 249
    10.9.4 Corticosteroids 249
    10.9.5 Chemotherapy 249
    10.9.6 Hematopoietic Stem Cell Transplantation 250
    10.9.7 Other Immunosuppressant Therapies 250
    10.9.8 Biologic Therapy 250
    10.9.9 Surgery 250
    10.9.10 Plasmapheresis 250
    10.9.11 Supportive Care 251
    10.9.12 Other Therapeutic Measures . . 251

10.10 Prognosis 251

10.11 Concluding Remarks 252

References 252

Supported in part by Grants CA 62242 and CA 91561 from the National Institutes of Health.

10.1   Introduction

Cryoglobulins were discovered as a laboratory epiphe-nomenon in a patient with multiple myeloma in 1933 by Wintrobe and Buell. As more is understood about vasculitis, viral infection, and lymphoproliferation (be-nign and malignant), it becomes evident that a connec-tion exists among these disorders. In fact, in all of these conditions there is dysfunction of the lymphoid com-partment–unchecked and misdirected stimulation and proliferation. Cryoglobulins are by-products of these aberrations, which in their own right produce organ dysfunction. An understanding of cryoglobulins and the cells that produce them along with their interactions with tissue matrix, systemic cytokines, and the remain-der of the immune system may provide insight into ba-sic control pathways and the earliest steps of malignant transformation.

The descriptive term "cryoglobulin" was coined by Lerner and Watson, in 1947, after careful study of cold-induced precipitation of these immunoglobulins. In the 1960s, Meltzer and Franklin (1966) delineated a distinct syndrome of purpura, arthralgias, asthenia, re-nal disease, and neuropathy – often in the context of im-mune complex deposition or vasculitis (or both). Brouet et al. (1974) popularized a system to classify cryoglobu-linemia on the basis of the components of the cryopre-cipitate: type I, isolated monoclonal immunoglobulins; type II, a monoclonal component, usually IgM, possess-ing activity toward polyclonal immunoglobulins, usual-ly IgG; and type III, polyclonal immunoglobulins. This classification provided a framework for clinical correla-tions. Associated conditions, including lymphoprolif-erative disorders (LPDs), connective tissue disorders, infection, and liver disease, were observed in some, but not all, patients (Table 10.1). In several large series (Brouet et al. 1974; Gorevic et al. 1980; Monti et al. 1995a), 34% to 71% of cases of cryoglobulinemia were not associated with other specific disease states and were termed "essential" or primary.

10.2   Epidemiology

The actual prevalence of cryoglobulinemia is difficult to estimate because of its clinical polymorphism and be-cause of the necessity of separating the laboratory phe-nomenon of cryoglobulins from the symptomatic dis-ease state. As many as 51% of normal individuals have detectable mixed cryoglobulins at a concentration less than or equal to 80 µg/mL. Certain conditions, includ-ing liver disease, infection, connective tissue disorders, and LPDs, promote the generation of cryoglobulins. These patients are said to have secondary cryoglobu-linemia (Fig. 10.1). Although only a minority have symptoms referable to their cryoglobulins, serum cryo-globulins are found frequently in individuals with cir-rhosis (up to 45%), alcoholic hepatitis (32%), autoim-mune hepatitis (40%), subacute bacterial endocarditis (90%), rheumatoid arthritis (47%), IgG myeloma (10%), and Waldenström macroglobulinemia (19%) (Dispenzieri and Gorevic 1999).

The presence of cryoglobulins can serve as a harbin-ger of undiagnosed chronic infections, including sub-acute bacterial endocarditis, Lyme disease, and Q fever. Cases have been reported of cryoglobulinemia asso-ciated with hepatitis A, hepatitis B virus, *Hantavirus*, cytomegalovirus, Epstein-Barr virus, human T-lympho-cytic virus I, hepatitis G virus, and human immunode-ficiency virus (Dispenzieri and Gorevic 1999). The rela-tionship between cryoglobulinemia and LPDs is com-plex; cause can be difficult to dissect from effect. At a minimum, approximately 9% of all cases, or 31% of all secondary cases, of symptomatic cryoglobulinemia are diagnosed as LPDs, and another 6% to 28% develop symptomatic lymphoma at follow-up (Invernizzi et al. 1979; Monteverde et al. 1995; Pozzato et al. 1994; Zignego et al. 1997).

An association of hepatitis C virus (HCV) with es-sential mixed cryoglobulinemia (EMC) was reported in 1990 (Ferri et al. 1994), and it has become apparent that more than half (42% to 100%) of patients with MC are infected with HCV (Agnello et al. 1992; Dam-macco et al. 1994; Disdier et al. 1991; Ferri et al. 1994; Galli et al. 1995; Misiani et al. 1992). In 2002, less than 10% of cases of cryoglobulinemia could be classified as essential (Trejo et al. 2001).

The median age at diagnosis is the early to mid 50s. There is a female predominance of cryoglobulinemia of greater than 2 to 1. No race preference has been noted, but the incidence is higher in regions where hepatitis C occurs at higher frequencies (e.g., southern Europe).

The most common causes of death include renal fail-ure, infection, LPDs, liver failure, cardiovascular com-plications, and hemorrhage (Brouet et al. 1974; Gorevic et al. 1980; Monti et al. 1995a; Singer et al. 1986).

Table 10.1. Cryoglobulinemia: clinical and experimental associations

Infections

Viral	Lyme disease (±erythema chronicum migrans)
EBV	Post-intestinal bypass with arthritis
CMV	Q fever
HBV	Fungal
HAV	Coccidioidomycosis
Adenovirus	Parasitic
HCV	Kala-azar
HIV	Toxoplasmosis
Bacterial	Tropical splenomegaly syndrome
Subacute bacterial endocarditis (±nephritis)	Echinococcosis
Lepromatous leprosy (±erythema nodosum)	Malaria
Acute poststreptococcal nephritis	Schistosomiasis
Syphilis	Trypanosomiasis

Autoimmune diseases

Systemic lupus erythematosus	Inflammatory bowel disease
Nephritis, hypocomplementemia	Celiac disease, ulcerative colitis,
Drug-induced lupus (procainamide)	regional enteritis
Rheumatoid arthritis	Endomyocardial fibrosis
Extra-articular disease, Felty syndrome, synovial fluid	Pulmonary fibrosis
Polyarteritis nodosa (HBsAg positive and negative)	Cutaneous vasculitis
Kawasaki syndrome	Pemphigus vulgaris
Sjögren syndrome	Erythema elevatum diutinum
Scleroderma	Cold-induced urticaria
Sarcoidosis	Epidermyolysis bullosa acquisita
Thyroiditis	Erythema multiforme
Henoch-Schönlein purpura	POEMS syndrome
Behçet syndrome	Pyoderma gangrenosum
Polymyositis	

Lymphoproliferative disorders

Macroglobulinemia (primary and secondary)	Biliary cirrhosis
Lymphoma (Hodgkin and non-Hodgkin)	Chronic hepatitis
Chronic lymphocytic leukemia	
Immunoblastic lymphadenopathy	
Hairy cell leukemia	

Table 10.1 (continued)

Renal cell diseases

  Proliferative glomerulonephritis

Liver diseases

  Cirrhosis (Laënnec, postnecrotic)

Familial (symptomatic, asymptomatic)

Essential

Experimental

  Pneumococcal vaccines

  Streptococcal (A and C) hyperimmunization

  NZB/NZW, MRL/1, BXSB mice

CMV, cytomegalovirus; EBV, Epstein-Barr virus; HAV, hepatitis A virus, HBsAg, hepatitis B surface antigen; HBV, hepatitis B virus; HCV, hepatitis C virus; HIV, human immunodeficiency virus; POEMS, polyneuropathy, organomegaly, endocrinopathy, M protein, and skin changes.
From Dispenzieri and Gorevic (1999). By permission of Elsevier Science.

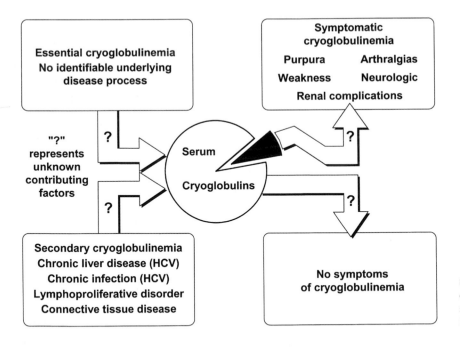

Fig. 10.1. Relationship among underlying diseases, cryoglobulins, and symptoms of cryoglobulinemia. *HCV,* hepatitis C virus

10.3   Etiology

Cryoglobulinemia is driven primarily by 4 classes of disease: liver disease (predominantly HCV), infection (again predominantly HCV), connective tissue disease, and LPD. The interactions among these predisposing conditions, the symptomatic clinical condition called cryoglobulinemia, and the vasculitic symptoms thereof are complex. An acquired imbalance of the immune system results in poorly regulated production of IgM-rheumatoid factors (RFs), which results in immune complexes and pathologic conditions.

10.3.1 Physical and Chemical Factors (Physical Properties of Cryoglobulins)

Cryoglobulins can be formed by 1 class of Ig – type I – or may form as a result of association of 2 or more different isotypes – types II and III. Cryoprecipitation of Ig light chains has been reported infrequently (Brouet et al. 1974). Precipitation of cryoglobulins depends on temperature, pH, cryoglobulin concentration, and weak noncovalent factors. RF activity – anti-Fc activity – is detectable in the sera in 87% to 100% of patients with MC (Brouet et al. 1974; Monti et al. 1995b) compared with 70% to 90% of patients with rheumatoid arthritis. In type III cryoglobulinemia and in rheumatoid arthritis, the RF is polyclonal, whereas in types I and II cryoglobulinemia, it is monoclonal.

Type I cryoglobulins, which are most often IgG or IgM, self-aggregate and precipitate because of primary, secondary, and tertiary structural properties that lead to the formation of intermolecular noncovalent bonds at low temperatures. In contrast, "mixed cryoglobulins" are composed of 2 immunoglobulins, 1 of which has RF activity. IgM typically serves as the RF. On occasion, the oligoclonal IgG may have anti-idiotype activity for the IgM RF as well, further increasing the avidity of the formed molecular complex. Along with antigen-antibody complexes within cryoprecipitates, complement components, fibronectin, and lipoproteins have been found. Although hepatitis B virus, Epstein-Barr virus, and bacterial products may be present, by far the most frequent pathogen within cryoprecipitates is HCV (Dispenzieri and Gorevic 1999).

HCV RNA, HCV-specific proteins, and anti-HCV antibodies are found in the supernatant of the cryoprecipitate and in the cryoprecipitate itself in 42% to 98% of patients with EMC (Agnello et al. 1992; Dispenzieri and Gorevic 1999; Misiani et al. 1992). Cryoprecipitates contain 20 to 1,000 times more HCV RNA than is present in the supernatant (Lunel et al. 1994). The IgG component to which the IgM-RF fraction binds is directed against the HCV proteins. Data suggest that although the virus itself is not required for the physiochemical reaction of cryoprecipitation, it likely contributes to an immune reaction and to reticuloendothelial system dysfunction that are conducive to production and persistence of antibodies – including natural autoantibodies – which are capable of cryoprecipitation (Lunel et al. 1994). Speculation abounds – but not concrete data – on how HCV may stimulate the immune reactivity, thereby causing cryoglobulins to be generated, with resulting immune complex deposition.

The primary mechanism of damage in cryoglobulinemia is related to immune complex deposition, which results in vasculitis, nephritis, or vascular occlusion. Impaired clearance of cryoglobulins and noncryoprecipitable immune complexes may contribute to the pathogenesis. High concentrations of monoclonal RF or other immune complexes may interfere with the function of Fc receptors of the reticuloendothelial system, thereby retarding clearance from the circulation and favoring deposition in tissues. Alternatively, there may be intrinsic abnormalities of reticuloendothelial and monocyte function. Abnormalities in complement concentration and function may also impair clearance or neutralization of the immune complexes or the pathogen associated with them (Dispenzieri and Gorevic 1999).

10.3.2 Cross-Reactive Idiotypes and Oligoclonal B Cells

All of the diseases that predispose individuals to cryoglobulinemia induce a seemingly nonspecific stimulation of B cells, resulting in polyclonal hypergammaglobulinemia. When this wide variety of antibodies is produced, antibodies to autoantigens may also result. A strong B-cell stimulus disrupts the sequence of idiotype-anti-idiotype interactions in animal models, resulting in both immunosuppression and idiotype-anti-idiotype immune complexes. This may serve as a model for what occurs in cryoglobulinemia (Fig. 10.2).

Conservation of light and heavy chain usage in IgMκ immunoglobulin serves as the RF in cryoglobulinemia (Fong et al. 1988). In the 1970s, Kunkel and associates demonstrated that the RF of approximately 60% of all patients with types I and II cryoglobulin shared a cross-reactive idiotypic (CRI) antigen named Wa; another 20% had the Po CRI (Agnello et al. 1995). The molecular basis of Wa is the preferential usage of the germinal gene humκv325 (human κ variable gene). This genetic region spans the nucleotides encoding for 96 amino acids including complementarity determining region (CDR) 1, CDR2, and CDR3. VκIIIb (the humκv325 gene product) usage occurs in 72% of monoclonal IgMκRFs in contrast to the 8% usage in IgM immunoglobulins not known to have autoantibody activity (Gorevic and Frangione 1991). Further studies using the antibody

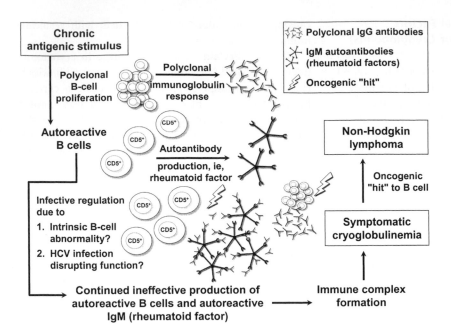

Fig. 10.2. Simplified model of continuum of antigenic stimulus to cryoglobulin to lymphoproliferative disorder. *HCV*, hepatitis C virus

17.109, which recognizes VκIIIb, have shown that this high rate of preferential usage of the variable region is shared by the autoantibodies observed in Sjögren syndrome, but not in rheumatoid arthritis (Dispenzieri and Gorevic 1999).

In addition, these monoclonal RFs do not appear to undergo somatic hypermutation, suggesting that their continued production may be the consequence of an antigen-independent proliferation of autoreactive B-cell clones. In normal individuals, IgM-RF precursor B cells represent up to 1 to 3 per 1,000 circulating normal B cells. They are generally CD5[+] B cells. Both early in ontogeny and during acute immunologic challenges, CD5[+] B cells and RF have important regulatory functions. CD5[+] B cells typically respond to T-cell independent antigens and produce low-affinity IgM antibodies. The IgM-RF–producing B cells in the peripheral blood of patients with mixed cryoglobulins, however, are CD5[-], but those infiltrating the liver and the bone marrow are CD5[+] (Dispenzieri and Gorevic 1999).

Whether there is an intrinsic property of these VκIII IgM-RF–producing cells that predisposes them to transform from clonal expansion to low-grade malignancy is unknown. Two observations may support this proposition: 1) there is an increased incidence of lymphoma in cryoglobulinemia (Invernizzi et al. 1979; Monteverde et al. 1995; Pozzato et al. 1994; Zignego et al. 1997); and 2)

in vitro B-chronic lymphocytic leukemia cells have the capacity to produce monoclonal RF, commonly sharing the same VL and VH gene rearrangements as found in cryoglobulinemia and Waldenström macroglobulinemia. Dispenzieri and Gorevic (1999) suggested that the tendency of humκv325-encoded light chains to have autoantibody properties may contribute to continuous proliferation of the B cells producing them, thereby rendering these humκv325-bearing cells susceptible to abnormal clonal expansion and malignant transformation.

Therefore, in the context of cryoglobulinemia, there appears to be a continuum in the lymphoid compartment from the polyclonal and oligoclonal to monoclonal proliferation observed in autoimmune disease and chronic infections to low-grade LPDs to frank lymphoma.

10.3.3 Relationships Among Predisposing Conditions and Cryoglobulinemia

10.3.3.1 Hepatitis C Virus

HCV serves as a chronic stimulus. Cryoglobulins are present in up to 50% of infected patients (Dispenzieri and Gorevic 1999). HCV is associated with autoimmune phenomena even in the absence of cryoglobulinemia, and it may predispose patients to lymphoma (De Rosa

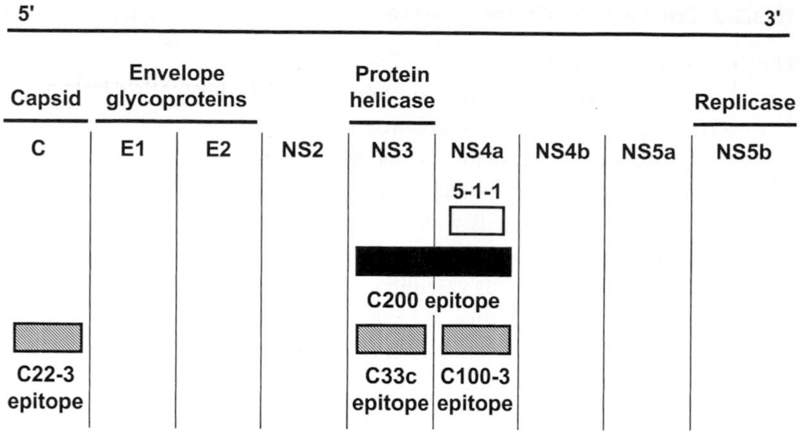

Fig. 10.3. Schematic structure of hepatitis C virus (HCV) and the origin of several cloned proteins used for serologic diagnosis of HCV. C, E1, and E2 refer to the structural genes. NS2 through NS5 refer to the nonstructural genes. The epitopes listed correspond to the antigenic determinants used to detect HCV serologically. The first-generation anti-HCV immunoassay recognizes the C100-3 polypeptide. The second-generation immunoassay detects antibodies to the HCV polypeptides, C33c, C100-3, and C22-3. Finally, the recombinant immunoblot assay detects antibodies to the recombinant HCV antigens 5-1-1, C100-3, C33c, and C22-3

et al. 1997; Ferri et al. 1994; Luppi et al. 1998; Yoshikawa et al. 1997; Zignego et al. 1997; Zuckerman et al. 1997).

HCV is a single-stranded, positive-sense, 9.5-kilobase RNA virus that is a member of the Flaviviridae family (Fig. 10.3). At least 6 major distinct genotypes have been recognized. The 2 popular methods of classifying genotypes are those of Simmonds and of Okamoto (Dispenzieri and Gorevic 1999). Listing Simmonds nomenclature first, followed by the corresponding Okamoto designation in parentheses, the most common genotypes include 1a (I), 1b (II), 2a (III), 2b (IV), and 3 (V). Among patients with MC, the genotypes 2a and 1b are common (Dispenzieri and Gorevic 1999). The risk of developing cryoglobulinemia is lowest in patients with the 1a genotype, whereas the presence of the 2a genotype in patients with MC is associated with absence of clinical and biochemical signs of liver disease. Other risk factors for cryoglobulinemia in HCV patients are female sex, alcohol consumption of more than 50 g/d, detectable serum HCV RNA, longer duration of hepatitis, higher serum concentration of gamma globulin, higher RF values, and extensive liver fibrosis or cirrhosis (Lunel et al. 1994; Dispenzieri and Gorevic 1999).

Humoral and cellular immune responses are directed to multiple HCV-encoded proteins and to multiple epitopes on these antigens. Antibodies specifically directed to the hypervariable region of HCV are thought to have neutralizing activity, but genotype factors and unknown patient factors affect antibody production. Gerotto et al. (2001) identified inserted residues at codon 385 (at the hypervariable region 1) of the HCV genome in 29% of patients with MC. These mutations were not found in any of the HCV patients without MC. They proposed that these mutations, which occur in a region containing immunodominant epitopes for neutralizing antibodies and binding sites for B lymphocytes, may be selected for interaction with (and stimulation of) host cells. Although extensive genetic variation exists in HCV, deletions and additions are rare (Gerotto et al. 2001), making their observation more provocative. Anti-hypervariable region antibodies are more prevalent in patients with HCV genotype 2a than 1b, which is concordant with the clinical observation that patients with 2a infection have less severe disease (Origgi et al. 1998) and a higher response rate to interferon (IFN)-α therapy than do individuals with genotype 1b.

Even in the absence of cryoglobulins, patients with HCV are predisposed to extrahepatic manifestations, including autoimmune phenomena such as membranoproliferative glomerulonephritis, nonerosive polyarthritis, autoantibody production, and porphyria cutanea tarda. Other phenomena likely associated with HCV are autoimmune hepatitis, B-cell non-Hodgkin lymphoma, and sicca syndrome.

10.3.3.2 Connective Tissue Disease

The incidence of cryoglobulinemia – most commonly type II or III – associated with specific connective tissue disease has been quite variable (Table 10.2). Twenty-five percent of patients with systemic lupus erythematosus (SLE) have detectable cryoglobulins (Garcia-Carrasco et al. 2001), and in individuals with systemic sclerosis, cryoglobulins have been detected in 12.5% of cases (Invernizzi et al. 1983). Cutaneous vasculitis, RF, hypocomplementemia, and HCV infection are more prevalent in SLE patients who have cryoglobulins than in those who do not (Garcia-Carrasco et al. 2001). Measurable amounts of cryoglobulins, usually polyclonal, can be found in up to 46% of patients with active rheumatoid arthritis, and the risk of extra-articular manifestations, including vasculitis, is significantly higher in patients with cryoglobulins. As many as 37% of patients with Sjögren syndrome have serum cryoglobulins (Invernizzi et al. 1983; Ramos-Casals et al. 1998); conversely, 5% to 15% of patients with MC have Sjögren syndrome (Brouet et al. 1974; Gorevic et al. 1980; Monti et al. 1995a).

Interesting observations have been made in patients with Sjögren syndrome. In one series, Sjögren patients with mixed cryoglobulins were 7 times more likely to have lymphoma develop than their cryoglobulin-negative counterparts (86% versus 12.5%). These same patients have a higher prevalence of leukocytoclastic cutaneous vasculitis (56% versus 8%, $P < 0.001$), hypocomplementemia (75% versus 2%, $P < 0.001$), and antibodies to HCV (47% versus 8%, $P < 0.001$) (Ramos-Casals et al. 1998). Both MC and Sjögren syndrome patients have polyclonal hypergammaglobulinemia, autoantibody production, circulating immune complexes, abnormal Fc-receptor-specific reticuloendothelial system clearance, depressed and abnormal T-cell function (Gorevic and Frangione 1991), and preferential usage of κ light chains of the VκIIIb sub-subgroup and heavy chains of the VH1 family (Shokri et al. 1991). Another thread of this intricate web of associations is the Sjögren-like syndrome, which can be observed as an extrahepatic manifestation of HCV (Ramos-Casals et al. 2001).

10.3.4 Putting the Associations Together

A recognized model for progression from chronic antigenic stimulation to benign to malignant lymphoproliferation is *Helicobacter pylori* and mucosa-associated lymphoid tissue (MALT) lymphoma. HCV, Sjögren syndrome, cryoglobulinemia, and immunocytoma may follow this model. This can be explored through the relationships between HCV and B cells and the shared, restricted, immunoglobulin usage among these 4 entities.

HCV is both a lymphotropic and a hepatotropic virus. Putative receptors by which the virus may enter cells include CD81 and the low-density lipoprotein receptor (Dispenzieri and Gorevic 1999). In HCV$^+$ patients with MC, HCV RNA is detected in the peripheral blood mononuclear cells in up to 81% of cases (Dispenzieri and Gorevic 1999) and in bone marrow cells in up to 100% of cases (Galli et al. 1995; Pozzato et al. 1994). Both in patients with and without mixed cryoglobulins, intrahepatic HCV-infected B cells develop monoclonal and oligoclonal B-cell expansions in close to 50% of specimens tested. Higher titers of serum RF are observed in patients with these clonal expansions (Sansonno et al. 1998). Clonal immunoglobulin gene rearrangements can be detected by reverse transcription polymerase chain reaction in all HCV-positive patients with type II MC and in 24% of HCV-infected patients without cryoglobulinemia (Franzin et al. 1995). Productive t(14;18) translocations with resultant *bcl*-2 overexpression occur in about 16% to 26% of HCV-positive patients without symptomatic cryoglobulinemia and in 71% to 86% of their cryoglobulin-positive counterparts (Kitay-Cohen et al. 2000; Zignego et al. 2000). The *bcl*-2 proto-oncogene is able to inhibit apoptosis, leading to extended survival, thereby contributing to the apparent B-lymphocyte expansion.

Furthermore, patients with cryoglobulinemia who develop lymphoma have been found to have genomic sequences of HCV in their sera, peripheral blood mononuclear cells, and lymphoma specimens (Ferri et al. 1994; Sansonno et al. 1998). The non-Hodgkin lymphoma subgroup most commonly observed in patients with HCV is lymphoplasmacytoid lymphoma or immunocytoma. An increased rate of HCV infection has been reported in idiopathic B-cell non-Hodgkin lymphomas by many (De Rosa et al. 1997; Ferri et al. 1994; Luppi et al. 1998; Yoshikawa et al. 1997; Zignego et al. 1997; Zuckerman et al. 1997), but not all, investigators (Table 10.3) (King et al. 1998; McColl et al. 1997). About 32% of cases of lymphoplasmacytoid lymphoma or immunocytoma are HCV$^+$ (Silvestri et al. 1996). Moreover, about 10% of patients with monoclonal gammopathy (multiple myeloma and monoclonal gammopathy of undetermined significance) are HCV$^+$ (De Rosa et al. 1997; Silvestri et al. 1996). The incidence in Waldenström

Table 10.2. Clinical features of cryoglobulinemia at diagnosis

Author	N	F:M	Essential cryo[a], %	Cryo type, %			LPD, %	Liver[b], %	Sicca, %	Skin, %	Raynaud, %	Renal, %	Arthralgia, %	Neuro, %
				I	II	III								
Meltzer et al.	29	3:1	41	59	←41→		31	72[c]	17[c]	92[c]	–	25[c]	92[c]	17[c]
Brouet et al. (1974)	86	–	34	25	25	50	44	–	9	55	50	21	35	17
Gorevic et al. (1980)	40	1.7:1	100	0	32	68		70	15	100	25	55	72	12
Tarantino et al. (1981)[d]	44	1:7	82	–	–	–	0[e]	14	2	59	7	100	57	7
Singer et al. (1986)	16	–	–	12	63	25	6	–	–	94	–	63	63	56
Monti et al. (1995b)	891	2:1	72	6	62	32	6	39	5	76	19	20	–	21
Ferri et al.	150	3:1	–	–	←100→		8	69	34	89	34	29	83	33
Trejo et al. (2001)[f]	206	–	–	–	–	–	10	–	–	51	11	39	40	14
Rieu et al. (2002)	49	1.7:1	12	6[g]	49	33	0	43	35	82	35	24	51	55

Cryo, cryoglobulinemia; LPD, lymphoproliferative disease; neuro, neurologic disease.

[a] Essential cryo refers to cryoglobulinemia without any identified predisposing condition. These values do not represent actual incidence, but rather the makeup of the population analyzed for symptoms.

[b] Liver refers to abnormal results of liver function tests or hepatomegaly or both.

[c] Symptoms of the essential mixed (types II and III) cryoglobulinemia population only.

[d] Series restricted to patients with renal involvement.

[e] Patients with multiple myeloma, Waldenström macroglobuinemia, and infection were excluded from this study by design.

[f] Only patients with a cryocrit ≥1% were included. The percentages were calculated from the 206 symptomatic patients described by the authors.

[g] No typing of 12% of patients.

Table 10.3. Lymphoma and hepatitis C virus (HCV)

Author	Site	B-NHL cohort, n	HCV in lymphoma, %	Control cohort, n	HCV in controls, %
Pioltelli et al.	Udine, Italy	126	21	94 (>60 y)	9.6
De Rosa et al. (1997)	Naples, Italy	91	23	93	5.4
Ferri et al.	Pisa, Italy	18	33	40	2.5
Luppi et al. (1998)	Modena, Italy	157	22	143:HD, PCD, T-NHL	13
McColl et al. (1997)	Glasgow, Scotland	72	0	38:CLL	0
Cucuianu et al. (1999)	Poland	68	29		5
Zuckerman et al. (1997)	Los Angeles, USA	120	22	258	5
King et al. (1998)	Missouri, USA	73	1.4	20:HD	0
Izumi et al. (1997)	Tochigi-Ken, Japan	29	17	18:non-B-cell NHL	0
Yoshikawa et al. (1997)	Kahihara, Japan	55	16	25	4
Overall		809	18	729	6.5

CLL, chronic lymphocytic leukemia; HD, Hodgkin disease; NHL, non-Hodgkin lymphoma; PCD, plasma cell dyscrasia.

macroglobulinemia has been reported to be as high as 61% (De Rosa et al. 1997).

There is remarkable homology among the antigen-combining site (variable region) of the RFs in patients with HCV, HCV-associated lymphoma, and cryoglobulinemia (Chan et al. 2001; De Re et al. 2000; Fong et al. 1988; Ivanovski et al. 1998; Sasso et al. 2001). Similar degrees of homology are seen between the immunoglobulin receptors in the lymphoproliferation of patients with Sjögren syndrome and of the lymphomas of HCV-infected individuals with or without type II MC (De Re et al. 2002).

The HCV genome cannot be inserted into the human genome because it is an RNA virus without a DNA intermediate as part of its replicative cycle. HCV RNA and structural proteins, however, are found in stromal cells surrounded by lymphoproliferative processes (De Vita et al. 2000), potentially serving as an antigenic stimulus to the B cells, and within the lymphoma itself (De Re et al. 2000; Sansonno et al. 1998). Specific antibodies against the HCV E2 antigen prefer-

entially use the V(H)1-69 gene locus (Chan et al. 2001; De Re et al. 2000), which is the same heavy chain variable region used in 71% of RFs that have the humκv325 light chain sequence (Fong et al. 1988), in 33% of cryoglobulins (Sasso et al. 2001), in about half of HCV-associated cryoglobulins (Sasso et al. 2001), and in more than 50% of HCV-associated immunocytomas (Ivanovski et al. 1998). These connections suggest that the combination of chronic antigenic stimulation, ineffective regulation by autoreactive B cells (which make restricted RF), and continued proliferation of B cells produces an oncogenic mutation(s), which transforms the lymphoid proliferation to a malignant lymphoma (Fig. 10.2).

10.3.5 Genetics

Although more than half of patients with MC are infected with HCV, less than half (13%–54%) of patients with HCV infection have cryoglobulins detected by laboratory testing, the majority (67%–91%) of which are type III (Dispenzieri and Gorevic 1999). Moreover, of these HCV-positive individuals with detectable cryoglobulins, only 27% have clinical signs consistent with the syndrome of cryoglobulinemia (Lunel et al. 1994). Whether this variability in expression is intrinsic to the host or to the virus species is unknown. Some data suggest that host HLA type may play a role. The DRB1*11, DR3, and B8 alleles occur with higher prevalence in individuals who have HCV with MC than in controls. DQB1*0301 has been associated with effective clearance of circulating HCV (Dispenzieri and Gorevic 1999). Human leukocyte antigen-DR7 appears to protect against the production of type II MC.

10.4 Clinical Presentation

Involvement of the skin, the peripheral nerves, the kidneys, and the liver is common (Tables 10.2 and 10.4). On autopsy, however, widespread vasculitis may be seen involving small- and medium-sized vessels in the heart, gastrointestinal tract, central nervous system, muscles, lungs, and adrenals (Gorevic et al. 1980). Symptoms of hyperviscosity may develop (Fig. 10.4 a). The interval between the onset of symptoms and diagnosis varies considerably, with a range of 0 to 10 years (Gorevic et al. 1980).

Overlap exists among the clinical features of types I, II, and III cryoglobulinemia (Tables 10.2 and 10.4). In general, type I is usually asymptomatic. When symptomatic, it most often causes occlusive symptoms rather than vasculitis like types II and III (Brouet et al. 1974; Gorevic et al. 1980). Type II cryoglobulinemia is more frequently symptomatic than is type III, 61% versus 21% (Donada et al. 1998b), and is associated with a higher incidence of purpura, Meltzer's triad (purpura, arthralgias, and asthenia), renal involvement, cryocrit >3%, and low C4 values (Monti et al. 1995a).

A distinction has also been made between the symptoms of primary (or essential) and secondary MC, suggesting that there is a higher incidence of Raynaud phenomenon, Meltzer triad, and neuropathy in the EMC group (Monti et al. 1995a). The distinction between essential and secondary MC has become ambiguous since the recognition of associations of HCV and clonal lymphocyte proliferation with MC (Ferri et al. 1994; Monteverde et al. 1995; Pozzato et al. 1994; Zignego et al. 1997). In fact, the incidence of HCV infection in essential and

Table 10.4. Contrasting symptoms and signs of types of cryoglobulinemia

Sign or symptom	Type I[a]	Type II[b]	Type III[c]
Purpura	+	+++	+++
Gangrene or acrocyanosis	+++	+ to ++	+/–
Arthralgias >> arthritis	+	++	+++
Membrano-proliferative glomerulonephritis	+	++	+
Neuropathy	+	++	++
Liver disease	+/–	++	+++

[a] Most often associated with lymphoproliferative and plasmaproliferative diseases; much less frequently seen with hepatitis C virus infection.

[b] Most often associated with hepatitis C virus infection, followed by lymphoproliferative disease and then chronic liver disease of other causes and connective tissue disease.

[c] Most often associated with hepatitis C virus infection, followed by chronic liver disease of other causes, and then connective tissue disease; least commonly associated with lymphoproliferative disease.

secondary MC is the same when the secondary disease associations are either chronic liver disease or LPDs. The incidence of HCV infection may be lower in the group of patients with MC due to connective tissue disease (Monti et al. 1995a). The clinical manifestations and cryoglobulin values in HCV-positive and HCV-negative patients do not differ significantly; only arthralgias and increased transaminase values are significantly more frequent in the former group (Rieu et al. 2002). LPDs are common at presentation and over time.

10.4.1 Skin

Purpura is the most frequent symptom of MC, being present in 55% to 100% of patients (Brouet et al. 1974; Gorevic et al. 1980; Monti et al. 1995a; Singer et al. 1986) (Table 10.4 and Fig. 10.4 b). The incidence varies from 15% to 33% in type I, 60% to 93% in type II, and 70% to 83% in type III. Petechiae and palpable purpura are the most common lesions, although ecchymoses, erythematous spots, and dermal nodules are possible

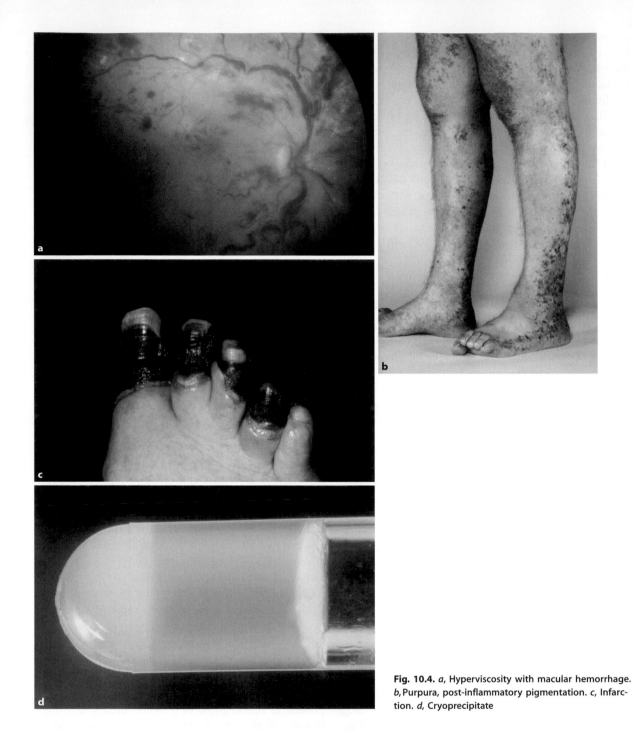

Fig. 10.4. *a*, Hyperviscosity with macular hemorrhage. *b*, Purpura, post-inflammatory pigmentation. *c*, Infarction. *d*, Cryoprecipitate

in as many as 20% of patients. Bullous or vesicular lesions are distinctly uncommon (Brouet et al. 1974). Successive purpuric rashes, which may be preceded by a burning or itching sensation, occur most commonly on the lower extremities, gradually extending to the thighs and lower abdomen. Occasionally, the arms are involved, but the face and the trunk are generally spared (Brouet et al. 1974). Head and mucosal involvement, livedoid vasculitis, and cold-induced acrocyanosis of the helices of the ears are more frequently observed in type I, as are infarction (Fig. 10.4c), hemorrhagic crusts, and ulcers, which occur in 10% to 25% of all patients (Dispenzieri and Gorevic 1999). Showers of purpura last for 1 or 2 weeks and occur once or twice a month. Cold precipitates these types of lesions in only 10% to 30% of cases (Brouet et al. 1974). Raynaud phenomenon occurs in about 19% to 50% of patients (Brouet et al. 1974; Gorevic et al. 1980; Monti et al. 1995a; Singer et al. 1986), and in a quarter of these, the symptoms may be severe, including necrosis of fingertips (Brouet et al. 1974). Skin necrosis, urticaria, and livedo, which are all rare, are more commonly associated with exposure to cold (Brouet et al. 1974). Urticaria and cutaneous ulcers may be more prevalent in patients with HCV genotype 2 (Origgi et al. 1998). Postinflammatory hyperpigmentation of the lower extremities occurs in about 40% of patients (Dispenzieri and Gorevic 1999).

Vasculitis, inflammatory or noninflammatory purpura, noninflammatory hyaline thrombosis, and postinflammatory sequelae were seen at relative frequencies of 50%, 15%, 10%, and 10%, respectively, in a Mayo Clinic series evaluating the cutaneous manifestations of 72 patients with cryoglobulinemia (Table 10.5). Noninflammatory hyaline thrombosis was relatively more common in patients with type I cryoglobulinemia (Dispenzieri and Gorevic 1999). The vasculitis is characterized by an inflammatory infiltrate surrounding and involving blood vessel walls with fibrinoid necrosis, endothelial cell hyperplasia, and hemorrhage, whereas the inflammatory and noninflammatory purpura are characterized by perivenular hemorrhage without vessel wall destruction. Intravascular deposition of eosinophilic periodic acid-Schiff–positive hyaline material is present in cases of noninflammatory hyaline thrombosis. Postinflammatory histopathologic findings are diverse and include infarction, necrosis, granulation tissue, fibrosis, and hemosiderosis. Deposition of immunoglobulin and complement (IgG, IgM, and C3) is common (Gorevic et al. 1980). Abnormalities in the uninvolved skin, including basement membrane alterations and deposits in vessel walls, may be found in patients with EMC.

10.4.2 Arthralgias

Arthralgias are common, affecting 35% to 75% of patients with cryoglobulinemia, with the highest incidence in type III cryoglobulinemia (Table 10.4). The small distal joints are affected more than the larger proximal joints. The polyarthralgia is symmetrical and often exacerbated by the cold. Frank arthritis is rare (Brouet et al. 1974; Gorevic et al. 1980; Monti et al. 1995a; Singer et al. 1986; Trejo et al. 2001).

10.4.3 Nervous System

Peripheral neuropathy is the more frequent presentation, although central nervous system involvement may occur (Brouet et al. 1974; Gorevic et al. 1980). In the largest clinical series, peripheral nerve involvement is described in 17% to 56% of patients (Brouet et al. 1974; Gorevic et al. 1980; Monti et al. 1995a; Singer et al. 1986; Trejo et al. 2001) (Tables 10.2 and 10.4). The incidence may be highest in type III cryoglobulinemia (Brouet et al. 1974; Monti et al. 1995a). Infection with HCV subtype 1b may also be a risk factor (Origgi et al. 1998). Mild peripheral neuropathy has been described in at least 80% of patients with MC screened with an electrophysiologic assessment. Sensory features usually precede motor ones (Brouet et al. 1974). The presentation may be as an acute or subacute distal symmetric polyneuropathy or a mononeuropathy multiplex with a chronic or chronic-relapsing evolution.

The neuropathy in EMC is most often characterized by axonal degeneration. Epineurial vasculitis is often found on sural nerve biopsy (Table 10.5) (Dispenzieri and Gorevic 1999). Demyelination may be present, either as the primary process or due to axonal degeneration. Even in the absence of active signs of vasculitis and of immunoperoxidase staining for immunoglobulins, endoneurial vessels may be extensively damaged, with abnormally thick endothelial cells and redundant basal membranes, suggesting ischemia as a mechanism in essential type II cryoglobulinemia. The mild distal neuropathy with relatively minor neurologic deficit may coincide with occlusion of the microcirculation of the vasa nervorum by intravascular deposits of cryoglobulins, whereas the severe, distal, symmetrical sensorimotor neuropathy or overlapping mononeuritis multiplex may be associated with necrotizing vasculitis. HCV viral particles are not seen by immunofluorescent staining, even in HCV-associated disease.

Table 10.5. Characteristic pathologic findings in cryoglobulinemia

Microscopic	Immunohistochemical	Electronmicroscopy	Reaction with anti-HCV antigens
Bone marrow			
Monomorphic small lymphocytes, sometimes with plasmacyloid features; paratrabecular only > interstitial only > both	CD5 positive; *bcl*-2 oncogene product overexpressed; low expression of Ki67		Involvement
Kidney			
Membranoproliferative glomerulonephritis (60%–80%) Endocapillary proliferation; subendothelial deposits Infiltration of leukocytes, mainly monocytes Intraglomerular hyaline thrombi (25%)	IgM, IgG, and C3 common C1q and C4 less common	Intraluminal and subendothelial deposits composed of a fibrillar or crystalloid material; fibrils 100 to 1,000 nm; cross section 62 to 63 nm	HCV-related proteins in glomerular capillaries/tubulointerstitial arterioles No HCV RNA or HCV-related proteins in glomeruli
Mesangial proliferative glomerulonephropathy (20%) Vasculitis with fibrinoid necrosis (32%)			
Skin			
Vasculitis (50%), inflammatory and noninflammatory purpura (15%), noninflammatory hyaline thrombosis (10%), and postinflammatory histopathologic findings (10%)	IgM, IgG, and complement fractions at the sites of vascular damage	Characteristic fibrils	Intraluminal deposits Deposits within vessel walls and perivascular space
Nerve			
Axonopathy with endoneurial microangiopathy Epineurial vasculitis: lymphocytes and monocytes surrounding arterioles Necrotizing vasculitis	Occasionally Ig and complement may be detected in endoneurial capillaries	Tubular deposits in endoneurium in the walls and lumina of the vasa nervorum	Potentially contradictory evidence: present by RT-PCR in 1 study and not present by immunofluorescence in another

10.4.4 Renal

Approximately 21% to 29% of patients with MC have renal involvement (Brouet et al. 1974; Trejo et al. 2001). The incidence of renal injury is highest in patients with type II cryoglobulins (Cordonnier et al. 1983; Monti et al. 1995a) (Table 10.4). Although renal and extrarenal manifestations can occur concurrently, renal involvement usually follows the onset of purpura by approximately 4 years (D'Amico 1998; Gorevic et al. 1980). Proteinuria greater than 0.5 g/day and hematuria are the most common features of renal disease at diagnosis (50%) (Tarantino et al. 1995), whereas nephrotic syndrome and acute nephritic syndrome affect

Table 10.5 (continued)

Microscopic	Immunohistochemical	Electronmicroscopy	Reaction with anti-HCV antigens
Liver			
Chronic persistent hepatitis, chronic active hepatitis, or cirrhosis	Portal lymphoid infiltrates: mostly $CD3^+/CD5^+$ T cells, also $CD5^+/bcl-2^+/Ki67^-$ B cells)		HCV in lymphocytes and hepatocytes
Periportal or lobular lymphoid infiltrates			
Microvesicular and macro-vesicular steatosis, ductular damage			
Occasionally vasculitis			

HCV, hepatitis C virus; RT-PCR, reverse transcription polymerase chain reaction.
Modified from Dispenzieri and Gorevic (1999). By permission of Elsevier Science.

approximately 20% and 25% of patients, respectively (D'Amico 1998; Tarantino et al. 1995). Arterial hypertension occurs in more than 80% of patients at the onset of renal disease (Tarantino et al. 1995). The nephrotoxicity of the cryoglobulins in patients with type II cryoglobulinemia cannot be explained by the amount or size of IgM-IgG complexes or the concentration of cryoglobulins in the serum (D'Amico 1998). Although cryopathic membranoproliferative glomerulonephritis (MPGN) portends a poor prognosis (Cordonnier et al. 1983; Gorevic et al. 1980; Invernizzi et al. 1983; Tarantino et al. 1995), progression to end-stage renal failure due to sclerosing nephritis is uncommon (Tarantino et al. 1995). Tarantino et al. (1995) reported that of 105 patients with MC-associated MPGN, whom they had followed for a median of 11 years from the onset of the disease, only 15% progressed to end-stage renal failure, whereas 43% died of cardiovascular, hepatic, or infectious causes. In their multivariate analysis, age greater than 50 years, purpura, splenomegaly, cryocrit values higher than 10%, C3 plasma concentrations lower than 54 mg/dL, and serum creatinine values higher than 1.5 mg/dL were independent risk factors for death or dialysis (Tarantino et al. 1995). Normal complement levels have been associated with long survivals without therapy (Gorevic et al. 1980).

MPGN is responsible for approximately 80% of all renal lesions in type II cryoglobulinemic nephropathy (Table 10.5) (D'Amico 1998). Type I MPGN is characterized by a markedly hypercellular glomerulus, infiltrated with numerous leukocytes, mainly monocytes (D'Amico 1998). There is thickening of the glomerular basement membrane, with a double-contoured appearance. Intraglomerular deposits, usually in a subendothelial location, may fill the capillary lumen, especially in patients with an acute rapidly progressive deterioration of renal function. These large eosinophilic, periodic acid-Schiff–positive intraluminal deposits, which are called "intraluminal thrombi," are usually amorphous, immune complex-like deposits. On electron microscopy, they appear as organized, finely fibrillar, cylindric, or immunotactoidlike structures. The immunoglobulin deposits found in the glomerular deposits are identical to those found in the serum cryoglobulin on immunohistochemistry and on electron micrography. These cylinders are 100 to 1,000 nm long and have a hollow axis, appearing in cross sections like annular bodies with a diameter of 62 to 63 nm (Cordonnier et al. 1983; Tarantino et al. 1995). Isolated massive deposits are limited to those with monoclonal components, i.e., types I and II (Brouet et al. 1974).

A less common presentation – occurring in about 20% of cases – is that of a mild mesangial proliferative glomerulonephropathy. Leukocyte infiltration is moderate or absent, and immune complex deposition is scanty (D'Amico 1998). Studies in mice suggest that mesangial deposits precede hyaline thrombi, suggesting that endoluminal immunodeposits result once the clearance capacity of the mesangium is exceeded. Approximately one-third of patients with cryoglobulinemic glomerulonephritis have acute vasculitis of the small- and medium-sized arteries, with fibrinoid necrosis of the arteriolar wall and monocytic infiltration (Tarantino et al. 1995).

10.4.5 Liver

Approximately 39% of patients with symptomatic cryoglobulinemia (Monti et al. 1995a) and as many as 77% with MC (Gorevic et al. 1980) have documented liver abnormalities at diagnosis (Tables 10.2 and 10.4). Furthermore, hepatomegaly and splenomegaly are present in up to 70% and 52%, respectively (Gorevic et al. 1980; Meltzer and Franklin 1966; Tarantino et al. 1981). Liver failure is the cause of death in 2.5% to 7.6% (Gorevic et al. 1980; Monti et al. 1995b; Tarantino et al. 1995) of patients and 5.6% to 29% of all reported deaths (Gorevic et al. 1980; Monti et al. 1995b; Tarantino et al. 1995). Patients with HCV subtype 1b appear to have a higher rate of chronic liver disease and lower rates of response to interferon therapy than patients with 2a (Origgi et al. 1998).

Histologic findings include portal fibrosis, chronic persistent hepatitis, chronic active hepatitis, chronic active hepatitis with cirrhosis, and postnecrotic cirrhosis (Table 10.6) (Dispenzieri and Gorevic 1999). Most specimens are characterized by diffuse lymphocytic infiltrate ranging from minimal periportal to extensive infiltration with nodule formation. These changes correlate with the severity of other pathologic findings. Plasma cell infiltration may be seen in several specimens (Donada et al. 1998b). Even in the absence of cryoglobulinemia, patients with chronic HCV infection have portal lymphoid infiltrates with features of B follicles composed of oligoclonal populations of B cells (Magalini et al. 1998). The severity or duration of HCV infection may have a role in the pathogenesis of cryoglobulinemia (Lunel et al. 1994). As the liver disease evolves to cirrhosis in cryoglobulinemia patients, the lymphoid aggregates become less prominent in number and size (Monteverde et al. 1995), the likelihood of finding a monotypic component to the cryoglobulin decreases, and the serum concentration of cryoglobulins decreases (Monteverde et al. 1997).

Furthermore, there are reports of resolution of liver histopathologic features on serial biopsy associated with clinical improvement and disappearance of serum cryoglobulins (Invernizzi et al. 1983; Monteverde et al. 1995).

Table 10.6. Suggested approach to classify the cryoglobulinemic syndrome by the Gruppo Italiano di Studio delle Crioglobulinemie

Cryocrit > 1% for at least 6 months
At least 2 of the following: purpura, weakness, arthralgias
C4 < 8 mg/dL
Positive RF in serum (to be distinguished as monoclonal or polyclonal)
Secondary if associated with: CTD, chronic liver disease, LPD, infections
Essential if without any underlying conditions
Assessment of the extent of the vasculitic process: hepatic and renal involvement, peripheral neuropathies
Identification of microlymphoma-like nodules in bone marrow

CTD, connective tissue disease; LPD, lymphoproliferative disease; RF, rheumatoid factor.
From Invernizzi et al. (1995). By permission of the journal.

The lymphoid population in the liver may show the histologic and immunophenotypic findings of lymphoplasmacytoid lymphoma or immunocytoma, and the lymphoid elements frequently arrange in pseudofollicular structures in the liver, with morphologic features similar to those previously reported in chronic HCV without cryoglobulinemia (Monteverde et al. 1995). The polytypic and monotypic B-cell infiltrates, which occur in the portal tracts of the HCV^+/type III cryoglobulin and HCV^+/type II cryoglobulin patients, respectively, express the CD5 antigen (Monteverde et al. 1995). These liver lymphoid nodules contain B cells, predominantly with a $CD5^+$/*bcl*-2$^+$/Ki67$^-$ phenotype – i.e., with low proliferative and apoptotic rates (Monteverde et al. 1997).

10.4.6 Other

Because cryoglobulinemia is a multisystem disease, often manifested as a vasculitis, all organs are at risk. Some authors have made the distinction between a polyarteritis nodosa-type and an MC vasculitis in the context of HCV. The former involves the medium-sized vessels, whereas the latter involves the small vessels. Muscle and cardiac involvement have been described on biopsy and autopsy (Gorevic et al. 1980; Meltzer and Franklin 1966). Abdominal pain occurs in 2% to 20% of patients (Brouet et al. 1974; Gorevic et al. 1980; Tarantino et al. 1981). Pain can be severe enough to warrant hospitalization and consideration of surgical exploration. Antemortem diagnosis of abdominal vasculitis is not common, but on autopsy vasculitis has been observed involving the small- and medium-sized vessels in the gastrointestinal tract (Gorevic et al. 1980). Although not described in the larger series of cryoglobulinemia, lung involvement is common, but often subclinical (Dispenzieri and Gorevic 1999). Forced expiratory flow and diffusing capacity of the lung for carbon monoxide are frequently decreased, and signs of interstitial involvement may be seen on x-ray. Associated pulmonary complications of MC include bronchiolitis obliterans with organizing pneumonia, severe pulmonary hemorrhage, and diffuse pulmonary vasculitis. Granular sludge in conjunctival and retinal vessels occurs fairly frequently, especially in those with monoclonal cryoglobulins (Brouet et al. 1974; Wintrobe and Buell 1933), and may be related to hyperviscosity. Lymphadenopathy is present in approximately 17% of patients (Gorevic et al. 1980).

10.5 Classification and Staging: Clinical and Pathologic

The only recognized staging system for defining and characterizing symptomatic cryoglobulinemia is offered by the Gruppo Italiano di Studio delle Crioglobuliniemie (GISC) group (Invernizzi et al. 1995) (Table 10.6). This same group offers a coding system to measure response (Migliaresi and Tirri 1995). Others have applied the Birmingham vasculitis activity score, the disease extent index, and complement C3c levels to assess disease activity and response to treatment (Lamprecht et al. 2000).

10.6 Diagnosis

10.6.1 Laboratory Tests

By definition, all patients with cryoglobulinemia have serum cryoglobulins. Their type or quantity does not reliably predict whether or which symptoms will be present. However, concentrations of cryoglobulins tend to vary by type, with the majority of cases of type III

being less than 1 mg/mL; of type II, greater than 1 mg/mL; and of type I, greater than 5 mg/mL (Brouet et al. 1974). About 95% of the monoclonal IgMs have an accompanying κ light chain, and the remainder have a λ chain (Dispenzieri and Gorevic 1999). Rarely, the monoclonal component of the MC can be IgA or IgG.

On serum protein electrophoresis, polyclonal hypergammaglobulinemia is the most frequent finding, although patterns of hypogammaglobulinemia may be seen too (Gorevic et al. 1980). Even in type II cryoglobulinemia, only 15% have a visible monoclonal spike on SPEP (Gorevic et al. 1980). Serum IgM values are frequently increased; cryoprecipitable IgM may comprise up to one-third of the total serum IgM concentration. Hyperviscosity occurs only occasionally (Meltzer and Franklin 1966). Marked depression of complement CH50, C1q, and C4 in the presence of relatively normal C3 values is usual (Gorevic et al. 1980; Trejo et al. 2001). Neither C4 concentration nor cryoglobulin values correlate with overall clinical severity, although for individual patients the cryoglobulin value can sometimes serve as a marker for disease activity (Ferri et al. 1986; Gorevic et al. 1980). RF may also decrease with response to therapy. An increased erythrocyte sedimentation rate and a mild normochromic, normocytic anemia are fairly common (Gorevic et al. 1980). Cytopenias (Meltzer and Franklin 1966) have been described, as have pseudoleukocytosis and pseudothrombocytosis. On peripheral blood films cryoprecipitate may form cloudlike structures. The antinuclear antibody result may be positive in as many as two-thirds of patients and in as many as one-third of the HCV-positive patients (Trejo et al. 2001). Because HCV is frequently concentrated in cryoglobulins (Agnello et al. 1992), serial measurements of plasma or serum HCV RNA in these patients are not reliable. High values of soluble CD30 are found in patients with cryoglobulinemia and appear to correlate with response to interferon (Lamprecht et al. 2000).

10.6.2 Laboratory Detection

Because cryoglobulins are cold-induced reversible precipitates of immunoglobulin, their collection and processing are critical (Dispenzieri and Gorevic 1999). A minimum of 10 to 20 mL of blood is required, and the specimen must be allowed to clot at 37 °C for 30 to 60 minutes before centrifugation. The serum supernatant is kept at 4 °C for as long as 7 days and inspected daily for cryoprecipitate. Types I and II cryoglobulins are usually apparent by the next day (Fig. 10.4 d). In contrast, type III cryoglobulins may require several days before a precipitate is visible. Precipitates are usually flocculent, but they may be gelatinous or crystalline. If a precipitate forms, it should be resolubilized at 37 °C to prove that it is indeed a cryoglobulin and washed a minimum of 3 to 6 times. Cryocrit measurements are the volume percent of the unwashed precipitate as compared to serum supernatant. This is a fairly inaccurate measurement because precipitated salts or other proteins may be present before washing. Other popular alternatives include total protein determination, immunoglobulin measurement by nephelometry, and area under the curve on protein electrophoresis. Methods to evaluate the composition of the cryoglobulin include immunoelectrophoresis, immunofixation, immunoblotting, and capillary electrophoresis. There is controversy as to whether immunoblotting or immunofixation allows for the most effective characterization.

10.7 Differential Diagnosis

The differential diagnosis of cryoglobulinemia includes connective tissue diseases, vasculitis, and HCV with autoimmune features.

10.8 Second Malignancies

The association of cryoglobulinemia and other B-cell LPDs and plasmaproliferative disorders dates back to Wintrobe's description of reversible cryoprecipitability of serum in a patient with multiple myeloma (Wintrobe and Buell 1933). In cryoglobulinemia, there is often difficulty in distinguishing whether the LPD is a primary or secondary malignancy. Different series reported different proportions of associated LPD (Table 10.2). Invernizzi et al. (1979) first recognized a significant evolution to LPD in their long-term follow-up studies, and their observations formed the basis for the GISC report. This multicenter cooperative report on 913 Italian patients may be most representative given its size and design. Approximately 8.9% of all patients, or 31% of all secondary patients with symptomatic cryoglobulinemia, had a diagnosis of LPD at diagnosis of cryoglobulinemia. Of these, 27% were type I; 68%, type II; and 5%, type III (Monti et al. 1995 a). These percentages are likely under-

estimates because not all patients had intensive investigation for a clonal disorder. In a small study of 35 type II MC patients, the distribution of EMC and secondary LPD was 63% and 23%, respectively, before bone marrow sampling, but 20% and 66%, respectively, after (Mussini et al. 1991). In yet another study, 25% of patients with chronic HCV and clinically active MC had evidence of a monoclonal B-cell population consistent with B-cell non-Hodgkin lymphoma by bone marrow morphology, flow cytometry, or molecular studies (Rasul et al. 1999).

Results of bone marrow studies must be interpreted with caution. In cryoglobulinemia, reactive bone marrow with lymphocytosis is common (Mazzaro et al. 1996; Monteverde et al. 1995; Pozzato et al. 1994) (Table 10.6). In 2 studies that used flow cytometry, the incidence of clonal LPD within the bone marrow of patients with essential type II cryoglobulinemia was 30% to 39% (Mazzaro et al. 1996; Pozzato et al. 1994). The presence of a monoclonal component in the cryoprecipitate of a type II cryoglobulin indicates that at least a small B-cell clone should be detectable. This proves to be the case; immunoglobulin gene rearrangements were positive in the peripheral blood in 25% to 100% (De Vita et al. 2000; Mazzaro et al. 1996) of cases, depending on the sensitivity of the assay – Southern blot or polymerase chain reaction. Proving clonality may be considered necessary for a diagnosis of malignancy, but whether it is sufficient is a matter of controversy. Whether the clonal lymphocytes detected in type II cryoglobulinemia truly represent a low-grade lymphoma or rather a potentially premalignant condition is unknown.

In a small series, only 1 of 5 patients who had polymerase chain reaction studies on bone marrow before and after transformation to overt lymphoma had the lymphoma originate from 1 of the dominant B-cell clones that were overexpanded in the putative neoplastic baseline bone marrow lesions (De Vita et al. 2000). This observation suggests that the underlying immunologic environment is permissive for emergence and recession of B-cell clones (oligoclones), some of which may derive an advantage and transform into an overt B-cell malignancy.

Symptomatic lymphoma develops in 6% to 28% of patients with type II cryoglobulinemia after 4 to 10 years of follow-up (Invernizzi et al. 1979; Monteverde et al. 1995; Pozzato et al. 1994; Zignego et al. 1997). Fifty percent of the cases are intermediate- to high-grade lymphoma (Monteverde et al. 1995), and the remainder are low-grade lymphoma. The most common histologic diagnosis among the low-grade lymphomas is immunocytoma (76%) (Mussini et al. 1991), followed by MALT and centrocytic follicular lymphoma (Luppi et al. 1998). Factors contributing to the evolution from polyclonal proliferation to asymptomatic clonal B-cell LPD to symptomatic lymphoma are not understood, although clues may be provided by an understanding of cross-reactive idiotypes and observations in patients with HCV infection.

10.9 Treatment

Cryoglobulinemia has a fluctuating course with spontaneous exacerbation and remission. This feature makes controlled clinical trials essential in evaluating the response to therapy. Unfortunately, such studies are rare in the field of cryoglobulinemia. With the exception of the IFN-a trials of the 1990s (Dammacco et al. 1994; Ferri et al. 1993; Lauta and De Sangro 1995; Mazzaro et al. 1995; Misiani et al. 1994) and the small low antigen diet trial performed in the 1980s (Ferri et al. 1989), the remainder of the information regarding the treatment of symptomatic cryoglobulinemia is anecdotal. On the one hand, there are several accepted or standard treatments that have no randomized trials to support their practice; on the other hand, there are several reported strategies that have questionable, if any, benefit (Table 10.7). Finally, there are therapies like H$_1$ and H$_2$ blockers and penicillamine, which had sound scientific grounds for consideration but have been shown to have no clear clinical benefit (Dispenzieri and Gorevic 1999; Gorevic et al. 1980). Treatments in the first 2 categories are discussed to provide the practicing clinician with as much information as possible to deal with the all too frequent

Table 10.7. Treatment strategies for moderately to severely symptomatic cryoglobulinemia

Treatment	Response	Quality of data
Interferon	Effective	RCT
Ribavirin	PU	A
Low antigen diet	PU (mild disease)	RCT
Plasmapheresis, plasma exchange, cryoapheresis, and cryofiltration	PU	A
Prednisone 1 mg/kg IV, methylprednisolone 1 g/wk or 1 g/d×3 days	PU	A
Chlorambucil	PU	A
IV CTX 750 mg/m^2 per mo, oral 1–2 mg/kg per day	PU	A
Melphalan	PU	A
Oral azathioprine 100 mg/day	PU	A
CSA 2.5 mg/kg per day	PU	A
Colchicine 1 mg/day	PNU	A
IV Ig	V[a]	A
Cladribine and fludarabine	V	A
Splenectomy	V	A
Chloroquine	PNU	A
H$_1$ and H$_2$ blockers	PNU	A
Penicillamine	PNU	A

A, anecdotal or single-armed trial; CSA, cyclosporine; CTX, cyclophosphamide; IV, intravenous; PNU, probably not useful; PU, probably useful; RCT, randomized controlled trial; V, variable.

[a] One case report of precipitating acute renal failure and another of systemic vasculitis.

From Dispenzieri and Gorevic (1999). By permission of Elsevier Science.

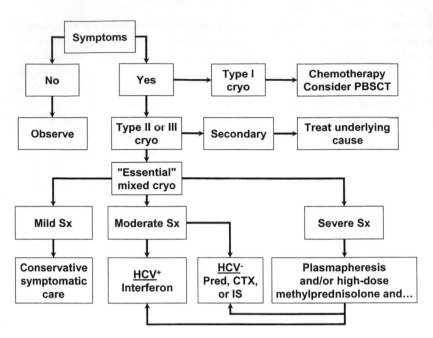

Fig. 10.5. Treatment schema. If interferon fails, try combination therapy with interferon-α and ribavirin, as long as no contraindications for ribavirin. *cryo*, cryoglobulins; *CTX*, cyclophosphamide; *IS*, immunosuppressant; *PBSCT*, peripheral blood stem cell transplant; *pred*, low-dose prednisone; *Sx*, symptoms

patient with refractory symptomatic cryoglobulinemia. Figure 10.5 outlines a strategy for managing patients with symptomatic cryoglobulinemia.

For years, the paradigm in approaching symptomatic cryoglobulinemia has been to use protective measures against cold, bed rest, analgesics, low-dose steroids, and low antigen content diet for mild disease (purpura, asthenia, arthralgia, and mild sensory neuropathy) and to use plasmapheresis, high-dose steroids, and cytotoxic therapy for severe disease (glomerulonephritis, motor neuropathy, systemic vasculitis).

Since the connection has been made between HCV and MC, immunosuppressive therapy is viewed in a less favorable light, and IFN is generally considered to be first-line therapy for HCV$^+$ patients who are in nonemergent situations (Dammacco et al. 1994; Ferri et al. 1993; Lauta and De Sangro 1995; Mazzaro et al. 1995; Migliaresi and Tirri 1995; Misiani et al. 1994). IFN-α response rates as high as 89% can be expected in HCV$^+$ patients with symptomatic MC (Table 10.8). The role of IFN in symptomatic type I cryoglobulinemia is unknown, although anecdotal benefits have been reported (Cohen et al. 1996). For those individuals with symptomatic type I cryoglobulinemia, cytotoxic therapy appropriate for their LPD is still the therapy of choice. Similarly, treatment of the underlying connective tissue disease or infection would be first-line therapy. Table 10.7

is a list of different therapeutic strategies that have been reported anecdotally. Table 10.8 is a compilation of the more important IFN trials. The importance of not overtreating patients cannot be emphasized sufficiently. Retrospective studies do not demonstrate any clear benefit of treatment over observation. This may be owing to the low effectiveness of our treatments or the fact that corticosteroids, immunosuppressive drugs, and plasmapheresis have routinely been reserved for only those patients with the most severe disease (Tarantino et al. 1995). Clinical trials are needed to clarify these issues.

10.9.1 Treatment of Life-Threatening Disease

The use of cytotoxic therapy, high-dose corticosteroids, and plasmapheresis in cryoglobulinemia with "uncontrolled features" has been the dogma, although no randomized clinical trials support this strategy. Most authors have reported the use of plasmapheresis and plasma exchange in combination with cytotoxic agents or corticosteroids (Ferri et al. 1986; Geltner et al. 1981). According to case reports, responses may be seen in 60% to 100% of patients (Ferri et al. 1986; Geltner et al. 1981). Skin manifestations and arthralgias are usually the quickest to respond, whereas the degree of nerve and renal responses depends on the acuity of their oc-

Table 10.8. Interferon trials

Author	N	Therapy	Induction doses	Rx time, mo	FU, mo	RR,[a] %	CR, %	PR, %	Comments
Randomized trials									
Ferri et al.	26	IFN vs. predni-sone	2 MU qd×1 mo, then qod for 5 mo; max pred 10 mg/d	Cross-over at 6 mo	NS	77 0	NS	NS	Rebound after IFN dc
Misiani et al. (1994)	53	IFN vs. prior Rx	1.5 MU qd×1 wk, then 3 MU tiw vs. no therapy or stable low-dose prednisone (≤ 0.2 mg/kg per d)	5.5	7.4	60 0[b]	NS	NS	Relapse in all patients when IFN dc
Dammacco et al. (1994)	65	IFN IFN/pred Pred No therapy	IFN 3 MU tiw Prednisone 16 mg/d	12	13	66 71 22 13	53 53 17 6.7	13 18 5.5 6.7	Most rapid and durable RR with IFN/pred
Lauta and De Sangro (1995)	33	IFN/pred vs. Pred	IFN 3 MU/day until CR or >minor resp at 6 mo followed by 3 MU tiw; predni-sone 10 mg/day	Indef	14 mo	83 27	50 0	33 27	
Mazzaro et al. (1995)	36	IFN vs. IFN	3 MU tiw × 6 mo vs. 3 MU tiw × 12 mo	6 12	NS	78 89	28 39	50 50	12 Mo → better RR & higher long-term response 22% vs. 11%
Early open trials									
Bonomo et al. (1987)	7	IFN	3 MU qd	4–12		100	NS	NS	First IFN trial, done before HCV
Casato et al. (1991)	18	IFN	3 MU qd×3 mo, then qod for >12 mo	Vari-able	30	77	61	17	Before HCV
Migliaresi and Tirri (1995)	24	IFN	3 MU tiw	12	18	67	54	13	Relapse in 85% within 6 mo of IFN dc
Cohen et al. (1996)	20	IFN	3 MU tiw[c]	6	12	60	NS	NS	92% relapse <1 y after IFN dc

CR, complete response; dc, discontinue; FU, follow-up, HCV, hepatitis C virus; indef, indefinitely, IFN, interferon-α; max, maximum; NS, not stated; PR, partial response; pred, prednisone; qd, daily; qod, every other day; resp, response; RR, response rate; Rx, treatment; tiw, 3 times per week; vs., versus.

[a] All responses are clinical responses, which refer to symptomatic responses as defined by both clinical symptoms or signs and laboratory results known to correlate with symptomatic disease. HCV response is an antiviral response that is frequently measured in IFN trials.

[b] HCV response was also measured.

[c] Other concomitant therapies allowed for severe disease.

From Dispenzieri and Gorevic (1999). By permission of Elsevier Science.

currence, with poorer responses occurring in chronic cases. With combination immunosuppressive therapy and plasma exchange, reversal of catastrophic complications such as encephalopathy and acute glomerulonephritis (Ferri et al. 1986) has been documented. High-dose pulsed methylprednisolone is also a favored therapeutic intervention for acute events (D'Amico 1998).

10.9.2 Interferon-α

The bulk of the experience with IFN-α to treat cryoglobulinemia is in patients with MC (types II and III), and its use predates the association of cryoglobulinemia and HCV. From responses to IFN seen in other LPDs, Bonomo et al. (1987) treated 7 patients with type II idiopathic MC with daily recombinant IFN and observed a reduction of circulating cryoglobulins and improvement of the clinical pattern within the first month. This prompted a prospective trial of IFN in 18 patients with idiopathic type II MC. A 77% response rate was achieved (Casato et al. 1991). Five randomized trials followed, evaluating the efficacy of IFN in patients with symptomatic type II MC (Dammacco et al. 1994; Ferri et al. 1993; Lauta and De Sangro 1995; Mazzaro et al. 1995; Misiani et al. 1994). All studies demonstrated a beneficial effect, with clinical response rates of 60% to 89%, but relapses occurred in a majority of patients within 6 months of discontinuation (Dammacco et al. 1994; Lauta and De Sangro 1995; Mazzaro et al. 1995; Migliaresi and Tirri 1995; Misiani et al. 1994). Dammacco et al. (1994) enrolled 65 patients onto a 4-arm randomized trial comparing natural IFN (nIFN) alone to nIFN with prednisone to prednisone alone to no therapy. Clinical response rates of 66%, 71%, 22%, and 13% were seen in the respective arms (Table 10.8).

Purpuric lesions and liver function abnormalities tend to respond rapidly (within weeks) to therapy with IFN. The neuropathy appears to be the slowest to respond (Casato et al. 1991; Migliaresi and Tirri 1995), followed by the nephropathy (Migliaresi and Tirri 1995). Although no randomized data exist, in the case of acute nephritis most authors suggest initially supplementing IFN with corticosteroids or plasmapheresis or both (D'Amico 1998). Both peripheral neuropathy (personal observation and Casato et al. 1991) and ischemic manifestations may be exacerbated by IFN (Cid et al. 1999).

If no response occurs after 3 to 4 months, it is unlikely that any will occur (Migliaresi and Tirri 1995). Responses to treatment often correlate with clearance of HCV RNA from the serum (Dammacco et al. 1994; Ferri et al. 1993; Misiani et al. 1994). Responders have significant decrements in cryocrit values, IgM values, RF activity, and alanine transaminase (Dammacco et al. 1994; Migliaresi and Tirri 1995; Misiani et al. 1994), but cryoglobulins may persist even after resolution of vasculitic symptoms (Casato et al. 1991). Complement values usually do not correct (Dammacco et al. 1994; Migliaresi and Tirri 1995; Misiani et al. 1994), although slow correction of the C4 value was observed at 12 months (Lauta and De Sangro 1995; Migliaresi and Tirri 1995). There is a report of documented regression of a B-cell clone in a patient with HCV-associated cryoglobulinemia and a chronic lymphocytic leukemia with marginal zone phenotype (Casato et al. 2002). The beneficial effect of IFN in cryoglobulinemic vasculitis is not mediated solely by its antiviral effects. Other mechanisms must have a role, given documented responses to IFN in patients without evidence of HCV infection (Casato et al. 1998). Potential mechanisms may include antiproliferative effect against the lymphocytes producing the components of the cryoprecipitate, more efficient clearance of circulating immune complex by the reticuloendothelial system by its effect on macrophages, inhibition of immunoglobulin synthesis, immunoregulatory activity on T-cell function, and up-regulation of expression of human leukocyte antigens (Agnello et al. 1992; Dammacco et al. 1994).

Factors associated with a poorer response to therapy or rapid relapse include liver cirrhosis, advanced age, male sex, high amounts of HCV RNA at the onset of therapy, genotype 1b, absence of antibody response to HCV NS5A region, low apolipoprotein A-I values, and high interleukin-6 values (Cresta et al. 1999; Dammacco et al. 1994; Dispenzieri and Gorevic 1999; Mazzaro et al. 1995; Migliaresi and Tirri 1995). The values of cryoglobulins or RF or the results of liver function tests do not seem to affect treatment outcome (Dammacco et al. 1994; Mazzaro et al. 1995; Migliaresi and Tirri 1995).

Higher dose – daily versus thrice weekly (Bonomo et al. 1987; Casato et al. 1991) – and longer duration of therapy – minimum of 1 year of therapy – may result in more rapid (Bonomo et al. 1987; Casato et al. 1991) and durable responses (Migliaresi and Tirri 1995). The use of prednisone in the induction strategy may result in quicker and more durable responses, but care must be taken because serum HCV RNA values may increase with the use of prednisone (Dammacco et al. 1994). If relapse occurs while on therapy, resistance may be due to antibodies to interferon; reinduction may be possible with nIFN (Casato et al. 1991). Rebound of symptoms and of serologic parameters is common after IFN-a discontinuation, but initial treatment for 10 to 20 months may result in prolonged remissions in a minority of patients even after discontinuation of therapy (Ferri et al. 1993; Misiani et al. 1994).

10.9.3 Ribavirin

From the promising results observed in patients with chronic HCV infection, ribavirin, an oral guanosine nucleoside analog, has been used in patients with symptomatic HCV$^+$ MC as monotherapy and combined with IFN-a (Calleja et al. 1999; Durand et al. 1998). Although minor responses are seen with monotherapy, ribavirin is typically used in combination with IFN-a. Donada et al. (1998a) treated 17 patients with relapsed, HCV-associated, asymptomatic MC with combination ribavirin and IFN. Compared with relapsed patients without cryoglobulinemia, response rates were equivalent at 85% and 79%, respectively (Donada et al. 1998a), suggesting that this may be another strategy for patients with symptomatic cryoglobulinemia. More than 60% of patients with symptomatic MC who do not respond to IFN alone have some response to combined therapy, and 80% of patients who relapse on IFN-a alone respond to combined therapy (Calleja et al. 1999). The drug is tolerated well but often mild dose-related hemolysis occurs (Durand et al. 1998; Zuckerman et al. 2000).

10.9.4 Corticosteroids

Unfortunately, no randomized controlled data exist to support the use of corticosteroids. The best data regarding low-dose prednisone come from 2 of the 4 arms of the Dammacco et al. (1994) IFN-a trial (Table 10.8). The response rate for those patients treated with 16 mg prednisone per day was 22% compared with the spontaneous remission rate of 13% in patients given no therapy. This difference was not statistically significant but the sample size was small. Regardless, low-dose prednisone continues to be the mainstay of symptomatic mild to moderate disease, because it appears to improve arthralgias, fevers, and asthenia.

For patients with rapidly progressive glomerulonephritis, initial improvement in more than 90% of patients with pulsed high-dose methylprednisolone appears to be superior to the spontaneous improvement rates of 15% seen with no intervention (Dispenzieri and Gorevic 1999). Fever, arthralgias, abdominal pain, and leg ulcers respond promptly. Improvements in serum creatinine and in proteinuria are also seen within 1 week, with maximal benefit at 1 month. Purpura and weakness gradually improve with this strategy. High doses of corticosteroids are also used for rapidly advancing peripheral neuropathy.

10.9.5 Chemotherapy

Authors state the importance of using cytotoxic therapy in cryoglobulinemia with uncontrolled features or if there is rapid increase in cryoglobulins, although no clinical trial supports this strategy. Low-dose cyclophosphamide (2 mg/kg) and prednisone (1 mg/kg) may also provide benefit (Dispenzieri and Gorevic 1999).

Personal experience and case reports support the use of chlorambucil, another oral alkylating agent, to manage symptomatic cryoglobulinemia, especially type I. In a prospective open series (Geltner et al. 1981), 5 patients with MC with renal or neurologic and vasculitic manifestations were treated with combined modality therapy including chlorambucil. Treatment included chlorambucil, prednisone (1 mg/kg per day), and plasmapheresis (1 to 3 liters/week). Healing of cutaneous ulcers (3 of 3), improvement in renal function (4 of 4), and diminution of purpura (2 of 2) were observed. There was no significant improvement in peripheral neuropathy.

Melphalan is most commonly used to treat patients who have symptomatic type I cryoglobulinemia due to multiple myeloma. There have been case reports, however, of benefit in patients with type II cryoglobulinemia (Dispenzieri and Gorevic 1999). If the patient is considered to be a candidate for peripheral blood stem cell transplantation, melphalan-containing regimens should be avoided until after stem cell harvest. As with other alkylator therapy, the potential benefit of melphalan for treating symptomatic cryoglobulinemia must be weighed against the risk of developing myelodysplastic syndrome or acute leukemia.

The purine nucleoside analogs have some activity in patients with MC. In total, there was 1 patient in 5 who responded to fludarabine and 1 of 1 who responded to cladribine (Dispenzieri and Gorevic 1999).

10.9.6 Hematopoietic Stem Cell Transplantation

Although not formally studied, high-dose therapy with autologous stem cell transplantation can be considered for patients with symptomatic, refractory cryoglobulinemia, which is due to a plasmaproliferative disorder. There is an increased risk of lethal veno-occlusive disease in patients with chronic hepatitis C undergoing stem cell transplantation.

10.9.7 Other Immunosuppressant Therapies

Colchicine inhibits intracellular microtubule assembly, thereby reducing the cellular functions of monocytes, granulocytes, and lymphocytes. Through this mechanism, and perhaps others, it blocks mitosis, chemotaxis, adhesion, and immunoglobulin secretion. In an open study, Monti et al. treated 17 patients with symptomatic MC with colchicine (1 mg/day for 6 to 48 months). Clinically, there was improvement in purpura, weakness, and leg ulcers. There was some improvement in hepatic and renal function tests as well as in RF and cryocrit levels. This improvement was more marked during the first 6 to 12 months; during prolonged follow-up, there was relapse in the different variables, although they remained at better levels than at the beginning. Only the cryocrit showed a further reduction. Clearly, randomized trials are needed to establish colchicine's efficacy.

Cyclosporine inhibits immunocompetent lymphocytes in the G_0 and G_1 phase of the cell cycle. Anecdotal reports of improvement using cyclosporine exist. Caution is needed on cessation of therapy because there has been a report of enhancement of HCV replication on discontinuation of immunosuppressive therapy. However, cyclosporine has been used in patients with chronic HCV infection without serious complication or increased HCV viral load (Dispenzieri and Gorevic 1999).

10.9.8 Biologic Therapy

The use of intravenous gamma globulin to treat symptomatic cryoglobulinemia is controversial, at best. Theoretical explanations for its potential mechanism of action abound (including blockade of the reticuloendothelial system, clearance of unidentified viral antigens associated with the patient's cryoglobulin, and a potential direct immunosuppressive effect of the intravenous gamma globulin), but none is known or proven. There was a report of a 46-year-old man who had significant leukocytoclastic vasculitis that was refractory to oral cyclophosphamide, oral prednisone, high-dose pulsed methylprednisolone, colchicine, and plasmapheresis, who derived a quick, durable response to 0.4 mg/kg intravenous gamma globulin for 4 consecutive days. However, there are also reports of intravenous gamma globulin precipitating acute renal failure (Dispenzieri and Gorevic 1999).

10.9.9 Surgery

Dramatic reductions in the cryocrit and the cryoglobulinemic symptoms – including MPGN – have been reported (Dispenzieri and Gorevic 1999; Ubara et al. 2000) in several patients who underwent splenectomy for hypersplenism. In contrast, in the series from Meltzer and Franklin (1966) the 1 patient who underwent splenectomy died of acute renal failure. Because this intervention has not been thoroughly studied, and because of the high risk involved, this intervention should not be considered a standard therapy, but rather a potential intervention for patients without cirrhosis who have disease that is difficult to manage because of cytopenias due to hypersplenism.

10.9.10 Plasmapheresis

Plasmapheresis (and related procedures) has been used for many years for cryoglobulinemia without ever having been subjected to randomized controlled trials (Dispenzieri and Gorevic 1999; Ferri et al. 1986; Geltner et al. 1981). The generally accepted indications are acute, life-threatening events, including renal failure, nervous system involvement, and acute gangrenous digits. Plasmapheresis rapidly reduces the levels of circulating antibodies, immune complexes, and toxic substances. The removal of the circulating complexes may contribute to restoration of reticuloendothelial system functioning, and the action of plasmapheresis may modify the quality of the immune complexes.

If no concurrent immunosuppressive drugs are given, there tends to be a rebound phenomenon whereby the cryoglobulin returns to pretreatment levels within 1 week after treatment, with the steepest increase within the first 4 days. It is, therefore, not usually used as monotherapy. Some authors suggest that if the taper of the plasma exchange is gradual – over 6 to 24 months – relapses do not occur (Dispenzieri and Gorevic 1999; Ferri et al. 1986). A more typical approach in an emergency situation is to initiate plasmapheresis and interferon, corticosteroids, or cytotoxic therapy (Ferri et al. 1986; Geltner et al. 1981). The plasmapheresis can then be tapered over months, based on clinical tolerance. Complete resolution of acute glomerulonephritis, skin involvement, and encephalopathy has been observed when treatment is started early in the course of the disease. Skin and arthralgia manifestations are usually the quickest to respond, whereas the extent of nerve and renal responses depends on the acuity of their occurrence. According to case reports, responses can be seen in 60% to 100% of patients (Dispenzieri and Gorevic 1999; Ferri et al. 1986; Geltner et al. 1981).

The current recommendations for plasmapheresis include the exchange of 1.0 to 1.5 plasma volumes (40 to 60 mL/kg) during each session. The plasma or albumin saline solution should be warmed because acute renal failure has been reported when the plasma to be infused was not prewarmed. Options for the replacement fluid include 6% hetastarch in 0.9% sodium chloride injection, 5% albumin, fresh frozen plasma, and combinations thereof. Initially, exchanges are done daily or every other day for a total of 3 to 6 sessions, followed by a taper or maintenance therapy over the next 1 to 6 months (Ferri et al. 1986). Cryofiltration and cryoglobulinpheresis (or cryoapheresis) can also be used (Dispenzieri and Gorevic 1999).

10.9.11 Supportive Care

Symptomatic MC patients with proteinuria and renal disease have significant improvement in their proteinuria on captopril therapy. Although immunoregulatory and anti-inflammatory mechanisms have been pro-

posed, the benefit is most likely via the drug's ability to modify intraglomerular hemodynamics.

Erythropoietin deficiency due to renal insufficiency is common in patients with cryoglobulinemia. No formalized studies have been done in the symptomatic cryoglobulinemia population, but those patients with renal insufficiency, relative erythropoietin deficiency, and symptomatic anemia should be considered for therapy. There are no data on the effect of this drug on the underlying disease, but it is often a helpful supportive measure.

10.9.12 Other Therapeutic Measures

Conservative measures are most effective against mild disease (i.e., purpura, asthenia, arthralgia, sensory neuropathy). In a randomized crossover trial including 24 patients and conducted for 48 weeks, a low antigen diet decreased the cryocrit, circulating immunocomplexes, and γ-glutamyltransferase and aspartate transaminase concentrations and slightly improved symptom status for patients while on the low antigen diet. There was significant improvement in purpura and a trend toward improvement for weakness, fatigability, and arthralgias (Ferri et al. 1989). Even though the benefits were modest, such an intervention is not an unreasonable approach to offer to patients with mild disease. The premise of a low antigen diet was that macromolecular antigens are absorbed from the mucosa and contribute to the immune complex formation. The low antigen diet is similar to a restricted hypoallergenic diet. Food rich in putative macromolecular antigens, like meat, was restricted; vegetables, fruits, and rice were encouraged.

Because as many as 77% of patients have or develop renal insufficiency, protective renal measures should be taken, like avoidance of nephrotoxic drugs when possible, maintaining adequate hydration, and scrupulous attention to management of hypertension.

10.10 Prognosis

In a cohort study of EMC with a median follow-up of 11 years, the clinical pattern remained stable in about 40% of cases and progressed in the remainder: progressive renal disease in 37%, development of an LPD in 11%, and cirrhosis in another 11% (Invernizzi et al. 1979). The most frequent causes of death include renal failure, infection, LPDs, liver failure, cardiovascular complications, and hemorrhage (Brouet et al. 1974; Gorevic et al. 1980; Monti et al. 1995a; Singer et al. 1986).

10.11 Concluding Remarks

Cryoglobulinemia may be found in a spectrum of disorders spanning clear-cut B-cell neoplastic states in which cryoprecipitation manifests as ischemic or occlusive vasculopathy, to various immune-complex diseases in which vasculitis or glomerulonephritis or both may occur. Symptomatic cryoglobulinemia is many diseases, driven by and driving antibody-antigen responses, hepatic dysfunction, lymphoproliferation, and immune complexes. Distinguishing features that cause only some cryoglobulins to be symptomatic, elucidating the pathogenic mechanisms of HCV in cryoglobulin formation, and devising better therapies and more systematic evaluation of existing therapies are among the challenges for the future. Prognostication and classification in the 21st century continue to rely on Brouet's classification (types I, II, and III), but additional features will likely include presence or absence of HCV; HCV factors (genotype, titer); coexisting infections; B-cell clone burden; host factors; and immune system interactions (B- and T-cell idiotype networks, cytokines). Antiviral therapy is a reasonable option for HCV-associated cryoglobulinemia, but not all patients are HCV positive and only 60% to 80% of HCV$^+$ patients respond to IFN. In addition, not all patients tolerate IFN and, in those who do, the response is often brief once the treatment is discontinued. Only creative strategies, systematically studied, will provide long-awaited solutions.

References

Agnello V, Chung RT, Kaplan LM (1992) A role for hepatitis C virus infection in type II cryoglobulinemia. N Engl J Med 327:1490–1495

Agnello V, Zhang QX, Abel G, Knight GB (1995) The association of hepatitis C virus infection with monoclonal rheumatoid factors bearing the WA cross-idiotype: implications for the etiopathogenesis and therapy of mixed cryoglobulinemia. Clin Exp Rheumatol 13 Suppl 13:S101–S104

Bonomo L, Casato M, Afeltra A, Caccavo D (1987) Treatment of idiopathic mixed cryoglobulinemia with alpha interferon. Am J Med 83:726–730

Brouet JC, Clauvel JP, Danon F, Klein M, Seligmann M (1974) Biologic and clinical significance of cryoglobulins. A report of 86 cases. Am J Med 57:775–788

Calleja JL, Albillos A, Moreno-Otero R, Rossi I, Cacho G, Domper F, Yebra M, Escartin P (1999) Sustained response to interferon-alpha or to interferon-alpha plus ribavirin in hepatitis C virus-associated symptomatic mixed cryoglobulinaemia. Aliment Pharmacol Ther 13:1179–1186

Casato M, Lagana B, Antonelli G, Dianzani F, Bonomo L (1991) Long-term results of therapy with interferon-alpha for type II essential mixed cryoglobulinemia. Blood 78:3142–3147

Casato M, Lagana B, Pucillo LP, Quinti I (1998) Interferon for hepatitis C virus-negative type II mixed cryoglobulinemia. N Engl J Med 338:1386–1387

Casato M, Mecucci C, Agnello V, Fiorilli M, Knight GB, Matteucci C, Gao L, Kay J (2002) Regression of lymphoproliferative disorder after treatment for hepatitis C virus infection in a patient with partial trisomy 3, Bcl-2 overexpression, and type II cryoglobulinemia. Blood 99:2259–2261

Chan CH, Hadlock KG, Foung SK, Levy S (2001) V(H)1-69 gene is preferentially used by hepatitis C virus-associated B cell lymphomas and by normal B cells responding to the E2 viral antigen. Blood 97:1023–1026

Cid MC, Hernandez-Rodriguez J, Robert J, del Rio A, Casademont J, Coll-Vinent B, Grau JM, Kleinman HK, Urbano-Marquez A, Cardellach F (1999) Interferon-alpha may exacerbate cryoglobulinemia-related ischemic manifestations: an adverse effect potentially related to its anti-angiogenic activity. Arthritis Rheum 42:1051–1055

Cohen P, Nguyen QT, Deny P, Ferriere F, Roulot D, Lortholary O, Jarrousse B, Danon F, Barrier JH, Ceccaldi J, Constans J, Crickx B, Fiessinger JN, Hachulla E, Jaccard A, Seligmann M, Kazatchkine M, Laroche L, Subra JF, Turlure P, Guillevin L (1996) Treatment of mixed cryoglobulinemia with recombinant interferon alpha and adjuvant therapies. A prospective study on 20 patients. Ann Med Interne (Paris) 147:81–86

Cordonnier D, Vialtel P, Renversez JC, Chenais F, Favre M, Tournoud A, Barioz C, Bayle F, Dechelette E, Denis MC, Couderc P (1983) Renal diseases in 18 patients with mixed type II IgM-IgG cryoglobulinemia: monoclonal lymphoid infiltration (2 cases) and membranoproliferative glomerulonephritis (14 cases). Adv Nephrol Necker Hosp 12:177–204

Cresta P, Musset L, Cacoub P, Frangeul L, Vitour D, Poynard T, Opolon P, Nguyen DT, Golliot F, Piette JC, Huraux JM, Lunel F (1999) Response to interferon alpha treatment and disappearance of cryoglobulinaemia in patients infected by hepatitis C virus. Gut 45:122–128

Cucuianu A, Patiu M, Duma M, Basarab C, Soritau O, Bojan A, Vasilache A, Mates M, Petrov L (1999) Hepatitis B and C virus infection in Romanian non-Hodgkin's lymphoma patients. Br J Haematol 107:353–356

D'Amico G (1998) Renal involvement in hepatitis C infection: cryoglobulinemic glomerulonephritis. Kidney Int 54:650–671

Dammacco F, Sansonno D, Han JH, Shyamala V, Cornacchiulo V, Iacobelli AR, Lauletta G, Rizzi R (1994) Natural interferon-alpha versus its combination with 6-methyl-prednisolone in the therapy of type II mixed cryoglobulinemia: a long-term, randomized, controlled study. Blood 84:3336–3343

De Re V, De Vita S, Marzotto A, Rupolo M, Gloghini A, Pivetta B, Gasparotto D, Carbone A, Boiocchi M (2000) Sequence analysis of the immunoglobulin antigen receptor of hepatitis C virus-associated non-Hodgkin lymphomas suggests that the malignant cells are derived from the rheumatoid factor-producing cells that occur mainly in type II cryoglobulinemia. Blood 96:3578–3584

De Re V, De Vita S, Gasparotto D, Marzotto A, Carbone A, Ferraccioli G, Boiocchi M (2002) Salivary gland B cell lymphoproliferative disorders in Sjögren's syndrome present a restricted use of antigen receptor gene segments similar to those used by hepatitis C virus-associated non-Hodgkin's lymphomas. Eur J Immunol 32:903–910

De Rosa G, Gobbo ML, De Renzo A, Notaro R, Garofalo S, Grimaldi M, Apuzzo A, Chiurazzi F, Picardi M, Matarazzo M, Rotoli B (1997) High prevalence of hepatitis C virus infection in patients with B-cell lymphoproliferative disorders in Italy. Am J Hematol 55:77–82

De Vita S, De Re V, Gasparotto D, Ballare M, Pivetta B, Ferraccioli G, Pileri S, Boiocchi M, Monteverde A (2000) Oligoclonal non-neoplastic B cell expansion is the key feature of type II mixed cryoglobulinemia: clinical and molecular findings do not support a bone marrow pathologic diagnosis of indolent B cell lymphoma. Arthritis Rheum 43:94–102

Disdier P, Harle JR, Weiller PJ (1991) Cryoglobulinaemia and hepatitis C infection. Lancet 338:1151–1152

Dispenzieri A, Gorevic PD (1999) Cryoglobulinemia. Hematol Oncol Clin North Am 13:1315–1349

Donada C, Crucitti A, Donadon V, Chemello L, Alberti A (1998 a) Interferon and ribavirin combination therapy in patients with chronic hepatitis C and mixed cryoglobulinemia. Blood 92:2983–2984

Donada C, Crucitti A, Donadon V, Tommasi L, Zanette G, Crovatto M, Santini GF, Chemello L, Alberti A (1998 b) Systemic manifestations and liver disease in patients with chronic hepatitis C and type II or III mixed cryoglobulinaemia. J Viral Hepat 5:179–185

Durand JM, Cacoub P, Lunel-Fabiani F, Cosserat J, Cretel E, Kaplanski G, Frances C, Bletry O, Soubeyrand J, Godeau P (1998) Ribavirin in hepatitis C related cryoglobulinemia. J Rheumatol 25:1115–1117

Ferri C, Moriconi L, Gremignai G, Migliorini P, Paleologo G, Fosella PV, Bombardieri S (1986) Treatment of the renal involvement in mixed cryoglobulinemia with prolonged plasma exchange. Nephron 43:246–253

Ferri C, Pietrogrande M, Cecchetti R, Tavoni A, Cefalo A, Buzzetti G, Vitali C, Bombardieri S (1989) Low-antigen-content diet in the treatment of patients with mixed cryoglobulinemia. Am J Med 87:519–524

Ferri C, Marzo E, Longombardo G, La Civita L, Lombardini F, Giuggioli D, Vanacore R, Liberati AM, Mazzoni A, Greco F, Bombardieri S (1993) Interferon alfa-2b in mixed cryoglobulinaemia: a controlled crossover trial. Gut 34 Suppl:S144–S145

Ferri C, Caracciolo F, Zignego AL, La Civita L, Monti M, Longombardo G, Lombardini F, Greco F, Capochiani E, Mazzoni A, Mazzaro C, Pasero G (1994) Hepatitis C virus infection in patients with non-Hodgkin's lymphoma. Br J Haematol 88:392–394

Fong S, Chen PP, Crowley JJ, Silverman GJ, Carson DA (1988) Idiotypic characteristics of rheumatoid factors. Scand J Rheumatol Suppl 75:58–65

Franzin F, Efremov DG, Pozzato G, Tulissi P, Batista F, Burrone OR (1995) Clonal B-cell expansions in peripheral blood of HCV-infected patients. Br J Haematol 90:548–552

Galli M, Zehender G, Monti G, Ballaré M, Saccardo F, Piconi S, De Maddalena C, Bertoncelli MC, Rinaldi G, Invernizzi F, Monteverde A (1995) Hepatitis C virus RNA in the bone marrow of patients with mixed cryoglobulinemia and in subjects with noncryoglobulinemic chronic hepatitis type C. J Infect Dis 171:672–675

Garcia-Carrasco M, Ramos-Casals M, Cervera R, Trejo O, Yague J, Siso A, Jimenez S, de La Red G, Font J, Ingelmo M (2001) Cryoglobulinemia in systemic lupus erythematosus: prevalence and clinical characteristics in a series of 122 patients. Semin Arthritis Rheum 30:366–373

Geltner D, Kohn RW, Gorevic P, Franklin EC (1981) The effect of combination therapy (steroids, immunosuppressives, and plasmapheresis) on 5 mixed cryoglobulinemia patients with renal, neurologic, and vascular involvement. Arthritis Rheum 24:1121–1127

Gerotto M, Dal Pero F, Loffreda S, Bianchi FB, Alberti A, Lenzi M (2001) A 385 insertion in the hypervariable region 1 of hepatitis C virus E2 envelope protein is found in some patients with mixed cryoglobulinemia type 2. Blood 98:2657–2663

Gorevic PD, Frangione B (1991) Mixed cryoglobulinemia cross-reactive idiotypes: implications for the relationship of MC to rheumatic and lymphoproliferative diseases. Semin Hematol 28:79–94

Gorevic PD, Kassab HJ, Levo Y, Kohn R, Meltzer M, Prose P, Franklin EC (1980) Mixed cryoglobulinemia: clinical aspects and long-term follow-up of 40 patients. Am J Med 69:287–308

Invernizzi F, Pioltelli P, Cattaneo R, Gavazzeni V, Borzini P, Monti G, Zanussi C (1979) A long-term follow-up study in essential cryoglobulinemia. Acta Haematol 61:93–99

Invernizzi F, Galli M, Serino G, Monti G, Meroni PL, Granatieri C, Zanussi C (1983) Secondary and essential cryoglobulinemias: frequency, nosological classification, and long-term follow-up. Acta Haematol 70:73–82

Invernizzi F, Pietrogrande M, Sagramoso B (1995) Classification of the cryoglobulinemic syndrome. Clin Exp Rheumatol 13 Suppl 13: S123–S128

Ivanovski M, Silvestri F, Pozzato G, Anand S, Mazzaro C, Burrone OR, Efremov DG (1998) Somatic hypermutation, clonal diversity, and preferential expression of the VH 51p1/VL kv325 immunoglobulin gene combination in hepatitis C virus-associated immunocytomas. Blood 91:2433–2442

Izumi T, Sasaki R, Tsunoda S, Akutsu M, Okamoto H, Miura Y (1997) B cell malignancy and hepatitis C virus infection. Leukemia 11 Suppl 3:516–518

King PD, Wilkes JD, Diaz-Arias AA (1998) Hepatitis C virus infection in non-Hodgkin's lymphoma. Clin Lab Haematol 20:107–110

Kitay-Cohen Y, Amiel A, Hilzenrat N, Buskila D, Ashur Y, Fejgin M, Gaber E, Safadi R, Tur-Kaspa R, Lishner M (2000) Bcl-2 rearrangement in patients with chronic hepatitis C associated with essential mixed cryoglobulinemia type II. Blood 96:2910–2912

Lamprecht P, Moosig F, Gause A, Herlyn K, Gross WL (2000) Birmingham vasculitis activity score, disease extent index and complement factor C3c reflect disease activity best in hepatitis C virus-associated cryoglobulinemic vasculitis. Clin Exp Rheumatol 18:319–325

Lauta VM, De Sangro MA (1995) Long-term results regarding the use of recombinant interferon alpha-2b in the treatment of II type mixed essential cryoglobulinemia. Med Oncol 12:223–230

Lerner AB, Watson CJ (1947) Studies of cryoglobulins; unusual purpura associated with presence of high concentration of cryoglobulin (cold precipitable serum globulin). Am J Med Sci 214:410–415

Lunel F, Musset L, Cacoub P, Frangeul L, Cresta P, Perrin M, Grippon P, Hoang C, Valla D, Piette JC, Huraux J-M, Opolon P (1994) Cryoglobulinemia in chronic liver diseases: role of hepatitis C virus and liver damage. Gastroenterology 106:1291–1300

Luppi M, Longo G, Ferrari MG, Barozzi P, Marasca R, Morselli M, Valenti C, Mascia T, Vandelli L, Vallisa D, Cavanna L, Torelli G (1998) Clinicopathological characterization of hepatitis C virus-related B-cell non-Hodgkin's lymphomas without symptomatic cryoglobulinemia. Ann Oncol 9:495–498

Magalini AR, Facchetti F, Salvi L, Fontana L, Puoti M, Scarpa A (1998) Clonality of B-cells in portal lymphoid infiltrates of HCV-infected livers. J Pathol 185:86–90

Mazzaro C, Lacchin T, Moretti M, Tulissi P, Manazzone O, Colle R, Pozzato G (1995) Effects of two different alpha-interferon regimens on clinical and virological findings in mixed cryoglobulinemia. Clin Exp Rheumatol 13 Suppl 13:S181–S185

Mazzaro C, Franzin F, Tulissi P, Pussini E, Crovatto M, Carniello GS, Efremov DG, Burrone O, Santini G, Pozzato G (1996) Regression of monoclonal B-cell expansion in patients affected by mixed cryoglobulinemia responsive to alpha-interferon therapy. Cancer 77:2604–2613

McColl MD, Singer IO, Tait RC, McNeil IR, Cumming RL, Hogg RB (1997) The role of hepatitis C virus in the aetiology of non-Hodgkin's lymphoma: a regional association? Leuk Lymphoma 26:127–130

Meltzer M, Franklin EC (1966) Cryoglobulinemia: a study of twenty-nine patients. I. IgG and IgM cryoglobulins and factors affecting cryoprecipitability. Am J Med 40:828–836

Migliaresi S, Tirri G (1995) Interferon in the treatment of mixed cryoglobulinemia. Clin Exp Rheumatol 13 Suppl 13:S175–S180

Misiani R, Bellavita P, Fenili D, Borelli G, Marchesi D, Massazza M, Vendramin G, Comotti B, Tanzi E, Scudeller G, Zanetti A (1992) Hepatitis C virus infection in patients with essential mixed cryoglobulinemia. Ann Intern Med 117:573–577

Misiani R, Bellavita P, Fenili D, Vicari O, Marchesi D, Sironi PL, Zilio P, Vernocchi A, Massazza M, Vendramin G, Tanzi E, Zanetti A (1994) Interferon alfa-2a therapy in cryoglobulinemia associated with hepatitis C virus. N Engl J Med 330:751–756

Monteverde A, Ballare M, Bertoncelli MC, Zigrossi P, Sabattini E, Poggi S, Pileri S (1995) Lymphoproliferation in type II mixed cryoglobulinemia. Clin Exp Rheumatol 13 Suppl 13:S141–S147

Monteverde A, Ballare M, Pileri S (1997) Hepatic lymphoid aggregates in chronic hepatitis C and mixed cryoglobulinemia. Springer Semin Immunopathol 19:99–110

Monti G, Galli M, Invernizzi F, Pioltelli P, Saccardo F, Monteverde A, Pietrogrande M, Renoldi P, Bombardieri S, Bordin G, Candela M, Ferri C, Gabrielli A, Mazzaro C, Migliaresi S, Mussini C, Ossi E, Quintiliani L, Tirri G, Vacca A, Italian Group for the Study of Cryoglobulinemias (GISC) (1995a) Cryoglobulinaemias: a multi-centre study of the early clinical and laboratory manifestations of primary and secondary disease. GISC. Italian Group for the Study of Cryoglobulinaemias. QJM 88:115–126

Monti G, Saccardo F, Pioltelli P, Rinaldi G (1995b) The natural history of cryoglobulinemia: symptoms at onset and during follow-up. A report by the Italian Group for the Study of Cryoglobulinemias (GISC). Clin Exp Rheumatol 13 Suppl 13:S129–S133

Mussini C, Mascia MT, Zanni G, Curci G, Bonacorsi G, Artusi T (1991) A cytomorphological and immunohistochemical study of bone marrow in the diagnosis of essential mixed type II cryoglobulinemia. Haematologica 76:389–391

Origgi L, Vanoli M, Lunghi G, Carbone A, Grasso M, Scorza R (1998) Hepatitis C virus genotypes and clinical features in hepatitis C virus-related mixed cryoglobulinemia. Int J Clin Lab Res 28:96–99

Pozzato G, Mazzaro C, Crovatto M, Modolo ML, Ceselli S, Mazzi G, Sulfaro S, Franzin F, Tulissi P, Moretti M, Santini GF (1994) Low-grade malignant lymphoma, hepatitis C virus infection, and mixed cryoglobulinemia. Blood 84:3047–3053

Ramos-Casals M, Cervera R, Yague J, Garcia-Carrasco M, Trejo O, Jimenez S, Morla RM, Font J, Ingelmo M (1998) Cryoglobulinemia in primary Sjögren's syndrome: prevalence and clinical characteristics in a series of 115 patients. Semin Arthritis Rheum 28:200–205

Ramos-Casals M, Garcia-Carrasco M, Cervera R, Rosas J, Trejo O, de la Red G, Sanchez-Tapias JM, Font J, Ingelmo M (2001) Hepatitis C virus infection mimicking primary Sjögren syndrome: a clinical and immunologic description of 35 cases. Medicine (Baltimore) 80:1–8

Rasul I, Shepherd FA, Kamel-Reid S, Krajden M, Pantalony D, Heathcote EJ (1999) Detection of occult low-grade B-cell non-Hodgkin's lymphoma in patients with chronic hepatitis C infection and mixed cryoglobulinemia. Hepatology 29:543–547

Rieu V, Cohen P, Andre MH, Mouthon L, Godmer P, Jarrousse B, Lhote F, Ferriere F, Deny P, Buchet P, Guillevin L (2002) Characteristics and outcome of 49 patients with symptomatic cryoglobulinaemia. Rheumatology (Oxford) 41:290–300

Sansonno D, De Vita S, Iacobelli AR, Cornacchiulo V, Boiocchi M, Dammacco F (1998) Clonal analysis of intrahepatic B cells from HCV-infected patients with and without mixed cryoglobulinemia. J Immunol 160:3594–3601

Sasso EH, Ghillani P, Musset L, Piette JC, Cacoub P (2001) Effect of 51p1-related gene copy number (V1-69 locus) on production of hepatitis C-associated cryoglobulins. Clin Exp Immunol 123:88–93

Shokri F, Mageed RA, Kitas GD, Katsikis P, Moutsopoulos HM, Jefferis R (1991) Quantification of cross-reactive idiotype-positive rheumatoid factor produced in autoimmune rheumatic diseases: an indicator of clonality and B cell proliferative mechanisms. Clin Exp Immunol 85:20–27

Silvestri F, Barillari G, Fanin R, Zaja F, Infanti L, Patriarca F, Baccarani M, Pipan C, Falasca E, Botta GA (1996) Risk of hepatitis C virus infection, Waldenström's macroglobulinemia, and monoclonal gammopathies. Blood 88:1125–1126

Singer DR, Venning MC, Lockwood CM, Pusey CD (1986) Cryoglobulinaemia: clinical features and response to treatment. Ann Med Interne (Paris) 137:251–253

Tarantino A, De Vecchi A, Montagnino G, Imbasciati E, Mihatsch MJ, Zollinger HU, Di Belgiojoso GB, Busnach G, Ponticelli C (1981) Renal disease in essential mixed cryoglobulinaemia. Long-term follow-up of 44 patients. Q J Med 50:1–30

Tarantino A, Campise M, Banfi G, Confalonieri R, Bucci A, Montoli A, Colasanti G, Damilano I, D'Amico G, Minetti L, Ponticelli C (1995) Long-term predictors of survival in essential mixed cryoglobulinemic glomerulonephritis. Kidney Int 47:618–623

Trejo O, Ramos-Casals M, Garcia-Carrasco M, Yague J, Jimenez S, de la Red G, Cervera R, Font J, Ingelmo M (2001) Cryoglobulinemia: study of etiologic factors and clinical and immunologic features in 443 patients from a single center. Medicine (Baltimore) 80:252–262

Ubara Y, Hara S, Katori H, Tagami T, Kitamura A, Yokota M, Matsushita Y, Takemoto F, Yamada A, Nagahama K, Hara M, Chayama K (2000) Splenectomy may improve the glomerulopathy of type II mixed cryoglobulinemia. Am J Kidney Dis 35:1186–1192

Wintrobe M, Buell MV (1933) Hyperproteinemia associated with multiple myeloma with report of case in which extraordinary hyperproteinemia was associated with thrombosis of retinal veins and symptoms suggesting Raynaud's disease. Bull Johns Hopkins Hosp 52:156–165

Yoshikawa M, Imazu H, Ueda S, Tamagawa T, Yoneda S, Yamane Y, Takaya A, Fukui H, Nakano H (1997) Prevalence of hepatitis C virus infection in patients with non-Hodgkin's lymphoma and multiple myeloma. A report from Japan. J Clin Gastroenterol 25:713–714

Zignego AL, Ferri C, Giannini C, La Civita L, Careccia G, Longombardo G, Bellesi G, Caracciolo F, Thiers V, Gentilini P (1997) Hepatitis C virus infection in mixed cryoglobulinemia and B-cell non-Hodgkin's lymphoma: evidence for a pathogenetic role. Arch Virol 142: 545–555

Zignego AL, Giannelli F, Marrocchi ME, Mazzocca A, Ferri C, Giannini C, Monti M, Caini P, Villa GL, Laffi G, Gentilini P (2000) t(14;18) translocation in chronic hepatitis C virus infection. Hepatology 31:474–479

Zuckerman E, Zuckerman T, Levine AM, Douer D, Gutekunst K, Mizokami M, Qian DG, Velankar M, Nathwani BN, Fong TL (1997) Hepatitis C virus infection in patients with B-cell non-Hodgkin lymphoma. Ann Intern Med 127:423–428

Zuckerman E, Keren D, Slobodin G, Rosner I, Rozenbaum M, Toubi E, Sabo E, Tsykounov I, Naschitz JE, Yeshurun D (2000) Treatment of refractory, symptomatic, hepatitis C virus related mixed cryoglobulinemia with ribavirin and interferon-alpha. J Rheumatol 27:2172–2178

Acquired Fanconi Syndrome Associated With Monoclonal Plasma Cell Disorders

Martha Q. Lacy, M.D., Morie A. Gertz, M.D.

Contents

11.1 Introduction 257

11.2 Epidemiology 257

11.3 Screening and Prevention 258

11.4 Molecular Biology and Genetics 258

11.5 Clinical Presentation 259

11.6 Classification and Staging 259

11.7 Diagnosis 260

    11.7.1 Electrolyte
and Renal Abnormalities 260

    11.7.2 Predominance of Kappa Light
Chains 260

    11.7.3 Bone Findings 261

    11.7.4 Pathologic Findings 261

11.8 Differential Diagnosis 261

11.9 Second Malignancies 261

11.10 Therapy 261

11.11 Prognosis 262

11.12 Quality of Life and Rehabilitation . . . 262

11.13 Emergencies 262

References 262

Supported in part by National Institutes of Health grant CA 62242.

11.1 Introduction

The renal Fanconi syndrome consists of a generalized dysfunction of the proximal renal tubule, with impaired proximal reabsorption of protein, amino acids, glucose, phosphate, urate, and bicarbonate. Fanconi syndrome may be inherited or acquired. Examples of inherited renal Fanconi syndromes include Dent disease, oculocerebrorenal syndrome of Lowe, autosomal dominant idiopathic Fanconi syndrome, cystinosis, tyrosinemia, galactosemia, fructosemia, Fanconi-Bickel syndrome, mitochondrial disorders, Wilson disease, and X-linked hypophosphatemic rickets. Acquired Fanconi syndrome may be associated with interstitial nephritis, toxicity of certain drugs or heavy metals, Sjögren syndrome, toxic nephropathy, Refsum disease, or monoclonal plasma cell disorders. This article reviews Fanconi syndrome associated with monoclonal gammopathies.

11.2 Epidemiology

A monoclonal gammopathy of undetermined significance (MGUS) occurs in up to 2% of persons age 50 years or older (Kyle et al. 2002). Fanconi syndrome is a rare complication of MGUS. Fanconi syndrome is associated with monoclonal kappa light chains in the urine. Overt hematologic malignancies such as multiple myeloma, Waldenström macroglobulinemia, or other lymphoproliferative disorders occur in one-third of patients.

11.3   Screening and Prevention

Fanconi syndrome is an exceedingly rare complication of MGUS, and screening for it cannot be recommended routinely. Instead, clinicians should be aware of the entity and initiate appropriate diagnostic testing if a patient with MGUS presents with slowly progressive renal failure, electrolyte abnormalities, or bone pain.

11.4   Molecular Biology and Genetics

The critical role of the proximal renal tubule in the catabolism of light chains was shown in a rat model (Clyne et al. 1974). Investigators were able to induce proximal tubular lesions in rats by the intraperitoneal injection of human κ-type Bence Jones proteins. They found that approximately 80% of injected κ chains were reabsorbed by the proximal tubular cells, where they formed crystal-like structures with phagolysosomes.

In an elegant series of investigations, Aucouturier et al. (Aucouturier et al. 1993; Leboulleux et al. 1995; Rocca et al. 1995) showed that light chain toxicity in Fanconi syndrome is related to the resistance of the V domain to degradation in lysosomes of the proximal tubular epithelial cells. Initially, they investigated light chains from 1 patient with Fanconi syndrome (Aucouturier et al. 1993). The sequence of the patient's monoclonal κ chain was determined by cloning the κ cDNA sequences from bone marrow plasma cells. Analysis of tubular crystals by N-terminal sequencing and mass spectrometry showed the crystals were composed primarily of the V domain of the κ light chain together with a small proportion of the entire light chain, suggesting posttranscriptional degradation in the lysosomes. Protease treatment of the κ light chain yielded a fragment of the V domain that, in contrast to other κ light chains, was completely resistant to further proteolytic degradation. In addition, the patient's light chain displayed an unusual self-avidity.

These studies prompted further investigations by the same group. They studied light chains from 4 patients with Fanconi syndrome, 12 patients with cast nephropathy, and 4 control patients (Leboulleux et al. 1995). All the light chains from patients with Fanconi syndrome were of the κ type. Kinetic studies of light chain digestion by pepsin and cathepsin B showed generation of a protease-resistant 12-kDa fragment corresponding to the V domain of the light chain (Fig. 11.1). In contrast, digestion studies of the light

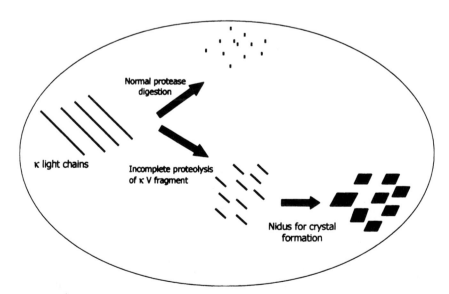

Fig. 11.1. Kappa light chains are endocytosed by lysosomes. Under normal conditions, they are completely degraded by proteases including pepsin and cathepsin D. In patients with Fanconi syndrome, protease-resistant 12-kDa fragments corresponding to the V domain are generated. These fragments avidly bind to other light chains and serve as a nidus for crystal formation. (From Lacy MQ, Gertz MA [1999] Acquired Fanconi's syndrome associated with monoclonal gammopathies. Hematol Oncol Clin North Am 13:1273–1280. By permission of Elsevier.)

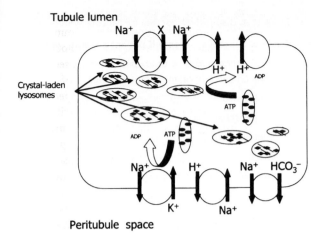

Tubule lumen

Peritubule space

Fig. 11.2. Crystal-laden lysosomes interfere with a broad range of apical membrane transporters. *ADP*, adenosine diphosphate; *ATP*, adenosine triphosphate. (From Lacy MQ, Gertz MA [1999] Acquired Fanconi's syndrome associated with monoclonal gammopathies. Hematol Oncol Clin North Am 13:1273–1280. By permission of Elsevier.)

chains obtained from patients with cast nephropathy had a variable pattern of protease resistance. All the light chains from myeloma patients without cast nephropathies were completely digestible. In addition, light chains from patients with Fanconi syndrome showed avidity for light chains but no reactivity with Tamm-Horsfall protein. The majority of the light chains from cast nephropathy patients bound to Tamm-Horsfall protein. Finally, the group demonstrated a preponderance of sequences of the VκI subgroup among patients with Fanconi syndrome (Rocca et al. 1995).

These studies suggest that complete proteolysis of the κ light chain cannot occur in vivo after endocytosis by the proximal tubule cells. This results in accumulation of the V fragment in the lysosomal compartment of the cells (Fig. 11.2). Reactivity with light chains from normal polyclonal IgG, which is continuously filtered by the glomerulus and reabsorbed in the proximal tubules, may serve as a nidus for crystal formation. The crystals interfere with a broad range of apical membrane transporters, including the Na-H exchangers and Na-linked exporters for glucose, phosphate, urate, and amino acids (Eiam-Ong et al. 1995; Leboulleux et al. 1995).

Decourt and colleagues (1999) designed an in vivo model in which murine hybridoma cell clones producing human Ig light chains were administered to mice. Depending on which monoclonal light chain was expressed, this model mimicked either myeloma cast ne-

phropathy or myeloma-associated Fanconi syndrome with light chain crystallization. They further showed that limited changes introduced through site-directed mutagenesis in the variable domain suppressed formation of intracellular crystals within tubular cells and that multiple peculiarities of the variable region were simultaneously needed to allow light chain crystallization. Their data suggest that specific somatic mutations of VκI genes are involved in nephrotoxicity and that subgroup-specific germline sequences are not sufficient to confer toxicity.

11.5 Clinical Presentation

Patients with Fanconi syndrome most often seek medical attention for back or bone pain, fatigue, or myalgias (Maldonado et al. 1975; Messiaen et al. 2000; Minemura et al. 2001; Rompala et al. 1998). Proximal muscle weakness is not uncommon. Symptoms frequently are confused with myeloma bone pain. Many patients with Fanconi syndrome are asymptomatic, and the finding of glycosuria, proteinuria, electrolyte abnormalities, or renal insufficiency triggers the work-up (Lajoie et al. 2000).

The primary cause of osteomalacia in Fanconi syndrome is proximal renal tubular phosphate wasting (Bergeron and Scriver 1992). The degree of osteomalacia correlates with the duration and severity of the hypophosphatemia (Bell 1990). However, osteomalacia may develop despite normal serum phosphorus values because these patients invariably have high fractional excretion of phosphorus (Clarke et al. 1995). This can eventually lead to secondary hyperparathyroidism. Parathyroid hormone concentrations were increased in 2 of 9 Fanconi syndrome patients with osteomalacia (Clarke et al. 1995). Low values of 1,25-dihydroxyvitamin D may be seen and are presumed to be due to low serum phosphorus, which is a potent stimulus of renal 1α-hydroxylase. Chronic acidosis is seen often in Fanconi syndrome and may contribute to the osteomalacia by decreasing conversion of amorphous calcium phosphate to hydroxyapatite (Bell 1990).

11.6 Classification and Staging

There is no universally accepted classification or staging system for Fanconi syndrome associated with monoclonal gammopathies. Fanconi syndrome may be found in association with overt hematologic malignant disease or with indolent processes such as MGUS or idiopathic Bence Jones proteinuria (IBJP). The most frequently associated malignancy is multiple myeloma (Bell 1990; Bergeron and Scriver 1992; Chan et al. 1987; Clarke et al. 1995; Costanza and Smoller 1963; Decourt et al. 1999; Dedmon et al. 1963; Dragsted and Hjorth 1956; Engle and Wallis 1957; Gailani et al. 1978; Harrison and Blainey 1967; Headley et al. 1972; Horn et al. 1969; Isobe et al. 1998; Leboulleux et al. 1995; Maldonado et al. 1975; Minemura et al. 2001; Orfila et al. 1991; Rao et al. 1987; Rompala et al. 1998; Sewell and Dorreen 1984; Short and Smith 1959; Sirota and Hamerman 1954; Truong et al. 1989; Uchida et al. 1990; von Scheele 1976; Yonemura et al. 1997). Fanconi syndrome has also been associated with primary amyloidosis (Finkel et al. 1973; Short and Smith 1959), Waldenström macroglobulinemia (Rompala et al. 1998), and chronic lymphocytic leukemia (Rao et al. 1987). Like MGUS and IBJP, Fanconi syndrome may predate a malignant diagnosis by many years. One report described Fanconi syndrome present for 16.5 years before the development of overt myeloma (Maldonado et al. 1975). In our experience at Mayo Clinic, only one-third of patients present with a malignant disease at the time Fanconi syndrome is diagnosed (Rompala et al. 1998). Only 1 patient in our series who did not have myeloma at diagnosis of Fanconi syndrome went on to develop overt myeloma 37 months later.

Table 11.1. Diagnostic algorithm for Fanconi syndrome

Consider Fanconi syndrome if patient presents with

Monoclonal gammopathy or idiopathic Bence Jones proteinuria (κ) and 1 or more of the following:

  Hypokalemia

  Hypophosphatemia

  Hypouricemia

  Renal insufficiency

  Bone pain due to osteomalacia

Confirm the diagnosis with

  Increased urine amino acids

  Glycosuria

  Phosphaturia

If clinically indicated, also consider

Kidney biopsy demonstrating crystal deposition

Bone marrow biopsy

  To demonstrate clonal plasma cells and crystal deposition

  To exclude coexisting malignancy

Treatment options

Phosphorus supplements ± calcitriol

Consider chemotherapy if:

  Symptomatic malignancy

  or

Progressive renal failure

11.7 Diagnosis

The diagnosis of Fanconi syndrome can be made when a patient with a monoclonal plasma cell disorder presents with aminoaciduria or with phosphaturia and glycosuria (Table 11.1).

11.7.1 Electrolyte and Renal Abnormalities

Mild and slowly progressive renal insufficiency is seen often in Fanconi syndrome (Maldonado et al. 1975; Messiaen et al. 2000; Rompala et al. 1998). Renal failure may stabilize or improve with chemotherapy (Gailani et al. 1978; Uchida et al. 1990; von Scheele 1976). Electrolyte abnormalities typically include hypokalemia, hypophosphatemia, and hypouricemia. The diagnosis is confirmed by the demonstration of aminoaciduria and

glycosuria. The renal dysfunction is a constellation of proximal tubule transport defects that results in broad failure of tubule reabsorption. The kaliuresis is not a direct effect but rather a consequence of the delivery of large amounts of bicarbonate past the distal nephron in conditions that favor aldosterone secretion (Eiam-Ong et al. 1995).

11.7.2 Predominance of Kappa Light Chains

Bence Jones proteinuria usually is present and is almost always of the κ type (Maldonado et al. 1975; Messiaen et al. 2000; Rompala et al. 1998). Rare patients have been reported with Fanconi syndrome associated with λ Bence Jones proteinuria (Isobe et al. 1998; Thorner et al. 1983). We observed that 22 of 23 patients (96%) with Fanconi syndrome had κ-type Bence Jones proteinuria

(Rompala et al. 1998), and a monoclonal protein was found in the serum in 60% of patients. Messiaen and colleagues (2000) studied the clinical, pathologic, and molecular features of light chain-associated Fanconi syndrome in a series of 11 consecutive patients. Ten patients had monoclonal κ light chains in the urine. The remaining patient had a monoclonal IgA κ light chain in the serum. Light chains from 9 patients were sequenced. All but 1 were in the VκI subgroup.

11.7.3 Bone Findings

Osteomalacia, with or without 1,25-dihydroxyvitamin D deficiency, has been seen in patients with acquired Fanconi syndrome and is a result of prolonged hypophosphatemia (Clarke et al. 1995; Lee et al. 1972; Rao et al. 1987). Radiographs are often normal but may show demineralization, fractures, or pseudofractures (Clarke et al. 1995; Maldonado et al. 1975). Lytic lesions suggest fully developed multiple myeloma. When radiographs are normal, the presence of osteomalacia may be suggested by an increased serum alkaline phosphatase concentration (Clarke et al. 1995; Maldonado et al. 1975; Rao et al. 1987).

11.7.4 Pathologic Findings

Kidney biopsy specimens viewed by light microscopy may reveal cytoplasmic crystals in proximal tubule cells (Costanza and Smoller 1963; Engle and Wallis 1957; Gardais et al. 2001; Messiaen et al. 2000; Orfila et al. 1991; Truong et al. 1989) or tubulointerstitial nephritis without glomerular lesions. Immunofluorescence studies have shown that the crystals stain strongly for monoclonal light chain. These findings have been confirmed by electron microscopy and immunoelectron microscopic techniques (Orfila et al. 1991; Truong et al. 1989). Similar cytoplasmic crystalline inclusions are seen in bone marrow plasma cells and macrophages (Costanza and Smoller 1963; Maldonado et al. 1975; Sewell and Dorreen 1984). Messiaen and colleagues (2000) noted severe abnormalities of the proximal tubule epithelium in all biopsy specimens. Crystals were observed in 8 of the 11 specimens.

11.8 Differential Diagnosis

Renal dysfunction frequently is associated with monoclonal gammopathies. Fanconi syndrome is characterized by crystalline cytoplasmic inclusions in the plasma cells of the bone marrow and the renal tubular cells (Maldonado et al. 1975). This is in contrast to multiple myeloma, which often causes renal failure via myeloma cast nephropathy or hypercalcemia. Myeloma casts are large, dense, and waxy and found in the distal and collecting tubules. They are composed of monoclonal light chains with small amounts of albumin and Tamm-Horsfall protein (Kyle 1994). Nephrotic syndrome is the most common renal manifestation of primary systemic amyloidosis. Amyloid deposition is found in mesangial or glomerular basement membranes (Kyle 1994). Light chain deposition disease is characterized by deposition of monoclonal light chains in the renal glomerulus, leading to renal insufficiency and nephrotic syndrome (Kyle 1994).

11.9 Second Malignancies

It is important to avoid prematurely exposing patients to chemotherapy, except in the setting of severe progressive renal dysfunction or overt malignant disease. In 1 series (Rompala et al. 1998), chemotherapy caused significant mortality. Among the 21 patients who received chemotherapy, 4 patients (19%) developed secondary myelodysplastic syndrome or acute leukemia during follow-up. All 4 patients died of complications.

11.10 Therapy

Fanconi syndrome is an indolent disorder among patients without overt multiple myeloma. Complications such as renal insufficiency develop gradually, and patients rarely die of the disease. In the asymptomatic patient, it is appropriate to withhold potentially toxic chemotherapy. In the setting of progressive renal dysfunction or symptomatic malignant disease, chemotherapy such as melphalan and prednisone may be of benefit (Gailani et al. 1978; Uchida et al. 1990; von Scheele 1976).

Treatment with phosphorus, calcium, and calcitriol may improve bone pain and ameliorate osteomalacia. In the absence of overt myeloma, bone pain may be dramatically relieved by treatment with phosphorus, with or without calcitriol. Complete reversal of the osteomalacia has been demonstrated by repeat bone biopsies after treatment with phosphorus (Rao et al. 1987). Noninvasive methods of assessing treatment efficacy include following serum alkaline phosphatase and phosphate concentrations and 24-hour urine calcium excretion.

11.11   Prognosis

Overt hematologic malignancies such as multiple myeloma, Waldenström macroglobulinemia, or other lymphoproliferative disorders occur in one-third of patients (Messiaen et al. 2000; Rompala et al. 1998). Patients with an associated symptomatic malignancy or rapidly progressive renal failure may benefit from chemotherapy. The prognosis is good in the absence of overt malignant disease.

11.12 Quality of Life and Rehabilitation

Clinical manifestations include slowly progressive renal failure and bone pain due to osteomalacia. The osteomalacia is caused by chronic hypophosphatemia and may be exacerbated by secondary hyperparathyroidism and renal tubular acidosis. Treatment consists of supplementation with phosphorus, calcium, and vitamin D. The osteomalacia is often completely reversible with mineral supplementation.

11.13 Emergencies

Fanconi syndrome is an indolent disorder and is rarely if ever associated with emergencies. On rare occasions, it may be associated with critically low electrolyte concentrations such as hypokalemia, hypophosphatemia, or hypocalcemia. In such situations, intravenous replacement of blood electrolytes is warranted.

References

Aucouturier P, Bauwens M, Khamlichi AA, Denoroy L, Spinelli S, Touchard G, Preud'homme JL, Cogne M (1993) Monoclonal Ig L chain and L chain V domain fragment crystallization in myeloma-associated Fanconi's syndrome. J Immunol 150:3561–3568

Bell NH (1990) Osteomalacia and rickets. In: Becker KL (ed) Principles and practice of endocrinology and metabolism. JB Lippincott Company, Philadelphia, pp 484–490

Bergeron M, Scriver CR (1992) Pathophysiology of renal hyperaminoacidurias and glucosuria. In: Seldin DW, Giebisch G (eds) The kidney: physiology and pathophysiology, 2nd edn, vol 3. Raven Press, New York, pp 2947–2969

Chan KW, Ho FC, Chan MK (1987) Adult Fanconi syndrome in κ light chain myeloma. Arch Pathol Lab Med 111:139–142

Clarke BL, Wynne AG, Wilson DM, Fitzpatrick LA (1995) Osteomalacia associated with adult Fanconi's syndrome: clinical and diagnostic features. Clin Endocrinol (Oxf) 43:479–490

Clyne DH, Brendstrup L, First MR, Pesce AJ, Finkel PN, Pollak VE, Pirani CL (1974) Renal effects of intraperitoneal κ chain injection: induction of crystals in renal tubular cells. Lab Invest 31:131–142

Costanza DJ, Smoller M (1963) Multiple myeloma with the Fanconi syndrome. Am J Med 34:125–133

Decourt C, Rocca A, Bridoux F, Vrtovsnik F, Preud'homme JL, Cogne M, Touchard G (1999) Mutational analysis in murine models for myeloma-associated Fanconi's syndrome or cast myeloma nephropathy. Blood 94:3559–3566

Dedmon RE, West JH, Schwartz TB (1963) The adult Fanconi syndrome: report of two cases, one with multiple myeloma. Med Clin N Am 47:191–206

Dragsted PJ, Hjorth N (1956) The association of the Fanconi syndrome with malignant disease. Danish Med Bull 3:177–179

Eiam-Ong S, Laski ME, Kurtzman NA (1995) Diseases of renal adenosine triphosphatase. Am J Med Sci 309:13–25

Engle RLJ, Wallis LA (1957) Multiple myeloma and the adult Fanconi syndrome. I. Report of a case with crystal-like deposits in the tumor cells and in the epithelial cells of the kidney. Am J Med 22:5–23

Finkel PN, Kronenberg K, Pesce AJ, Pollak VE, Pirani CL (1973) Adult Fanconi syndrome, amyloidosis and marked κ-light chain proteinuria. Nephron 10:1–24

Gailani S, Seon BK, Henderson ES (1978) Kappa light chain-myeloma associated with adult Fanconi syndrome: response of the nephropathy to treatment of myeloma. Med Pediatr Oncol 4:141–147

Gardais J, Genevieve F, Foussard C, Delisle V, Zandecki M (2001) Is there any significance for intracellular crystals in plasma cells from patients with monoclonal gammopathies? Eur J Haematol 67:119–122

Harrison JF, Blainey JD (1967) Adult Fanconi syndrome with monoclonal abnormality of immunoglobulin light chain. J Clin Pathol 20:42–48

Headley RN, King JS Jr, Cooper MR, Felts JH (1972) Multiple myeloma presenting as adult Fanconi syndrome. Clin Chem 18:293–295

Horn ME, Knapp MS, Page FT, Walker WH (1969) Adult Fanconi syndrome and multiple myelomatosis. J Clin Pathol 22:414–416

Isobe T, Kametani F, Shinoda T (1998) V-domain deposition of λ Bence Jones protein in the renal tubular epithelial cells in a patient with the adult Fanconi syndrome with myeloma. Amyloid 5:117–120

Kyle RA (1994) Monoclonal proteins and renal disease. Annu Rev Med 45:71–77

Kyle RA, Therneau TM, Rajkumar SV, Offord JR, Larson DR, Plevak MF, Melton LJ III (2002) A long-term study of prognosis in monoclonal gammopathy of undetermined significance. N Engl J Med 346:564–569

Lajoie G, Leung R, Bargman JM (2000) Clinical, biochemical, and pathological features in a patient with plasma cell dyscrasia and Fanconi syndrome. Ultrastruct Pathol 24:221–226

Leboulleux M, Lelongt B, Mougenot B, Touchard G, Makdassi R, Rocca A, Noel LH, Ronco PM, Aucouturier P (1995) Protease resistance and binding of Ig light chains in myeloma-associated tubulopathies. Kidney Int 48:72–79

Lee DB, Drinkard JP, Rosen VJ, Gonick HC (1972) The adult Fanconi syndrome: observations on etiology, morphology, renal function and mineral metabolism in three patients. Medicine (Baltimore) 51:107–138

Maldonado JE, Velosa JA, Kyle RA, Wagoner RD, Holley KE, Salassa RM (1975) Fanconi syndrome in adults: a manifestation of a latent form of myeloma. Am J Med 58:354–364

Messiaen T, Deret S, Mougenot B, Bridoux F, Dequiedt P, Dion JJ, Makdassi R, Meeus F, Pourrat J, Touchard G, Vanhille P, Zaoui P, Aucouturier P, Ronco PM (2000) Adult Fanconi syndrome secondary to light chain gammopathy: clinicopathologic heterogeneity and unusual features in 11 patients. Medicine (Baltimore) 79:135–154

Minemura K, Ichikawa K, Itoh N, Suzuki N, Hara M, Shigematsu S, Kobayashi H, Hiramatsu K, Hashizume K (2001) IgA-κ type multiple myeloma affecting proximal and distal renal tubules. Intern Med 40:931–935

Orfila C, Lepert JC, Modesto A, Bernadet P, Suc JM (1991) Fanconi's syndrome, κ light-chain myeloma, non-amyloid fibrils and cytoplasmic crystals in renal tubular epithelium. Am J Nephrol 11:345–349

Rao DS, Parfitt AM, Villanueva AR, Dorman PJ, Kleerekoper M (1987) Hypophosphatemic osteomalacia and adult Fanconi syndrome due to light-chain nephropathy: another form of oncogenous osteomalacia. Am J Med 82:333–338

Rocca A, Khamlichi AA, Touchard G, Mougenot B, Ronco P, Denoroy L, Deret S, Preud'homme JL, Aucouturier P, Cogne M (1995) Sequences of VκL subgroup light chains in Fanconi's syndrome: light chain V region gene usage restriction and peculiarities in myeloma-associated Fanconi's syndrome. J Immunol 155:3245–3252

Rompala JF, Lacy MQ, Rajkumar SV, Greipp PR, Kyle RA, Gertz MA (1998) Acquired Fanconi's syndrome is an indolent disorder in the absence of overt multiple myeloma (abstract). Blood 92 Suppl 1:269b

Sewell RL, Dorreen MS (1984) Adult Fanconi syndrome progressing to multiple myeloma. J Clin Pathol 37:1256–1258

Short IA, Smith JP (1959) Myelomatosis associated with glycosuria and aminoaciduria. Scott Med J 4:89–93

Sirota JH, Hamerman D (1954) Renal function studies in an adult subject with the Fanconi syndrome. Am J Med 16:138–152

Thorner PS, Bedard YC, Fernandes BJ (1983) Lambda-light-chain nephropathy with Fanconi's syndrome. Arch Pathol Lab Med 107:654–657

Truong LD, Mawad J, Cagle P, Mattioli C (1989) Cytoplasmic crystals in multiple myeloma-associated Fanconi's syndrome: a morphological study including immunoelectron microscopy. Arch Pathol Lab Med 113:781–785

Uchida S, Matsuda O, Yokota T, Takemura T, Ando R, Kanemitsu H, Hamaguchi H, Miyake S, Marumo F (1990) Adult Fanconi syndrome secondary to κ-light chain myeloma: improvement of tubular functions after treatment for myeloma. Nephron 55:332–335

von Scheele C (1976) Light chain myeloma with features of the adult Fanconi syndrome: six years remission following one course of melphalan. Acta Med Scand 199:533–537

Yonemura K, Matsushima H, Kato A, Isozaki T, Hishida A (1997) Acquired Fanconi syndrome associated with IgG κ multiple myeloma: observations on the mechanisms of impaired renal acid excretion. Nephrol Dial Transplant 12:1251–1253

Subject Index

A

Acid phosphatase 101
Acute abdomen 144
Acute pulmonary edema 8
Acute renal failure 105
Adrenocorticotropic hormone 56
Adriamycin 83, 125, 215
AL (see Amyloidosis)
Albuminuria 69, 127, 160
Alcohol consumption 57
Alcoholic hepatitis 228
Alcoholism 36
Alkaline phosphatase 20, 169, 192, 198, 262
– concentration 174
Alkylating agent 48, 85, 215
Allergy-related disorders 57
Allogeneic stem cell transplantation 88
Allogeneic transplantation 126
Alopecia 138
a_2-globulin 3
a-HCD 135–143, 152
– age ratio 135
– incidence 134
– mortality 134
– sex ratio 134
– survivorship 135
a_2-plasmin inhibitor 178
Alzheimer disease 158
Amenorrhea 138
Amino acid 158
Aminoaciduria 69, 260
Amino terminal proteolysis 137
3-Aminothalidomide 126
Ampicillin 142
Amyloid cardiomyopathy 168, 171, 185
Amyloid fibril protein 158

Amyloid heart disease 180
Amyloid P 164, 165
Amyloid polyneuropathy 43
Amyloid purpura 161
Amyloidosis (AL) 2, 5–9, 20, 24, 45, 138, 157–159, 177, 210
– light chain 164
– urethral 167
Anemia 11, 60, 65, 112, 147, 152, 169, 222
– chemotherapy-induced 104
– hemolytic 211
Aneuploidy 120, 149, 160
Angiogenesis 77, 100
Angiography 175
Angioimmunoblastic lymphadeno-pathy 26
Angiotensin-converting enzyme inhibi-tor 129, 183
Anhidrosis 45
Ankylosing spondylitis 159, 167
Anorexia 175, 176
Anthracycline 76, 79, 94
Antiangiogenic agent 126
Antibiotic therapy 159
Antibody-antigen response 252
Anti-CD20
– antibody 95
– monoclonal antibody 143
Anticoagulation therapy 172
Antigen selection 121
Anti-HCV antibody 231
Anti-MAG antibody 38, 39, 45
Antiphospholipid antibody 26
Antistreptolysin O 30
Antithymocyte globulin 88
AP-1 58
Apolipoprotein A-I 168
Areflexia 41
Arrhythmias 198

Arterial thrombosis 179
Arthralgia 246, 249
Arthroplasty 167
Asbestosis 136
Ascites 138, 152
Asthenia 249
Autoantibody activity 231
Autoimmune cytopenia 147
Autoimmune hepatitis 228
Autoimmune illnesses 57
Autologous peripheral blood stem cell transplantation 188
Autologous stem cell transplantation 48, 84, 86, 87, 91
– for primary systemic amyloidosis 191, 192
Azathioprine 46, 48
Azotemia 127

B

Bacteremia 190
Bacterial endocarditis 228
BAD 59
Basophilic cytoplasm 99
B-cell chronic lymphocytic leukemia 213, 214, 232
B-cell lymphoma, follicular 213
B-cell lymphomatosis 44
B-cell lymphoproliferative disorder 136, 206, 211
B-cell malignancy 92
B-cell neoplasms 212
B-cell non-Hodgkin lymphoma 233, 244
Bcl-X_L 58
Bence Jones myeloma 60, 65
Bence Jones protein 4, 55, 70, 145, 158, 212, 258

Bence Jones proteinuria   13, 16–18, 23, 24, 69, 152, 163
β-globulin   140
β₂-microglobulin   86, 97, 98, 102, 120, 123, 185, 221, 222
Biclonal gammopathy   22
Bisphosphonates   103, 127
Blindness   221
Blood stem cells   78
Blood urea nitrogen   98
Bone biopsy   18, 117
Bone lesion   61
Bone marrow biopsy   21, 123, 165, 179, 200
Bone marrow damage   186
Bone marrow infiltration   104
Bone marrow labeling index   19
Bone marrow morphology   244
Bone marrow plasma cell   6, 14, 17–19, 98, 101, 102, 188, 258
– infiltration   96
– number   97
Bone marrow plasmacytosis   16, 67, 72, 199
Bone marrow transplantation   84, 88
Bone scanning   61
Bony metastases   103
Bowel obstruction   144
Bromodeoxyuridine   99
Bronchiectasis   167

C

Calcitonin   103
Calcitriol   261, 262
Calcium   261, 262
Calcium channel blocker   181
Captopril   251
Carcinoma of the colon   8, 30
Cardiac amyloidosis   160
Cardiac transplantation   182
Cardiomyopathy   162, 179, 198
– progressive infiltrative   170
Carmustine   77, 79, 80, 83, 125, 187, 215, 221
Carpal tunnel syndrome   40, 44, 162, 176
Castleman disease   26, 46, 69
Cathepsin D   258
CC-5013   95
CCT (combination chemotherapy)   79–82, 124
CD4   100
CD5   212
CD5 antigen   242
CD5⁺ B cell   232

CD9   123
CD10   64, 212, 213
CD11a   59
CD11b   122
CD16   101
CD19⁻   64, 116, 212
CD19⁺   116
CD19 expression   19
CD20   64, 68, 95, 122, 212
CD22   212
CD23   212
CD28   64, 122
CD30   243
CD34⁺   85, 86, 126, 129, 189
CD34 cell selection   188
CD38⁺   64, 116
CD38 expression   19
CD40   58
CD45   64
CD56   20, 59, 64, 101, 116, 122
CD81   234
CD117   123
CD138   64, 212
CDK (cyclin-dependent kinase)   59
CDK4   59
CDK4/CDK6   122
CDK6   59
Cell signaling   58
Cellular therapy   90
Cerebrospinal fluid   177
– examination   44
C_H1 151
C_H2 151
– domain   145
C_H3 151
– domain   145
CH50   243
Chemotherapy   86, 93, 124, 249
– adjuvant   115
– cytotoxic   185, 201
– systemic   201
Chlorambucil   46, 47, 213, 249
Chromosome 13   122
Chromosome 13q   19
Chromosome abnormality   19
Chronic active hepatitis   29
Chronic diarrhea   138
Chronic granulocytic leukemia   160
Chronic infected sinuses   159
Chronic inflammatory demyelinating poly-neuropathy (see CIDP)
Chronic inflammatory polyarthritis   159
Chronic Leukemia-Myeloma Task Force (see CLMTF)
Chronic lymphocytic leukemia   11, 12, 25, 148, 151, 260
Chronic myelocytic leukemia   27
Chronic myelogenous leukemia   92

Chronic osteomyelitis   159, 167
CIDP (chronic inflammatory demyelinating polyneuropathy)   44, 45, 47
Cigarette smoking   57
Circulating plasma cell   22
Cisapride   183
Cisplatin   77, 94, 95, 128
c-kit   64
Cladribine   218, 219
Clarithromycin   22
Clonal plasma cell disorder   159
CLMTF (Chronic Leukemia-Myeloma Task Force)   66, 71, 74
c-myc   59, 116, 121
Colchicine   184, 186, 250
– oral   167
Collagenous colitis   166
Combination chemotherapy (see CCT)
Congo red   158, 159, 165, 166, 172, 176, 198, 200
Connective tissue disorder   228, 230
Corticosteroid   27, 48, 56, 75, 78, 79, 90, 91, 93, 94, 103, 220, 246, 248, 249, 251
Cortisone   74
C-reactive protein (CRP)   97, 98, 102, 123, 164
Creatinine concentration   185
Crohn disease   167
Crow-Fukase syndrome   69
Cryofiltration   251
Cryoglobulinemia   8, 104, 172, 210, 222, 227ff., 242
Cryoglobulinemic nephropathy   241
Cryoglobulinpheresis   251
Cryoprecipitation   231, 252
CT   61, 139, 141, 153
C-terminal telopeptide   19
Cutaneous vasculitis   234
Cyclin D   121, 213
Cyclin D1   160
Cyclin-dependent kinase (see CDK)
Cyclophosphamide   46, 47, 56, 70, 74, 76, 78–80, 82, 85, 93, 95, 104, 125, 126, 128, 142, 143, 149, 153, 187, 189, 215, 219, 221, 250
Cyclosporine   29, 89, 250
Cystectomy, partial   167
Cytarabine   128
Cytokines   58
Cytomegalovirus   228
– infection   28, 29
Cytopenia   187, 221
Cytoplasmic light-chain isotype   19
Cytosine arabinoside   77, 94
Cytotoxic therapy   246

D

Dehydroepiandrosterone   22
Demyelinating neuropathy   40
Demyelination   43, 44
Dendritic cell vaccine   126
Deoxycoformycin   77
Dermabrasion   167
Desmopressin   26
Dexamethasone   74, 77, 78, 82, 90, 91, 93, 94, 125, 128, 185, 221
– high-dose   187
Dextran   30
Diabetes mellitus   36
Diagnostic x-ray exposure   57
Dialysis   125, 182, 189
Diarrhea   169
Diastolic heart failure   171
Dietary lectin   136
Diets   57
Digoxin   172, 181
Dimethyl sulfoxide (DMSO)   183
Diphenoxylate   183
Disialosyl gangliosides   39
Diuresis   105, 129
DNA replication   71
Donor lymphocyte infusion   88
Doppler studies   171, 180
Doxorubicin   56, 76, 78–80, 82, 94, 125, 142, 185–187, 215
Drug resistance   101
Drug toxicity   210
Duodenitis   176
Durie-Salmon system   123
– stage I disease   67
D-xylose test   140
Dyserythropoietic anemia   26
Dyspnea   178

E

Eastern Cooperative Oncology Group (see ECOG)
Echocardiography   169–171
ECOG (Eastern Cooperative Oncology Group)   72, 73, 98, 102, 170
Electromyography   41, 43
Electron micrography   241
Electrophoresis   6, 10, 55, 148
EMC   251
Encephalopathy   248, 251
Endocrinopathy   41
Endoplasmic reticulum   63

Endoscopy   141
Endothelial growth factor   38
Endothelial proliferation   39
Enterotoxin of *Vibrio cholerae*   136
Eosinophilia   148
Epineurial vasculitis   239
Epineurium   44
Epstein-Barr virus   117, 136, 228
Erythrocyte sedimentation rate   16, 55, 243
Erythropoiesis   60, 148
Erythropoietin   104, 210, 251
Escherichia coli   105
Esophagitis   176
Etoposide   75, 95, 128, 221
European Blood and Marrow Transplantation Group   87, 91, 92
Evans syndrome   147
Exton reagent   4
Extramedullary plasmacytoma (EMP)   111, 114–117

F

Factor VIII   65
Factor X deficiency   178
Familial Mediterranean fever (FMF)   184
Fanconi syndrome   62, 67, 174, 257–262
– acquired   69
Fibrinogen   168
Fibroblast growth factor receptor 3   121
Fibroblasts   58
Filgrastim   189
Finnish Leukaemia Study   104
FISH (fluorescence in situ hybridization)   98–100, 120, 160
FK506 immunosuppression   29
Flow cytometry   164, 244
Fludarabine   88, 215, 216, 218, 222
Fludrocortisone acetate   181
Fluorescence in situ hybridization (see FISH)
Fluorodeoxyglucose positron emission tomography   61
Furosemide   181

G

Gallium nitrate   103
γ-glutamyltransferase   174, 251
γ-HCD   134, 141, 145–149
– age ratio   144
– epidemiology   144
– etiology   144

– mortality   144
– sex ratio   144
– survivorship   144
Gastric lymphoid tumor   147
Gastritis   176
Gastroesophageal reflux   176
Gastrointestinal tract bleeding   188, 189
Gastrointestinal tract toxicity   186
Gaucher disease   27
Gaucher-like cells   63
Gene p16   59
GISC (Gruppo Italiano di Studio delle Crioglobulinimie)   243
Glomerulonephritis   10, 246, 251
– acute   248
– membranoproliferative   199
Glomerulonephropathy   241
Glomerulosclerosis   183
– nodular   198, 199
Glucocorticoid   74
Glycoprotein   164
Glycosuria   69, 260
Graft-versus-host disease (see GVHD)
Graft-versus-myeloma effect   87
Granular lymphocytes   20
Granulocyte-macrophage colony-stimulating factor   95, 126
Granulocytopenia   216
Growth retardation   138
Guillain-Barré syndrome   38
GVHD (graft-versus-host disease)   88, 89
Gynecomastia   42

H

H_1 blocker   245
H_2 blocker   127, 245
Haemophilus influenzae   105, 129
Hairy cell leukemia   218
Hantavirus   228
HCD (heavy chain disease)   2, 134
– protein   146
HCDD (heavy chain deposition disease)   200
HCV   233, 234, 236, 237, 246, 252
– infection   242, 250
HCV RNA   231, 248
HCV$^+$MC   249
HCV-encoded protein   233
HCV-specific protein   231
Heart failure   193, 198
Heavy chain deposition disease (see HCDD)
Heavy chain disease (see HCD)
Helicobacter pylori   142, 234
Hematologic malignancy   16
Hematopoietic stem cell   85, 186

– support 86, 101
– transplantation 84, 87, 96, 187, 192
Hematuria 167, 240
Hemolytic anemia 148
Hepatic cirrhosis 152
Hepatic dysfunction 252
Hepatitis C 29, 57, 232, 250
Hepatomegaly 42, 146, 162, 169, 174, 175, 181, 193, 210
Hepatosplenomegaly 6, 138, 152, 161
HIV (human immunodeficiency virus) 117, 228
Hodgkin disease 160, 168
Howell-Jolly body 174, 179
Human herpesvirus 8, 39, 57
Hyaline thrombosis 239
Hyperbilirubinemia 174
Hypercalcemia 56, 62, 63, 65, 67, 103, 104, 111, 112, 129, 261
– of malignancy 127
Hypergammaglobulinemia 67, 148, 243
Hyperimmunoglobulinemia 152
Hyperkalemia 129, 183
Hyperlipoproteinemia 28
Hypermutation 121
Hyperparathyroidism 24, 68, 259, 262
Hyperpigmentation 28, 42
Hyperprolactinemia 42
Hyperproteinemia 60
Hypersplenism 211, 250
Hypertrichosis 42
Hypertrophy
– asymmetric septal 171
– ventricular 170, 172
Hyperuricemia 129
Hyperviscosity 64, 104, 210, 215, 221, 238
– syndrome 26, 208
Hypogammaglobulinemia 123, 129, 148
Hypokalemia 260
Hypophosphatemia 69, 259, 260
Hyposplenism 175, 179
Hypothyroidism 128
Hypouricemia 69, 260

I

IBMTR/ABMTR 72, 73, 74
Idarubicin 76
Idiopathic Bence Jones proteinuria (IBJP) 260
Idiopathic proteinuria 197
Idiopathic thrombocytopenic purpura 14, 147
Idiotypic vaccination 92
IFN-α 245, 246, 248, 249

IgA 4, 8, 21, 23, 40, 46, 60, 135, 170, 211, 212
IgAκ 23
– protein 12, 15
IgD 3, 60
– MGUS 24
– myeloma 65
IgE 3
– myeloma 66
IgG 4, 6, 8, 18, 21, 23, 38, 40, 46, 60, 170, 211, 212
– myeloma 228
– protein 12
IgG1 29
IgG3 29
IgG3 M protein 30
IgGκ 23
– M protein 114
IgGλ protein 30
IgH gene 116
IgM 23, 47, 170, 209, 212, 221, 243
– antibody 38
– immunoglobulin 231
– lymphoma 57
– MGUS 206
– monoclonal gammopathy 178
– protein 7, 12, 15, 21, 211
– rheumatoid factor 230, 232
IL-1β 20, 58, 59, 75, 116, 117
IL-6 20, 58, 59, 75, 101, 115, 122
Ileocolonoscopy 139
IMiDs 71
Immune cell interactions 58
Immunoblastic lymphoma 139–142
Immunoblotting 148
Immunocytochemical detection 101
Immunocytoma 234
Immunodeficiency 136
Immunoelectron microscopic technique 261
Immunoelectrophoresis 2, 10, 14, 23, 24, 60, 244
Immunofixation 4, 14, 23, 41, 102, 111, 123, 152, 164, 221, 244
– of serum and urine 10, 163, 165, 171, 193
Immunofluorescence 65, 140, 164
Immunoglobulin 3, 115, 158
– isotype 96
– type 17
Immunoglobulin light chain amyloidosis (see also Primary amyloidosis) 157ff.
Immunohistochemistry 164, 241
Immunoperoxidase 65
– staining 239
Immunophenotype 122
Immunoproliferative disease, malignant 17
Immunoproliferative disorder 137

Immunoproliferative small intestinal disease (see IPSID)
Immunosuppression 28
Immunosuppressive drug 251
Immunosuppressive therapy 89, 246
Induction chemotherapy 124
Induction therapy 91
Interferon 90, 91, 251
– therapy 242
– trials 247
Interferon-α 47, 48, 56, 71, 77
Intergroupe Française du Myélome 84
Intergroupe Francophone du Myélome 126
Interleukin 58
International normalized ratio 123
Interstitial pulmonary fibrosis 138
Intestinal bleeding 169
Intestinal tumor 141
Intravenous gamma globulin (see IVIG)
Iodine-123 165
IPSID 136, 139, 141, 143
Isoleucine 172
IVIG (intravenous gamma globulin) 47

J

JAK-2 58
JAK-STAT 58
Juvenile rheumatoid arthritis 159

K

Kahler disease 55
Kaposi sarcoma 26
κ chain 152
κ immunoglobulin group 159
κ light chain 258, 260
Kidney 172–174, 197
– biopsy 261
– transplant 201
K-ras 59, 121
Kyphosis 62

L

Lactate dehydrogenase 97, 123
Laminectomy 103
Laparotomy 141, 143, 176

LCDD (light-chain deposition disease)   68, 69, 198–202
- diagnosis   198
- epidemiology   197
- etiology   197
Leprosy   159
Leukemia   90, 186
- acute   261
- secondary   124
Leukocyte alkaline phosphatase   20
Leukopenia   78
LFA-1   59
LFA-3   59
LHCDD (light- and heavy-chain deposition disease)   200
Lichen myxedematosus   28
Light- and heavy-chain deposition disease (see LHCDD)
Light-chain deposition disease (see LCDD)
Light-chain transcription   146
Lipopolysaccharides   136
Liver biopsy   174, 175
Liver failure   252
Liver function abnormality   248, 251
Liver transplantation   29
Lomustine   76, 77, 82
Loperamide   183
LPD (lymphoproliferative disorder)   69, 228, 237, 244, 246, 248, 251, 252, 257, 262
- malignant   2
Lupus erythematosus   27, 147, 152
Lyme disease   228
Lymphadenopathy   68, 146, 152, 210
Lymphocytic leukemia   57
Lymphocytic lymphoma   25
Lymphocytic proliferation   26
Lymphocytosis   147, 152, 244
Lymphoid disease   25
Lymphoma   5, 6, 8, 151
Lymphoplasmacytic cells   139
Lymphoplasmacytic disorder, malignancy   30
Lymphoplasmacytic lymphoma   207, 213
Lymphoproliferation   252
Lymphoproliferative disease   9, 24, 25, 197
Lymphoproliferative disorder (see LPD)
Lymphoproliferative malignancy   151
Lysozyme   168
Lytic bone disease   213
Lytic bone lesion   103, 123, 124, 126, 153

M

M protein   2–4, 6, 7, 11, 16, 18, 19, 21, 41, 74, 114, 115, 164, 193
Macroglobulinemia   5–7, 9, 11, 14, 16, 29, 57
Macroglossia   162
Macrophages   58
Macular detachment   221
MAF antibody   43
MAG (myelin-associated glycoprotein)   38
Malaria   167
MALT (mucosa-associated lymphoid tissue)   134, 139
- lymphoma   234
Mantle cell lymphoma   213, 214
MAP (mitogen-activated protein)   59
Marrow aplasia   95
Marrow fibrosis   64
Marrow toxicity   218
Mayo Clinic   6 ff., 22, 36, 48, 102, 165, 168, 170, 171, 180, 182
Mcl-1   58
Mediastinal nodes   138
Melphalan   22, 27, 46–48, 56, 70, 74, 76–80, 82, 86, 88, 90, 91, 94, 104, 124–126, 178, 185, 187, 189, 215, 221, 249, 261
Mesenteric lymph nodes   135, 139, 167
Metabolic acidosis   129
Methionine   46
Methotrexate   88, 89
Methylprednisolone   93, 94, 128, 187, 248
Metronidazole   142
MGUS (monoclonal gammopathy of undetermined significance)   4, 57, 122, 177, 257, 258, 260
- age ratio   37
- diagnosis   15
- neuropathy   38, 39, 43, 44
- race ratio   37
- sex ratio   37
- variants   21
Midodrine   182
MIP-1α   59
Mithramycin   103
Mitogen-activated protein (see MAP)
Mitoxantrone   76, 82, 94
Monoclonal gammopathy   150, 153, 163, 168, 234
- benign   5, 6, 16
- malignant   2
- of undetermined significance (see MGUS)
Monoclonal IgM paraproteinemia   206
Monoclonal immunoglobulin light chain   4, 18, 165
Monoclonal lymphoplasmacytosis   206

Monoclonal plasma cell   19
- disorder   260
Monoclonal (M) protein (see M protein)
Monoclonal urine protein   17
Monocytes   58
Morbidity, transplant-associated   126
Mott cells   63
MPGN (membranoproliferative glomerulonephritis)   241
MRI (magnetic resonance imaging)   19, 22, 61, 111, 112, 129
mRNA   137, 138, 146
μ-HCD   134, 151–153
- age ratio   150
- epidemiology   150
- etiology   150
- mortality   150
- race ratio   150
- sex ratio   150
- survivorship   150
Mucosa-associated lymphoid tissue (see MALT)
Mucosal ischemia, chronic   176
Multidrug-resistant phenotype (MDR-1)   20
Multifocal neuropathy   38
Multiple bone lesions   48
Multiple myeloma (MM)   2, 11, 18, 24, 28, 40, 41, 44, 46, 55, 64, 160, 163, 181, 197, 201, 214
- set domain   121
- smoldering   21
- standard therapy   70
- survival   96
Myasthenia gravis   147
Mycophenolate   88
Myelin-associated glycoprotein (see MAG)
Myelodysplasia   152, 187, 213, 220
Myelodysplastic syndrome   90, 104, 124, 189, 261
Myelofibrosis   27
Myelogenous leukemia, acute   213, 215
Myeloma Aredia Study Group   127
Myeloma bone disease   102
Myeloma cast nephropathy   172
Myeloma Trialists' Collaborative Group   71, 80, 83
Myelosuppression   86, 94, 96, 186, 219, 220
Myocardial infarction   49
Myocardium   170

N

Natural killer cells   20, 77
N-CAM   59

Neoplastic karyotype   120
Nephelometry   4, 164, 212, 244
Nephrectomy   175
Nephritis   231
– tubulointerstitial   261
Nephropathy   183, 261
Nephrotic syndrome   8, 179, 185, 190, 198, 240
Nephrotic-range proteinuria   193
Nephrotoxicity, avoidance of   127
Nerve biopsy   166, 177
Nerve conduction velocity   45
Nerve damage   36
Nervous system   239
Neuralgia   103
Neuropathy   193, 248
– classification   42
– idiopathic peripheral   162
– peripheral   168
NF-IL-6   58
NF-κB   58
NHL   92, 134, 141, 143, 234
Nodular lymphoma   25
Non-Hodgkin lymphoma (see NHL)
Nonmyeloablative allogeneic transplantation   88
Nonplasma cell disorders   12, 17
North American Intergroup Study   86
N-ras 59, 121
N-telopeptides of Type I collagen   102
Nuclear weapons   57

O

Octreotide   183
Oculocerebrorenal syndrome of Lowe   257
Oligoclonal B cells   231
Omm cells   146
Organomegaly   41
Oronasal bleeding   208
Orthopedic surgery   127
Orthostatic hypotension   169, 179
Osteoblasts   58
Osteoclasts   58
Osteolytic lesion   18
Osteomalacia   259, 261, 262
Osteopenia   62
Osteoporosis   7, 61, 127, 153
Osteosclerotic lesion   41, 42, 43, 61
Osteosclerotic myeloma (see also POEMS)   27, 37, 44
Ouchterlony test   55

P

p16   100, 207
p53   59
$p53$ suppressor gene   122
Paclitaxel   77
Pamidronate   102, 127
Pancytopenia   152, 186, 220
Papilledema   42, 46
Paraprotein   158, 210
Paraproteinemia   212
Paresthesia   176
PBSCT   125, 129
PCD (plasma cell dyscrasia)   43, 54, 63, 100, 166, 197
PCL (plasma cell leukemia)   59, 66, 84, 121–123
– etiology   120
PCLI (Plasma Cell Labeling Index)   99, 101, 102, 124, 180
Penicillamine   245
Pepsin   258
Peptichemo   82
Pericardiectomy   172
Peripheral blood stem cell   89
– transplantation (see PBSCT)   85, 192, 249
Peripheral neuropathy   40, 179, 181, 239
Peritransplantation mortality   188
Petechiae   237
Pharmacokinetics   126
Phosphaturia   69, 260
Phosphorus   261, 262
Phosphorylation status   58
Plasma cell disorder   12, 13, 15, 17, 45
Plasma cell dyscrasia (see PCD)
Plasma Cell Labeling Index (see PCLI)
Plasma cell leukemia (see PCL)
Plasma cell morphology   98
Plasma cell type   140
Plasma cells, median   169
Plasmacytoma   2, 11, 13, 43, 57
– radiosensitivity   114
– of the sacrum   7
Plasmapheresis   46, 48, 105, 246, 248, 250, 251
Pleural effusion   46, 138
Ploidy   120
$Pneumocystis\ carinii$ pneumonia   129, 216
Pneumonia   105
POEMS (polyneuropathy, organomegaly, endocrinopathy, M protein, skin changes)   27, 36, 40, 41, 44, 46–48, 69, 177
– age ratio   37
– etiology   31
– race ratio   37
– sex ratio   37
Polyarthropathy   167
Polyclonal hypergammaglobulinemia   67, 68, 231, 234
Polyclonal immunoglobulin   2
– reduction   16
Polycythemia   27, 160
Polymyalgia rheumatica   27, 162
Polyneuropathy   40, 41, 43, 47
Polyserositis   184
Posttransplantation period   189
Postural hypotension   45
Prednisone   22, 27, 46–48, 74, 76, 78–80, 82, 90–93, 124, 142, 143, 149, 153, 178, 185–187, 215, 248–250, 261
Primary amyloid neuropathy   36, 37, 39, 40, 44, 47, 48
Primary amyloidosis (see also AL, immunoglobulin light chain amyloidosis)   36, 57, 157, 161, 162, 197
– diagnostic pathway   193
Primary biliary cirrhosis   29
Primary refractory myeloma   85
Primary systemic amyloidosis   37, 40, 60, 69
Procarbazine   82, 142, 143
Protease resistance   259
Protein Ait   137
Protein C resistance   179
Proteinuria   63, 162, 167, 172–174, 249
Proteosome inhibitor   71, 127
Prothrombin   178
PS-341   95
Pseudo-obstruction   169
Psoriatic arthritis   167
Pulmonary embolism   103
Pulmonary hemorrhage   243
Pulmonary vasculitis   243
Purging   86
Purine nucleoside analogs   215, 216, 219, 220–222, 250
Purpura   237, 241
Purpuric lesion   248
Pyoderma gangrenosum   28

Q

Q fever   228

R

Radiation therapy   13, 51, 95, 114, 142
Radioisotope   126

Ras-MAP kinase pathway   58
Raynaud phenomenon   239
REAL (Revised European-American Lymphoma) classification system   54
Red cell rouleaux   211
Relapsed or refractory disease   93, 94
Renal amyloid   182
Renal biopsy   165, 183, 197
Renal blood flow   173
Renal dysfunction   261
Renal failure   125, 183
– acute   129
Renal insufficiency   62, 111, 162, 173
Renal tubular acidosis   262
Renal vein thrombosis   174
Reticulum cell sarcoma   24
Retinal hemorrhage   208, 221
Retinal vein occlusion   208
Retroperitoneal fibrosis   174
Rheumatoid arthritis   147, 150, 167, 228
Ribavirin   249
Riboflavin   30
Rituximab   47, 143, 219, 220, 222
RNA transcript   137
Russell bodies   63

S

Salvage chemotherapy   143
Schnitzler syndrome   28
Sclerotic bone lesion   46
Sebia Pentafix   3
SEER (Surveillance, Epidemiology, and End Results)   56
Serum albumin   96, 101, 102, 177
Serum alkaline phosphatase   184
Serum β_2-microglobulin   180, 181, 211
Serum creatinine concentration   10, 181
Serum M protein   209
Serum protein electrophoresis (SPEP)   2–4, 123, 140, 198
Sicca syndrome   233
Signal transduction   126
Sjögren syndrome   26, 147, 234, 236
Skin changes   41
Skin inflammation   167
Skin lesion   147
Solitary plasmacytoma of bone (SPB)   111–114
– pathogenesis   115
Southwest Oncology Group (see SWOG)
Sphincter dysfunction   45
Spinal nerve root   103
Splenectomy   221
Splenomegaly   68, 146, 210, 241

Standard intensity chemotherapy   97
Staphylococcus aureus   63, 129
STAT3   58
Steatorrhea   138, 163, 175
Stem cell collection   124, 126
Stem cell reconstitution   85
Stem cell transplant recipients   192
Stem cell transplantation   104, 129, 142, 182, 188, 193
Stilbamidine   55
Streptococcus pneumoniae   105, 129
Stroke   49
Stromal cell   58
Subacute bacterial endocarditis   228
Submandibular lymph nodes   162
Surface antigen   120
SWOG (Southwest Oncology Group)   71–74, 80, 90, 94
Syphilis   159, 167
Systemic amyloidosis   63, 67
Systemic lupus erythematosus (SLE)   234

T

Tachyarrhythmias   198
Tachycardia   182
Takatsuki syndrome   69
– Crow-Fukase syndrome   37
Tamm-Horsfall protein   63, 259, 261
Tamoxifen   48
T-cell immunodeficiency   28, 219
T-cell leukemia   26
T-cell lymphoma   28
T-cell lymphomatosis   44
Telomerase activity   20
Teniposide   77
Tetany   138
Tetracycline   142
Thalidomide   56, 77, 78, 93, 126–128, 220
Thoracic spine tumor   114
Thoracolumbar spine disease   112
Thrombocytopenia   64, 78, 152, 182, 210, 219
Thrombocytosis   187
Thromboembolism   178, 179
Thyroiditis   147
T-lymphocytic virus   228
Topotecan   77
Total body irradiation   187
Total Therapy II   95
TP53   122, 207
Transretinoic acid   48
Transthyretin (see TTR)
Triclonal gammopathy   23

Trimethoprim-sulfamethoxazole (TMP-SMX)   105
Trisomy 7   149
Trisomy X   160
Trisomy 21   149
TTR (transthyretin)   168, 172
Tuberculosis   159, 167
Tubular atrophy   199
Tubular cell   259
Tumor cell adhesion molecule   120
Tumor mass index   78
Tumor necrosis factor-α 58, 60
Tumor suppressor gene   122
Type I collagen   166

U

Ultrasonography   141
Uremia   64
Urethane   55
Urinary monoclonal light chain   181
Urinary tract infection   105
Urine   124
– M protein   14
Urine protein electrophoresis (UPEP)   78, 123, 243, 244
Urticaria   239

V

VAD   125
Val30Met mutation   168
Vascular occlusion   231
Vascular sclerosis   199
Vascular-derived endothelial growth factor (see VEGF)
Vasculitis   147, 231, 242
VCMP/VBAP   125
VDJ junction   145
VDJ recombination   121
VEGF (vascular-derived endothelial growth factor)   58, 69
Ventricular fibrillation   198
Vessel endothelial cell   58
Vincristine   47, 78–80, 82, 91, 94, 125, 128, 142, 143, 149, 153, 185–187, 215
Vitamin D   262
VLA-4   59
v-myc   115
von Willebrand disease   26
von Willebrand factor   30, 65

W

Waldenström disease 151
Waldenström macroglobulinemia (see WM)
Waldeyer ring 146
WHO (World Health Organization) 54
WM (Waldenström macroglobulinemia) 2,
36, 40, 60, 66–69, 148, 153, 170, 178, 205,
210, 213–217, 228, 236, 257, 260, 262
– age ratio 206
– epidemiology 206
– etiology 206
– genetics 207
– mortality 206
– race ratio 206
– screening/prevention 207
– sex ratio 206
– survivorship 206

X

Xanthoderma 30
Xanthotrichia 30
Xerostomia 165

Y

YAG laser therapy 177
Yttrium-aluminum-garnet (YAG) laser resection 167

Z

Zoledronic acid 127

Printing and Binding: Stürtz AG, Würzburg